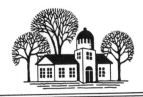

THE
HEALERS

THE HEALERS

THE RISE OF
THE MEDICAL
ESTABLISHMENT

John Duffy

McGRAW-HILL BOOK COMPANY

New York St. Louis San Francisco
Düsseldorf London Mexico
Sydney Toronto

To the memory of my brother,
Jim, a kindred spirit

Book design by Stanley Drate.
Copyright © 1976 by John Duffy. All rights reserved. Printed in the United States of America. No part of this publication may be reproduced, stored in a retrieval system, or transmitted, in any form or by any means, electronic, mechanical, photocopying, recording, or otherwise, without the prior written permission of the publisher.

1 2 3 4 5 6 7 8 9 B P B P 7 9 8 7 6

Library of Congress Cataloging in Publication Data

Duffy, John, 1915–
The healers.

Bibliography: p.
Includes index.
1. Medicine—United States—History. I. Title. [DNLM: 1. History of medicine, Modern—United States. 2. Education, Medical—History—United States. WZ70 AA1 D85h]
R151.D83   610'.973   76-13616
ISBN 0-07-018020-2

PREFACE

DURING the almost fifty years which have passed since Francis R. Packard wrote his two-volume history of American medicine, a great deal of historical research and publication has been done. In writing this volume I have relied upon both my studies and those of a good many of my friends and colleagues. I have also tried to view medicine objectively and place it in its social setting, although one can scarcely spend a lifetime studying the history of a profession or any other group without developing some empathy for it. Medicine and health embrace a wide range of topics and the problem of selection has been particularly difficult; hence knowledgeable readers may feel that their favorite figure or field of interest has either been omitted or slighted. They may also recognize that this history reflects the major interests of the author.

Throughout the past thirty-odd years I have read widely in medical journals and society transactions, public health records, newspapers, and the other sources for American medical and health history. My research notes cover virtually every state in the Union, but my familiarity with and extensive files relating to the history of Louisiana, New York, and Pennsylvania have led me to cite a good many examples from these states. The points they illustrate, however, have a much wider applicability. If I have given too little attention to the West, the explanation lies in the recency of its history. By the time the Western states were coming of age, American medicine had begun to merge with that of Western Europe and to lose its distinctive characteristics.

I have already acknowledged a large debt to my fellow historians, and I am equally obligated to a great number of librarians who have cheerfully helped me to dig out useful material. In the actual writing I was aided by two successive part-time research assistants, Dr. Peter Bruton and Mr. William Stowe, and by a gem of a secretary with a fine ear for the English language, Ms. Denise Senstad. A former undergraduate student who is now in medical school, Mr. Fernando Martinez, contributed a good many hours to the final checking, and, as usual, my wife Corinne untangled some of my prose.

CONTENTS

Publisher's Note

This volume is part of a McGraw-Hill publishing program on Aspects of American Life and Culture.

Editorial Consultants for this program are Harold M. Hyman, William P. Hobby Professor of American History, Rice University; and Leonard W. Levy, Andrew W. Mellon Professor of Humanities and History, Claremont Graduate School.

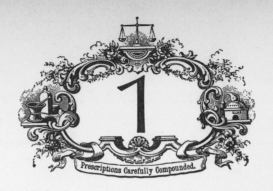

THE MYTH OF
INDIAN MEDICINE

O NE of the oldest and most enduring of American myths relates to Indian medical skills. The American attitude toward the Indians has always been one of ambivalence, fluctuating between seeing them as savage barbarians and Noble Red Men, yet we have consistently believed in the efficacy of Indian medicine. This idea was expressed by most early writers and became embedded in Romantic literature, thus accounting for the touring Indian medicine shows which were an integral part of the American scene well into the twentieth century. This same theme has been reiterated in recent publications, and the new emphasis upon the role of minorities in American history should provide a further impetus to refurbishing the myth.

The major difficulties in comprehending the culture of the North American Indians prior to the coming of the whites arise from the failure of the Indians to keep written records and from the fact that the first contacts with European culture sent shock waves throughout the many and varied Indian tribes. The explorers, missionaries, and soldiers who first described the Indian way of life were at the same time directly and indirectly modifying it. Moreover, these early Europeans judged the Indians in terms of the Europeans' own cultural development. French, Spanish, and English explorers in the sixteenth century obviously used far different criteria from those of Lewis and Clark, who described the Western tribes in the early nineteenth century. To complicate matters further, few Europeans recognized the wide cultural variations among the Indian tribes, a diversity which was at least as great as that of the European nations.

In part the myth of Indian medicine was based on the golden expectations of the early European adventurers. The incredible wealth captured by the Spanish in Central and South America convinced the explorers of North America that similar treasure troves awaited them, and these expectations were further incited by the seemingly boundless quantity of rich land. Among the wonders they hoped to find were botanical remedies. The New World offered a variety of exotics, and the healthy and robust natives gave proof that they were acquainted with plants of medicinal value. European medicine itself still relied largely upon botanical therapeutics, and the Indian use of herbals in religious rites was taken as evidence that the Indians were well versed in medicine.

To understand better the myth of Indian medicine one must realize that, prior to the advent of the whites, there is no question that the Indians were generally strong and healthy. The great endemic and epidemic diseases which plagued the peoples of the Euro-Asian land mass left the North American Indians untouched. All evidence clearly indicates that they were exempt from malaria, typhoid, typhus, smallpox, measles, scarlet fever, diphtheria, venereal diseases, and the host of other disorders besetting Europeans. The relatively sparse Indian population—approximately one million in the entire North American Continent—meant there were no sanitary problems, and the outdoor life and widely varied diet prevented nutritional diseases. The mobility of the Indians and their custom of isolating the sick and wounded tended to keep wound infections to a minimum. Indian women, to whom rickets was virtually unknown, seldom had pelvic problems, and their active life insured relatively easy births.[1]

The major Indian medical problem arose from trauma, occasional digestive complaints due to alternate periods of feasting and famine, and what were described as rheumatism and neuralgia resulting from constant exposure. The latter may have been rheumatoid or infectious arthritis. Pleurisy, lung inflammations, and bronchial disorders afflicted the Indians after the coming of the whites, but their existence in pre-Columbian days is debatable.

With a healthy population, a relatively balanced diet, an active outdoor life, and few if any infections, the Indians had a minimal need for therapeutics. European observers were struck by the tall stature and healthy bodies of the first Indians they encountered. As late as the nineteenth century Lewis and Clark described the Plains Indians as "tall in stature, straight and robust."[2] Yet the Indians, as do all people, suffered psychological stress, were subject to injury, and endured physical complaints. To meet these problems they had evolved an elaborate form of medicine which provided them with adequate support.

Indian medicine was closely identified with religion, and among most tribes it had achieved a stage between animism and monotheism which was characterized by a Great Spirit ruling over a host of lesser ones. These spirits were omnipresent and quick to take offense. The slightest misstep, such as inadvertently breaking one of the many taboos, could threaten an individual's social well-being and good health. The medicine man was essentially a religious leader, a priestly intermediary between the world of man and the world of spirits. He could invoke friendly spirits and ward off evil ones. His major function was to bring victory to the warriors, success to the hunters, rain from the sky, and good crops to the tribe. Since offended or malicious spirits often sought revenge by bringing sickness, the task of healing also fell to the medicine man.

Indian medicine is too complex for more than a cursory survey, but sickness was generally ascribed to an offended or malevolent spirit, to a spirit acting at human behest, or to the soul of a human being. In the latter case, for example, the sick individual might lose his soul in having offended the spirit of a dead individual. Whatever the case, the function of the medicine man was to divine which spirit was causing the trouble and either to propitiate the spirit or secure the intervention of a friendly spirit. In divining the spirit responsible for the sickness and in dealing with it, the medicine man relied primarily upon incantations, chants, dances, medicine bags, amulets, and all the other paraphernalia of magic and witch doctors everywhere. In connection with these rituals, he made use of herbs and herbal concoctions, and resorted to sucking, blowing, sprinkling, and bloodletting. In his quest for cause, the medicine man was more concerned with the patient's dreams than with his physical condition.

Although the emphasis was upon spiritual healing, a wide range of botanicals was used by the many Indian tribes. These herbals were boiled, pounded, or steeped in water and the resulting concoction administered orally and rectally. In most cases huge quantities of an infusion or decoction were poured down the throat of the sick person, with the result that the medicines almost invariably had an emetic effect—which may have saved some from overdoses of poisonous herbals! Undoubtedly some of these medicines were effective, but the reasons for using them were mystical rather than empirical. Although the sum total of herbals used by the Indians is large, most tribes were familiar with only a few. Even the use of these plants with a specific medicinal value varied from tribe to tribe, each of which might use them for a different ailment.

In dealing with dislocations, fractures, cuts, and abrasions, the Indians were fairly successful. Although certain tribes possessed more skill than others, in general they knew how to replace luxated bones, make crude splints for fractures, use bird down, moss, and other materials to stop hemorrhage, and wash out open wounds with clean water or herbal cococtions. They were skilled too in treating the pains of neuralgia and rheumatism—relying upon sweat baths, warm poultices, massage, and aromatic fumigations.

In terms of their medical problems, Indian medicine was quite adequate, and it did not compare too unfavorably with the medical practices of sixteenth- and seventeenth-century Europe. The major difference was that Western medicine had already begun the shift from a spiritual to a rational basis, whereas Indian medicine men still looked first to the world of the spirits. In the clash of cultures, the most significant impact of European civilization upon Indian medicine was to transform it from a religious procedure with empirical overtones to an empirical procedure with religious overtones.

The coming of the whites not only brought drastic changes in Indian medicine, but it led to even more significant alterations in Indian health. As indicated, the Indians had had virtually no experience with infectious disorders prior to the advent of the Europeans, and hence they had little immunological defense against white contagions. Consequently, smallpox, measles, tuberculosis, and venereal diseases, among others, wrought havoc among the Indian tribes. The one disease above all others responsible for destroying the Indians was smallpox. It paved the way for the Spanish conquest of Central and South America by killing an estimated three million natives in the early sixteenth century; it may have been responsible for the epidemic which depopulated New England in 1616 and facilitated the English settlement; and it was the chief factor in the virtual elimination of the Eastern Indians during the colonial period.[3] In 1679 Count de Frontenac referred to smallpox as the "Indian Plague," and from South Carolina in 1699 it was reported "to have swept away a whole neighboring [Indian] nation, all to 5 or 6 which ran away and left their dead unburied. . . ."[4]

The tragedy of the Indians lay in the hopelessness of their position. No matter what the occasion for contact with whites—trade, religion, or war—sickness and disease were the inevitable results. Every colonial war led to the widespread dissemination of smallpox, and invariably the Indians, whether allies or enemies, were the chief victims. The Indians did get a measure of revenge. Not infrequently smallpox, after passing through the Indian tribes, was returned to the whites with renewed virulence. The Indians also served as an intermediary, alternately passing the disease between the French Canadian and British settlements. Major outbreaks in the middle colonies were invariably spread via the Indians into the Great Lakes and St. Lawrence regions and vice versa. Probably one reason the New England colonies suffered less from smallpox than the middle colonies was their limited contacts with the major Indian tribes.[5]

One can scarcely leave the Indians without making some mention of the first definite use of what is now called germ warfare. Granting the colonial mixture of contempt and fear toward the Indians, it would be surprising if some form of crude germ warfare had not been used against them. The first recorded use of smallpox in this capacity came during Pontiac's Rebellion, 1763–64. Pontiac had organized a well-coordinated attack which destroyed nearly all the British frontier posts west of the Alleghenies. Hard put to meet the Indian threat, in the summer of 1763 General Jeffrey Amherst suggested to Colonel Henry Bouquet that smallpox be sent among the disaffected tribes. Bouquet replied: "I will try to inoculate the —— with Some Blankets that may fall in their Hands, and take care not to get the disease myself." Bouquet then added that he wished he could hunt them with dogs and Rangers, "who would I think effectually extirpate or remove that vermin." Subsequently, the British Army was billed by a private company for "Sundries got to Replace in kind those which were taken from people in the Hospital to Convey the Small-pox to the Indians." The "Sundries" consisted of two blankets and two handkerchiefs.[6]

Granting that somewhere between 700,000 and 1,000,000 Indians roamed the vast continent of North America and that in terms of their needs Indian medical practices were satisfactory, why was it that North America remained so sparsely populated? Some of the tribes had well-organized agricultural economies, and, all told, the various tribes represented many stages of cultural development. Based on the willingness of Indians to ally with whites in fighting their traditional tribal enemies during colonial days and the bitter tribal warfare of the nineteenth century, one may speculate that warfare represented a major source of population control. Drought, forest fires, and other natural disasters periodically reducing food production in the hunting areas must have often caused one or more tribes to encroach on the preserves of neighboring tribes, leading to wide-scale bloodshed. The lack of natural geographic boundaries and the concept of the adult male as a warrior and hunter may also have contributed to the perennial warfare.

Over and above tribal conflicts, one might expect a high infant mortality rate to characterize the Indians, particularly among those tribal groups dependent largely upon a hunting and fishing economy. Regrettably, we know little about conditions prior to the coming of the whites, but the recent emphasis upon the history of minority groups has already focused attention upon the early Indians and has resulted in several intensive studies of particular tribes during specific time periods. These studies should make for a better understanding of the Indian culture and may provide answers to some of the questions. In terms of Indian medicine, at least one recent publication has tended to refurbish the old mythology, but the net effect of this renewed interest in all aspects of Indian life should be beneficial.

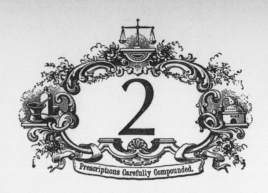

Prescriptions Carefully Compounded.

HEALTH CONDITIONS IN THE NEW WORLD

Tragic as was the impact of Europeans upon the health of the Indians, health conditions among the early settlers were little better if at all. The high hopes of the first colonists were quickly shattered by the harsh realities of wilderness living. By 1600 Europeans were already well acquainted with the rich fishing banks off the coast of North America, the lucrative fur trade, the vast forests and naval stores, and the untold quantities of land. Their expectations had been increased further by the bonanzas uncovered by the Spanish to the south. Thus it was that the New World held promise for everyone— fur, fishing, and timber trade for the merchants, adventure for the restless, hope of freedom for oppressed religious minorities, and land for all. Virginia was settled by adventurers, Plymouth by Pilgrims, and Massachusetts by an upward-striving middle class seeking both economic improvement and religious liberty; all of these factors played a role in the British settlement of North America.

Health conditions were grim for the first settlers. The leaders of the initial expeditions had little idea of what to expect or what equipment and food supplies were necessary. The London Company envisioned opening a trading post in Virginia comparable to the ones established by the East India Company in Asia, and they recruited adventurers rather than settlers, men who were ill-suited for the drudgery of turning a wilderness into cultivated land. Therefore, before the colony could establish a sound agricultural basis, thousands of lives were lost to hunger and disease. The Plymouth settlers were a little more realistic, but they too, when they left Holland and England, had little conception of what awaited them on the stern New England coast. Moreover, creating farm land out of wilderness was an almost impossible task for the small handfuls of sick and half-starved settlers who had landed with the first ships. With no farm animals and few implements, their diet was limited and inadequate; to return across the cruel sea was almost impossible, and so they were left to confront an equally cruel wilderness. Judging from the accounts of Plymouth and Virginia, one cannot help being impressed by man's tenacity and his ability to survive—qualifications which were tested to the fullest in the early seventeenth century.

A major factor in the high mortality rate among newcomers, and one that continued to winnow immigrants until well after the Civil War, was the dangerous and distressing ocean voyage, the length of which—sometimes six weeks, but more often eight to fourteen weeks—was entirely dependent upon the vagaries of weather and the skill of the captain. Owners and captains tended to crowd as many passengers as possible into their vessels and cut water and provisions to a minimum. Under these circumstances adverse winds, which unduly lengthened the voyage, meant literal starvation and thirst. The food consisted largely of dried and salted provisions, and as the long weeks at sea dragged by, scurvy and other dietetic disorders frequently appeared among crew and passengers. Jammed into small cabins or crowded into the holds for days on end during inclement weather, the passengers suffered all the torments of sea sickness and the inevitable crowd diseases— diarrheas, dysentery, typhus, typhoid, smallpox, measles, and so forth. Those who survived the voyage were in no condition to start clearing the wilderness.[1]

By the 1630s, when the large-scale settlement of Massachusetts was undertaken, the bitter experiences of the first settlements had taught a hard lesson. Farmers and craftsmen rather than soldiers and adventurers were now recruited, and they were supplied with the tools, implements, and livestock necessary to recreate a British farming economy in the New World. While the climate of Virginia and New England tended more to extremes than that of England, English domesticated plants, animals, and birds could readily be transplanted. In addition, the settlers learned from the Indians the value of New World products. In the long run North America offered many advantages, but it was to take over a hundred years before the colonists could capitalize upon them.

The incredible story of sickness and death in Virginia and Plymouth has been recorded many times. Suffice it to say that, out of the almost 9,000 newcomers who had arrived in Virginia by 1625, a census that year showed only 1,100 to 1,200 remaining. A few hundred had returned to England, but the vast majority had fallen prey to sickness and starvation. In Plymouth almost half of the settlers died during the winter of 1620–21, and a high rate of sickness and death characterized all the New England settlements until well into the 1630s.[2] The first and most obvious cause of this high mortality was starvation and nutritional deficiencies. Most settlers lacked the skill and knowledge to take advantage of the game, fish, and wild plants available to them, and the few that might have done so were inhibited by fear of the Indians and the unknown terrors of the forests. Thus the newcomers, arriving weak and debilitated after a long and arduous voyage, were compelled to subsist on the limited and dietetically unsound provisions they had brought with them. Scurvy was a major problem in nearly all the early settlements, and it is quite likely that beriberi and other deficiency diseases were present. Subacute or chronic scurvy would not have been recognized as such, but anyone making a long ocean voyage in the seventeenth century would have encountered well-developed cases. Lord Delaware, the Governor of Virginia, sailed for the West Indies in 1611 along with his physician, Dr. Lawrence Bohun, seeking relief from an obstinate case of scurvy. Dr. Bohun achieved a cure by prescribing oranges and lemons, "a sovereign Remedy for that Disorder."[3] While the term scurvy undoubtedly was a coverall name applied to many disorders, there can be no question that true scurvy was a major problem.

Dietetic diseases rarely killed, but they paved the way for a host of fatal and debilitating infections. The early records constantly speak of fevers, fluxes, bellyaches, smallpox, and a wide assortment of epidemic outbreaks described as burning, malignant, pestilential, summer, or winter fevers. Occasional references are also made to "calenture," a term applied to delirious fever and one frequently used as a synonym for yellow fever. The descriptive names flux or bloody flux were applied to bowel disorders and included any of the enteric complaints, ranging from a simple diarrhea through bacillary dysentery and typhoid fever.

Among the many fevers to trouble the colonists, malaria ranks high. By the late seventeenth and early eighteenth centuries, it had gained a strong foothold in North America, and it remained one of the major causes of morbidity and mortality throughout the rest of the colonial period. The distinctive alternations of fever and ague (chills), marked by clearly defined remissions, made the disease relatively easy to identify. If the anopheles mosquito was not already available in North America to spread the malarial parasite, it was exported from England and Holland; the open water caskets and water buckets on sailing vessels and the presence of infected passengers and crews would have facilitated the passage. More than likely, innocent and unsuspecting American mosquitoes were infected with the plasmodium by the early settlers.

The role of malaria in connection with the "burning fevers" which struck the first settlers in Virginia is an interesting question. Colonial historians, long familiar with malaria, continued well into the twentieth century to assume that this disease was the explanation for these burning fevers. Wyndham B. Blanton showed that early seventeenth-century Virginia records include only an occasional mention of fever and ague, and that those newcomers who successfully survived the "seasoning" tended to be healthy. The earliest sanitary law for Jamestown in 1610 forbade disposing slops, waste water, and human wastes within forty feet of the wells, an ordinance which shows how easily the shallow wells could have been contaminated.[4] We know typhoid was common in Europe, and that the disorder, unlike malaria, confers immunity following one attack. These facts, in conjunction with the association of the burning fevers with the water supply, makes typhoid the chief suspect for the enormous mortality during the early years of the Jamestown settlement.

Summer was the season for fluxes and fevers, while winter saw the perennial respiratory complaints. The combination of inadequate food, poorly ventilated homes, and overcrowded housing provided an ideal environment for respiratory infections. A report from Virginia in 1623 stated that constantly getting wet in the process of landing goods caused the settlers to "get such violent surfetts of cold upon cold as seldome leave them untill they leave to live." What was probably the first influenza epidemic in North America was described by John Winthrop in 1647 as an "epidemical sickness" involving "a cold, and light fever. . . ."[5]

In addition, colonial records show repeated onslaughts of "pleuretical disorders," "pleurisies," and "peripneumonies." Although the incidence of respiratory disorders was greater in the northern colonies, they were common to all regions. While these recurrent colds, coughs, influenzas, and other respiratory ailments were not as dramatic as the great pestilences such as smallpox and yellow fever, in the long run they constituted a more significant factor in colonial morbidity and mortality.[6]

The epidemic disease which received the greatest attention from the colonists throughout the entire pre-Revolutionary era was smallpox. This terrible disorder is exceedingly infectious, carries a high case fatality rate, and leaves a percentage of its survivors scarred and pitted for life. The name smallpox was coined in the sixteenth century to differentiate it from the pox, the name applied to syphilis. The incidence of smallpox rose steadily in Europe during the seventeenth century, and the disease probably peaked in the latter part of the eighteenth. It was repeatedly introduced into the American colonies, but did not become an endemic disease until the colonial wars of the mid-eighteenth century. The relative isolation of the British colonies from Europe and from each other limited the extent of the smallpox epidemics, restricting them generally to the major port cities. On the other hand, those who escaped added to the reservoir of non-immunes, and the long intervals between outbreaks, sometimes as much as fifteen to twenty years, meant that a large non-immune population tended to develop; hence, when the disease was reintroduced, the results were often devastating.

Precisely when smallpox was first introduced into North America is not clear, but the disease was present aboard the ships which brought the mass migration of Puritans to New England in the 1630s. On one vessel fourteen passengers died from smallpox and many more were sick. Minor outbreaks occurred in New England during the 1630s, although it was not until 1648–49 that the first general epidemic developed.

By the eighteenth century colonial port cities were large enough to sustain major epidemics—and none escaped. Probably because of its more effective quarantine laws, New England suffered only occasional attacks, but when smallpox did gain a foothold, the relatively high percentage of non-immunes among the population guaranteed a high case rate. For example, smallpox was epidemic in Boston in 1702, 1721, 1730, and 1752, and on each occasion the number of cases reached into the thousands. In 1721 the town had a population of slightly over 10,600. During the course of the epidemic approximately 6,000 individuals were seized with smallpox and of these about 900 died—over 8 percent of the total population.[7]

The pattern of smallpox attacks in the eighteenth century varied according to region. The middle colonies were repeatedly visited by smallpox, while New England seems to have gone untouched for relatively long periods. The southern colonies, as a result of their sparse population and comparative isolation, were affected least. Virginia, which had no major cities, had the fewest problems, while South Carolina, with its major port of Charleston, suffered more than any other southern colony. Whenever and wherever smallpox struck, it was capable of inflicting serious casualties. When the disorder returned to Charleston in 1760 after an absence of nearly twenty years, the result was a devastating epidemic which killed 730 citizens, approximately 9 percent of the city's population. Of the 8,000 inhabitants, approximately 6,000 caught smallpox. From today's vantage point it is difficult to conceive the horror and suffering of a major epidemic. With three quarters of the population seriously ill and many dying, the entire energies of the well were devoted to caring for the sick and burying the dead. As one newspaper correspondent wrote: "no Description can surpass its Calamity."[8] In 1730 and 1731 epidemic outbreaks occurred in Boston, Philadelphia, and New York. Late in 1731 Rip Van Dam, President of the New York City Council, in submitting a census covering ten counties reported a population of 50,242, but he added, "since the taking of said list I believe near eight hundred are lost by the small pox, and daily more dying." His figures are confirmed by the New York *Gazette*, which reported in mid-November that smallpox had killed 549 residents of New York City alone.[9]

Another disease which justifiably created terror and consternation among the colonists was yellow fever. Fortunately it was not a widespread problem until the end of the seventeenth century, as its ravages were restricted largely to major ports. From 1699 to 1702 Charleston, Philadelphia, and New York each experienced serious outbreaks. Describing the attack on Charleston in 1699 one observer wrote that nothing was done "but carrying Medicine, digging graves [and] carting the dead: to the great astonishment of all beholders."[10] These three epidemics successively wiped out 7 percent of Charleston's population, 5 percent of Philadelphia's, and 10 percent of the inhabitants of New York City. Charleston, because of its proximity to the West Indies, bore the brunt of the yellow fever attacks, but fortunately none were as serious as that of 1699. After 1761 yellow fever withdrew from the colonies, and for some unexplainable reason did not return until the 1790s. Although it was a malignant pestilence and created constant apprehension, it had only a limited impact upon colonial development.

Two other diseases deserve mention: diphtheria and scarlet fever. Both of these disorders appeared in relatively mild forms during the seventeenth century, and it was not until 1735 that they became serious threats. In that year a virulent and deadly form of diphtheria developed first in New England and then slowly spread southward through the other colonies. It was given many names— the throat distemper, throat "canker," and "cynanche trachealis"—and it was quickly recognized as a children's disease. Noah Webster spoke of it as the "plague among children," a fact which many colonists learned to their sorrow. The disease began its course in Kingston, New Hampshire, where not one of its first forty victims recovered. From there it spread to Hampton, where it wiped out all the children in twenty families. In the town of Hampton-Falls, in the course of one year the disease killed 210 out of a population of 1,200, and nearly all the victims were below the age of twenty. Dr. Ernest Caulfield, whose study of this diphtheria outbreak is a minor classic, estimated that the disease caused about

5,000 deaths during the five years it ravaged New England. The impact caused by the loss of 5,000 children in a population of 200,000 is hard to imagine.[11] Although New England suffered the heaviest losses, one can find equally grim accounts of diphtheria ravages in nearly every colony. This outbreak of diphtheria in the colonies was part of a great pandemic and marks the beginning of a new era in the history of diphtheria. After the initial onslaught, the disease did not again strike in such deadly fashion, but it remained to winnow the ranks of colonial children, and periodically it flared up into epidemic proportions.

Scarlet fever followed the pattern of diphtheria. There is evidence of the disease in the seventeenth century, but it was not until 1735, in conjunction with the diphtheria onslaught, that a highly fatal form of scarlet fever, called *scarlatina anginosa*, began spreading through the colonies. Although not as fatal as diphtheria, scarlet fever compounded the ravages of the former disease and helped to desolate colonial families. Colonial physicians tended to classify both diseases under the rubric of throat distemper, but several of them, including Dr. William Douglass of Boston, clearly identified two separate forms of throat disease, one of which we know as diphtheria and the other as scarlet fever.[12] The evidence of scarlet fever in the succeeding years of the colonial era is scant, and it does not appear to have been a significant epidemic disorder.

In reviewing the colonial period, it is clear that life was both short and grim, particularly for the earliest settlers, over whom starvation hovered constantly. Once the settlers had established themselves and adjusted to life in North America, health conditions showed a decisive improvement. Yet during the seventeenth and eighteenth centuries life expectancy was brief everywhere; death was a constant companion, and it was assumed that a good share of infants would not survive. The chilling inscriptions on New England tombstones reflected the ever-present awareness of death. While the Grim Reaper exacted his heaviest toll among infants, no age was exempt. Those colonial children who survived witnessed the deaths of parents, brothers, sisters, relatives, and friends close at hand. Death today takes place largely in aseptic hospitals, and the bodies are fast removed to funeral homes. In colonial days individuals died in their homes, suffering from bellyaches, "strangularies," cancers, bladder stones, and a host of other ailments.

Parents watched their children, besmeared with blood and pus, gradually strangle to death from diphtheria, or be swept away with the flux, measles, and so forth. Others died with their faces a mass of smallpox pustules, or else vomiting partially digested blood, the so-called "black vomit" of yellow fever. Some died quietly, but many groaned or cried aloud in agony during the final stages. The visibility and omnipresence of death was a major factor of life in colonial days, and it must have had a profound psychological impact upon the colonists.

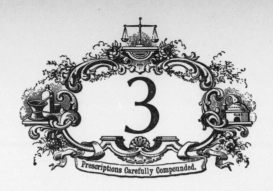

Prescriptions Carefully Compounded.

SEVENTEENTH-CENTURY COLONIAL DOCTORS

AN organized profession can only exist in a well-structured society, and the various English and Dutch settlements in America were in no position to support a medical profession until well into the eighteenth century. In the meantime medical care was provided from many sources, most notably minister-physicians and barber-surgeons. While religion played a significant role in the movement of Englishmen to the colonies, the chief factor was economic. Once it became evident that North America offered no quick and easy way to wealth, few university-trained physicians were willing to risk their comfortable careers. Physicians holding medical degrees were university men with good middle- and upper-class connections, and their clienteles were well-to-do. Colonial life, particularly in the seventeenth century, held little attraction for these relatively secure English gentlemen.

The lack of a physician class was not as serious as it might appear. In the first place, medicine was taught largely from a theoretical standpoint, and one could acquire a degree with little or no practical knowledge of anatomy or clinical medicine. Since "reading medicine"—a phrase which hung on until the end of the nineteenth century—was the way to a medical degree, any individual who wished, providing he was literate, could learn medicine. In early seventeenth-century England, where many dissenters were clashing with the established Anglican Church, prospective ministers often read both theology and medicine in order to have a profession to fall back on in the event they were dismissed from the church. In the colonies, nearly all educated men had acquired some medical knowledge, and they either practiced or gave occasional advice.

Since surgeons were looked upon as tradesmen in a class with barbers and were a relatively low-level income group, they were far more likely to be found in the ranks of immigrants, and most of the so-called doctors who came from Britain and the Continent in the seventeenth century fell into this category. Some came as settlers, but undoubtedly many were ship surgeons who elected to remain in the colonies. Along with the barber-surgeons came the apothecaries, midwives, *zieckentroosters*, and *krankenbezoekers*. In England and on the Continent, the customary fourteen years of study required for a doctor's degree meant that the number of trained medical men was always limited, and, as already noted, their relatively high social status led them to restrict their practice to the upper classes. The vast majority of people resorted to barber-surgeons, apothecaries, bloodletters, midwives, and a wide range of folk practitioners. The apothecaries, whose trade was compounding and selling drugs, always gave medical advice to their poorer customers, and in England they eventually gained the right to practice medicine. The same situation held true for the apothecaries in the colonies, but here the transition was even easier. Neither universities nor licensing agencies existed to prevent them—or anyone else who wished—from simply appropriating the title of doctor. Ironically, when trained physicians began arriving in the colonies in the eighteenth century, they were often compelled to open an apothecary shop. Occasionally they were forced into this action by the lack of an adequate pharmacy, but more frequently physicians had to enter the drug business in order to make a living.

The *zieckentroosters* and *krankenbezoekers* practiced in the Dutch colony of New Amsterdam and can be classified as the common man's physicians. Both groups originally sought to provide spiritual consolation for the sick and dying, but over the years they acquired some rudimentary medical and nursing skills. The midwives landed with the first women settlers, and they handled nearly all obstetrical work.[1] Doctors were summoned only in difficult cases, and not until the second half of the eighteenth century did any of them begin to take charge of normal births. Midwives did not restrict themselves to obstetrics. They served as nurses and pediatricians, and they often helped lay out the dead. Such training as they had was largely folklore, passed on from generation to generation, and the quality of care provided depended largely on the intelligence and common sense of the individual midwife.

The London Company which first colonized Virginia recognized the need for medical care. Several able physicians were members of the company, and more than likely they were responsible for the specific instructions relating to health matters which were given to the expedition leaders. These concerned the location of the colony, the type and number of physicians and apothecaries, and the building of hospitals. The first group of settlers to arrive in Virginia included a gentleman chirurgeon (or surgeon), Henry Wotton, who was listed as chirurgeon general, and another chirurgeon, Will Wilkinson, whose social status is indicated by the way his name is listed along with the bricklayer and barber. The first physician, Dr. Walter Russell, arrived in 1608, and the second, Dr. Lawrence Bohun, was brought by Lord Delaware in 1610. Leaving the colony in 1611, Dr. Bohun was mortally wounded when his ship was attacked by a Spanish man-of-war on his return in 1620. Bohun's replacement was Dr. John Pott, described as "a Master of Arts and . . . well practised in Chirurgerie and Phisique. . . ." Dr. Pott was an able medical practitioner, and, besides accumulating a substantial estate, he was a member of the Governor's Council and for one year served as temporary governor.[2]

During the years in which the London Company controlled Virginia, 1607–24, it provided the colony with a number of able physicians, surgeons, and apothecaries. Whatever mistakes the company may have made, the incredibly high death rate during the early years was not for want of medical care, for the company's physicians and surgeons were well versed in the prevailing medical knowledge. Once the British Crown took over, however, the colony became dependent upon its own resources and the few medical practitioners willing to emigrate. As a result, for the rest of the seventeenth century none of the colony's physicians measured up in terms of their training or education with Drs. Russell, Bohun, and Pott. Medical practice henceforth was largely in the hands of colonial doctors who had acquired their training through an apprenticeship or by self-education. To this group should be added the occasional ship surgeons or apothecaries who elected to settle in Virginia.

The early medical history of Massachusetts bears a close resemblance to that of Virginia. According to Henry R. Viets, the medical historian of Massachusetts, the best-trained physician for almost a hundred years, Deacon Dr. Samuel Fuller, arrived on the *Mayflower* in December 1620. His exact educational background is not clear, but he received part of his education in Leyden, a leading medical center. Although Fuller had received a sound theological training and held the title of deacon, he was usually referred to as Dr. Fuller by the colonists. His medical reputation in the 1630s led Governor Endicott of Salem to ask Governor Bradford for Fuller's services, and Fuller was later sent to Charleston to help Governor Winthrop's settlers. Judging by the comments of the governors, Dr. Fuller may have helped to draw the diverse New England colonies together. As an interesting aside, Fuller's third wife, who came to Plymouth in 1623, was a midwife, possibly the first to practice her profession in the colonies.[3]

The second physician worth noting in Massachusetts was Mr. Giles Fermin, who had studied medicine at Cambridge but apparently did not take a medical degree. He arrived in the colony in 1632 and returned to England for good in 1644. His one claim to fame lies in a brief reference to his having "made an anatomy," a phrase which refers to a dissection rather than simple demonstration with a skeleton. It may have been the urging and example set by Mr. Fermin which led the Massachusetts General Court in 1647 to recommend that "such as studies physick or chirurgery may have liberty to reade anatomy, and to anatomize once in foure yeares some malefactor." Except for a few leaders, medicine was seldom a lucrative profession in the colonies, a fact which Fermin soon discovered. In 1639 he wrote that he was "strongly sett upon to studye divinitiae . . . for physick is but a meene helpe."[4]

After the initial New England settlement, medicine fell into the domain of governmental leaders and ministers, aided by schoolmasters, apprentice-trained doctors, midwives, and folk practitioners. The lack of trained physicians in the Massachusetts Bay Settlement forced Governor John Winthrop to use the medical knowledge he had gained through his reading. So great was the demand for his medical services that he wrote to friends in England seeking further advice on herbals and general medical practice.

Among the best of the early minister-physicians was the Reverend Thomas Thacher. Thacher migrated to America around the age of fifteen, and in 1635 began studying under Charles Chauncy, who later became the second president of Harvard. Like many of his colleagues, Chauncy had probably received some instruction in medicine at Cambridge. His student Thacher subsequently was ordained a minister and followed his preceptor in combining ministerial duties with the practice of medicine. Ironically for a staunch Puritan, his reputation was gained as a physician rather than as a theologian. In 1677 Thacher published a broadside entitled *A Brief Rule to Guide the Common People of New England how to order themselves and theirs in the Small Pocks, or Measles* in which he advised his readers to make the patient comfortable, provide a moderate diet and ample liquids, and avoid excessive medication. In a day when large-scale bloodletting, purging, and bleeding characterized medical practice, Thacher's advice was unusually perceptive. He published his article at a time when smallpox was spreading through New England, and his sound advice must have been welcomed. Despite his own reputation in the field of medicine, at the conclusion of his essay Thacher modestly disclaimed professional knowledge, stating: "I am, though no Physitian, yet a well wisher to the sick. . . ."[5]

The list of seventeenth-century New England preachers who ministered to the physical as well as the spiritual needs of their flocks is a long one, and only one or two other examples need to be cited. John Eliot, the Apostle to the Indians, discovered very quickly that medicine was an effective means for gaining the confidence of potential converts. Michael Wigglesworth, whose grim poem *The Day of Doom* was widely acclaimed and speaks volumes for the Puritan psyche, also sought to alleviate the physical ills of his congregation. Since those ministers selected as successive presidents of Harvard College represented the more able and better-educated ones, they nearly all shared a common interest in medicine. President Charles Chauncy had some acquaintance with medicine, which he subsequently imparted to his six sons, all of whom became ministers and physicians. President Henry Dunster petitioned the General Court to allow students of physic to perform anatomies on the bodies of executed criminals. Apparently the College was already offering some instruction in medicine, since Dunster was also seeking funds for medical books. The general interest in medicine is shown by the fact that between 1642 and 1689 some twenty-seven Harvard graduates became physicians.[6]

The colony of New York, which differed from Virginia and the New England colonies in that it was established as a private company under a paternalistic government, escaped the sickness and starvation of its English counterparts. The Dutch, having learned from the English experience, were better prepared for the New World, and the locations of their settlements were generally healthful. While the colonists did not escape occasional epidemics of smallpox and other diseases, the colony on Manhattan and those along the Hudson River experienced only minimal health problems throughout the seventeenth century. As early as 1630 a midwife arrived in New Amsterdam, followed a year later by the first of the barber-surgeons. Within a few years the colony's barber-surgeons were objecting to the practice of ship surgeons treating patients while in port, and they successfully petitioned the Director-General and Council to give them the exclusive right to treat wounds and to shave all persons within the town. The Council also decreed that "Ship-Barbers" were not to practice medicine on shore without the consent of the barber-surgeons "or at least of Doctor La Montagne." Dr. Johannes La Montagne, a Huguenot refugee who had received his education at the University of Leyden, arrived in 1637. In addition to being the first physician with a formal medical degree, La Montagne was an able individual, and his medical skill and general ability eventually gained him a seat on the Council.[7]

Possibly because New York was a more cosmopolitan city, it was able to attract better-trained physicians and surgeons than was the case with the other colonies. The career of Samuel Megapolensis indicates that Holland's role as a leading medical center was another contributing factor. Megapolensis graduated from Harvard College and then took degrees in theology and medicine at the

University of Utrecht. On his return to New York he assumed the pastorate of a church and joined many of his contemporaries in combining a ministerial and medical practice. Incidentally, he was one of the commissioners who negotiated the transfer of New Amsterdam to the English in 1664. Another prominent university-trained physician in the midcentury was Dr. Adriaen Van der Donck. He had considerable intellectual curiosity and made some keen observations on the New World medicinal plants and mineral resources and upon the medical practices among the Indians. He also joined with other prominent colonists in complaining to Holland in 1649 about conditions in New Amsterdam. One of the specific grievances was the lack of a hospital.[8] Even though New York appears to have been better supplied with physicians than the other colonies, the ministerial practice of medicine was quite common.

The polyglot population of New York City by the end of the century was reflected in the diverse nationalities of its medical men. When the Provincial Council requested an autopsy on the body of Governor Henry Sloughter in 1691, six physicians and surgeons assisted in the task. The group was headed by Dr. Johannes Kerfbyle and included one Scotsman, one German, two Englishmen, and one Frenchman.[9] In glancing over the early medical history of New York, the similarities with the other colonies are probably greater than were the differences. Early medical care was provided by empirics, barber-surgeons, midwives, occasional physicians, and the omnipresent minister-physicians. Later, apprentice-trained doctors began to assume a more important role, but at the same time the colony was beginning to attract a few well-educated physicians. It was this higher percentage of doctors with medical degrees which differentiated New York from the other American colonies. New Yorkers as of 1700 appear to have had relatively fewer medical problems—and probably better medical care—than the other colonists.

Although ordinances relating to sanitation, water supplies, and provisions were soon enacted in the colonies, virtually no attempts were made to regulate the practice of medicine. The first hesitant steps in this direction were taken to guard the public against fraud and/or excessive fees. In 1630–31 a Bostonian was fined for selling a purported cure for scurvy, and a Virginia law first passed in 1639 and reenacted in 1645 provided for the arrest of any physician making an unreasonable charge. This same law permitted the court to censure a physician refusing assistance to the sick or neglecting his patients. In 1649 the Massachusetts General Court expressed its concern by requiring all medical practitioners, including midwives, to operate within "the known, approved Rules of Art. . . ." The General Court stated that it did not intend to discourage medical practitioners from the lawful use of medical skill but rather "to incourage and direct them in the right use thereof. . . ." When the Duke of York took control of New Amsterdam in 1664 and issued a new legal code, a law similar to the 1649 Massachusetts one was included. However sound the intent of these laws, they were vaguely worded and no provision was made for their enforcement. The only references to the licensing of physicians occur in certain county records in Massachusetts which show that occasional licenses to practice medicine were issued. No specific qualifications were required of the applicants, however, and it is safe to assume that in Massachusetts, as in the other colonies, anyone who wished could establish a medical practice.[10]

Despite the lack of regulation, seventeenth-century America was not overrun by quacks, bloodletters, traveling lithotomists, itinerate cataract couchers, and the other empirics who flooded Europe. Nor was the shortage of trained physicians a serious handicap. Ministers, governmental leaders, and prominent laymen were generally well educated, and, as indicated earlier, knew as much about the prevailing medical theories as orthodox physicians. Since they had not been indoctrinated in medicine they were far more likely to take an empirical or pragmatic approach to their patients, permitting common sense to take precedence over theory. The colonial doctors who learned their medicine via the apprentice system were also imbued with an empirical approach to medicine. They read their mentors' medical books, but they acquired most of their knowledge through experience and observation.

All physicians, whether or not they held a medical degree, were compelled to practice surgery along with medicine—and often to compound their own drugs. Frontier conditions and the fluidity of American society did not permit any sharp distinction between physicians and surgeons. This is not to say that social distinctions did not exist. A university-trained physician was a gentleman, and, even though he might engage in surgery out of necessity, he held himself above the common surgeon who had acquired his knowledge through an apprenticeship. If the gentleman physician did not bring capital to the colony, he usually acquired some in short order and was far more likely to be honored by an appointment to the Governor's Council. Yet, because society was fluid, an intelligent and able surgeon could rise in the social order, acquire a respectable estate, and gain a measure of acceptance in society.

An important factor in eliminating the distinction between physicians and surgeons was the general use of the term doctor. It is not clear precisely when it came into general use, but certainly by the end of the seventeenth century medical practitioners of all sorts were beginning to assume the title. By this date, too, gentlemen physicians in the southern colonies were adopting the perukes and periwigs of European society. However dashing the long curls hanging down to the shoulders may have looked, the wigs must have been hot, uncomfortable, and dirty. In partial compensation, beards were out of fashion, and gentlemen were now clean shaven. The yards of plaited linen which made up the ruffs of Elizabethan days and the tight-fitting doublets were no longer fashionable. The well-dressed physician now appeared in his heavy periwig, cravat, vest, knee breeches, garters and buckles. His coat, which reached down to the knees, was quite often elaborately embroidered. Colonial caste lines were not as rigid as in the mother country, but the well-to-do did their best to maintain them.

By the end of the seventeenth century the worst hardships and suffering were over. While the relative number of university-trained physicians was lower than during the first settlements, the slack had been taken up by minister-physicians, apprentice-trained doctors, and barber-surgeons, most of whom were supplying medical care at least comparable to that found in Europe. The few physicians with medical degrees were too scattered to unite for professional purposes, and a medical profession awaited the establishment of medical schools, societies, and licensure laws late in the colonial period.

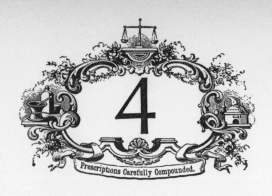

MEDICINE IN EIGHTEENTH-CENTURY COLONIAL AMERICA

By 1700 the British foothold on the American continent was well established. The struggling settlements in New England and Virginia were becoming prosperous towns and communities, reproducing in part the social structure of the mother country. The accumulating wealth led to caste lines' becoming sharper as the well-to-do sought to emulate the so-called "better classes" of England. The emergence of a leisure class facilitated the development of professions, and slowly doctors and lawyers began to form professional organizations. Those young colonials interested in medicine turned first to the British and European medical schools; then, as a consciousness of American nationality began to develop and American communities became large enough to support medical institutions, hospitals and medical schools made their appearance. By the time of the Revolution one hospital and two medical schools were firmly established, a number of local medical societies were functioning, and several colonies had enacted medical licensure laws.

MEDICINE AND THE MEDICAL PROFESSION

It may be misleading to speak of an American medical "profession" at this time, since as late as the nineteenth century it was still fighting to attain a measure of professional respectability; nonetheless, by the mid-eighteenth century, individual doctors were being accorded the respect and income commensurate with professional status. They were also conscious of the need for mutual support, and it was in this same period that the first tentative steps toward establishing professional societies were taken. The movement toward professionalization was receiving an impetus from developments in medicine itself. The majority of physicians in the seventeenth century had held to a vague humoral concept of disease which assumed that sickness resulted from an imbalance of the four basic bodily humors. This imbalance was caused by an excess of a particular humor, by a fermentation or putrefaction of one of them, or by an alteration in the movement of the humors. This century of genius, however, witnessed remarkable discoveries in science and these were to have a direct impact upon eighteenth-century medicine.

The advances in mathematics and astronomy which culminated in Isaac Newton's promulgating one basic principle to explain the workings of the universe sent medical philosophers off on a fruitless quest for the one fundamental principle of health. In consequence, the eighteenth century became preeminently an age of medical theorizing in which the proponents of vitalism, solidism, tonism, and tension vied with one another. The first new medical theories to evolve were the seventeenth-century iatrophysical and iatrochemical schools. The iatrophysical school sought to explain the functioning of the human body in terms of mechanical principles. It saw locomotion, respiration, and digestion as purely mechanical processes and envisioned the body as a machine motivated by a "life force" circulating through the nerves to motivate the muscles. The iatrochemists believed digestion was a chemical process in which glands acted upon the food to modify fermentation. They asserted that all things in the body were reduced to acids or alkalis, and that the aim of medicine was to correct imbalances. Sickness, then, was the result of abnormal chemical reactions, which, if unchecked, could produce morbid phenomena such as gallstones and urinary calculi.

Most American practitioners were too pragmatic to pay much attention to the arguments raging in Europe, and they continued to operate upon the Galenical or humoral theory. The better-educated colonial physicians were inclined to accept the modified humoral theory taught by the great English physician Dr. Thomas Sydenham. He maintained that particles of morbific or peccant matter entered the body via the air and vitiated the humors by producing fermentation or putrefaction. The resulting sickness could be cured by eliminating this morbific matter by purging, sweating, vomiting, and so forth. Sydenham also revived the Hippocratic concept of epidemic constitutions, *i.e.*, that epidemics were caused by inexplicable changes in the earth's atmosphere. The irony of all the new seventeenth- and eighteenth-century medical theories was that they simply rationalized the traditional practice of bleeding, blistering, purging, vomiting, and sweating. Whether restoring the humoral or chemical balance, or eliminating morbific substances, the treatment was the same, varying only according to the preferences of the individual practitioner.

In the mid-eighteenth century the more moderate ideas of the famous Dutch clinician, Hermann Boerhaave, had some impact on American medical practice. Boerhaave was an eclectic willing to borrow from any system who reverted to the Hippocratic idea of observing the patient and who believed it the function of the physician to assist nature in effecting the cure. Dr. David Ramsay, an early historian, wrote that in 1760 the "practice of physic . . . was regulated in Carolina by the Boerhaavian system." Unfortunately the moderating influence of Sydenham and Boerhaave was eclipsed later in the century by the extreme views of John Brown and Benjamin Rush—a development which did little to help the medical profession and, as will be seen in subsequent chapters, proved even worse for the patients.[1]

By twentieth-century standards, little of colonial medical practice could be classified as moderate. In addition to wholesale bloodletting and purging, the use of nauseating substances (the well-known *dreckapotheke*) was widely accepted. A purported cure for smallpox consisted of bleeding, a soft diet, and the administration of a variety of drugs including syrup of white poppies and sheep's "Purles" in water. A poultice of cow's dung, milk, and bread was also to be applied to the throat and was to be used inwardly for "Defluxion." Cotton Mather, who kept well abreast of the latest medical developments, was an ardent advocate of the use of dung and urine. Human excreta, he declared, was "a Remedy for Humane Bodies that is hardly to be paralleled," and urine had virtues far beyond all the waters of medicinal springs. The prescription for a patient suffering from rheumatism in 1720 illustrates the relentless fight of man against disease. On the first day the patient was to be purged twice. On the second day he was to be bled 12 to 14 ounces of blood, preferably from the foot. A day or so later the patient was to be purged twice more. In the meantime, the prescription read: "On those Days he doth not Purge, and Bleed, Give one of the powders In the morning and another In the Evening, mixt In some Diet Drink made with Equal Parts Horse Redish Roots, and Bark of Elder Roots, Pine Budds, or the Second Bark, wood or Toad Sorrel, make it strong with the Ingredient." If nothing else, the cure surely took the patient's mind off his rheumatism.[2]

Even a casual survey of the horrendous medical prescriptions makes one shudder at the implications in the phrases "brisk purging" or "copious bleeding." Colonial records abound with complaints of patients dying from the effects of excessive purging or vomiting. An Anglican missionary in 1709 described the death of a colleague in the following terms: "This Gentleman had the misfortune to take Physick of a pretended Phisitian which work't so violently that it gave him 100 vomits and as many stools, brought the Convulsions on him, which soon carried him off, and caused him to purge till he was Interr'd." In 1733 the New York *Gazette* reported that the wife of a local silversmith had been treated by a physician who "appointed her a portion of Physick; after the receiving of which, she fell to vomiting to such a degree" that death came two days later. William Douglass, probably the best-trained physician in early eighteenth-century Boston, asserted that New England medical practice "was very uniform, bleeding, vomiting, blistering, purging, anodyne, etc. if the illness continued, there was repetendi, and finally murderandi." The practitioners, he added, "follow Sydenham too much in giving paragoricks, after catharticks, which is playing fast and loose."[3]

The same drastic therapy characterized the southern colonies. In the Carolinas during the late colonial period the lancet (for bloodletting) was used freely for pleurisies and rheumatisms, while patients with febrile complaints were first purged and vomited, and then given sudorifics to sweat the poisons out of the system. Cinchona bark (from which quinine is derived) was administered for intermittent fevers or malaria. According to one observer, there was a strong prejudice against cinchona bark, and the physicians were often compelled to disguise it. Cinchona was one of the few specifics available to eighteenth-century physicians, but administering the crude bark made it difficult to standardize the dosage. This fact, combined with the adverse side effects of quinine, may well account for the popular suspicion of the bark.[4] If Carolina doctors restricted their use of the bark to cases of intermittent and remittent fevers, they were scarcely typical of colonial physicians. The success of cinchona in these fever and agues led to its general use as an antifebrile. As late as the 1830s and 1840s southern physicians were using massive doses of quinine to treat yellow fever patients—a form of therapy which merely added to the patient's medical problems.

SURGERY

Surgery, despite all the advances in anatomical knowledge and certain technical improvements, was still limited largely to emergency situations. Fractures, luxations, amputations, wounds, abrasions, lancing boils, dressing ulcers, catheterizing, extracting teeth, giving enemas, and letting blood formed the major part of the surgeon's work. The more able ones occasionally operated for urinary calculi (bladder stones) or performed paracentesis (surgical puncture of a cavity for the aspiration of a fluid), but these were considered major operations. The *South Carolina Gazette* in 1732 reported that, when a British naval surgeon drew ten quarts of water from the abdomen of a seaman, the operation was watched by the surgeons of all his Majesty's ships in the harbor. By 1766 colonial surgeons were becoming more venturesome, as indicated in a fee bill issued by the New Jersey Medical Society. Listed among the charges for medical and surgical services were trepanning (or removing a portion of the skull), extracting of cataract, "extirpation of the tonsils," correction of "Harelip" and "Wryneck," amputations of the limbs and breasts, excision of tumors, paracentesis, and cutting for the stone (lithotomy). The last operation was performed by Dr. John Jones of Newark in 1767. According to the newspaper account, this successful lithotomy was performed "before several very eminent Gentlemen in the Practice of Physick and Surgery."[5]

One can only speculate on how many doctors were capable of or willing to attempt these operations. It is safe to assume, however, that in the days before anesthetics, only the most desperate of patients would be willing to submit to them. Other than dealing with injuries and providing routine services such as opening abscesses, surgical intervention remained uncommon throughout the colonial period. The account book of Dr. William Fleming of Virginia for 1768 typifies the customary surgical practice.[6]

"Drawing tooth from Negro Wench . . . . £0=2=6"

"Opening a Tumor & Dressing . . . . £3=0=0"

"Opening his breast and Extracting pin . . . . £2=8=2"

"Amputating leg & Dressing . . . . £8=0=0"

As the New Jersey fee bill cited earlier shows, medicine and surgery continued to go hand in hand. Many physicians handled surgical work only out of necessity and kept these services to a minimum. Others, with greater manual dexterity and an inclination toward surgical intervention, gradually gained a reputation in this area and attracted surgical patients. The same held true of obstetrics, which by the time of the Revolution had become almost a specialty for a handful of colonial physicians: Dr. William Moultrie in Charleston, William Shippen, Jr. in Philadelphia, and James Lloyd of Boston, to name a few. Even though their interests led them into surgery or obstetrics, these men considered themselves physicians first of all; specialism in the modern sense was a much later development.

REGULARS AND IRREGULARS

By the mid-eighteenth century medicine was still in the hands of a diverse group of practitioners, but a distinct professional body was beginning to emerge. These physicians, known as the "regulars," constituted the best of the four main categories of medical practitioners. The "regulars" were a rather amorphous group representing the better-trained and more intelligent individuals. As Whitfield Bell points out, the regulars achieved this status by a combination of formal preparation, ethical conduct, and demonstrated success in medical practice. hysicians with medical degrees from British or European universities ordinarily were accepted without question. Skilled practitioners who had served an apprenticeship under a first-rate physician and had later studied in Britain or the Continent, as was the case with James Lloyd (1728–1810) of Boston, were also included among the regulars. The same held true for students with American college degrees who subsequently read medicine with an established physician. Occasionally individuals whose sole training had been an apprenticeship, but whose medical skill had won them general approbation, were also accepted into the ranks of the regulars. Membership was both informal and arbitrary, and no sharp caste line divided the regulars from the lesser rank of doctors. Yet the regulars were the physicians whose advice was requested by municipal and colony authorities during the recurrent epidemics, and the health officers and port physicians were usually chosen from their ranks.[7]

As the eighteenth century wore on, there was a growing professional consciousness among the regulars. Recognizing each other's ability, they began drawing together to exchange professional information and to give each other mutual support. Aside from intellectual curiosity and a growing desire to improve their medical skill, economic competition from the large numbers of lesser qualified practitioners supplied a major motive in the formation of professional societies. This competition came chiefly from the second category, the run-of-the-mill apprentice-trained practitioners who probably constituted the majority of colonial doctors. The better ones, as already noted, frequently sought additional training and moved upward. The qualifications of the doctors in this category varied widely, but many of them were conscientious individuals who rendered good service. In 1751 a newspaper obituary of Dr. Roelof Kierstede of New York City described him as a "Gentleman eminent in his Profession, altho' not skill'd in the technical Terms thereof, which often drew on him the Contempt of his Brethren; yet his great Knowledge in Simples, his extensive Charity and successful Cures to poor People, has made his Memory precious to them, and his death a real public loss."[8] To offset the Kierstedes were probably an even larger number of poorly equipped practitioners, only vaguely acquainted with anatomy and the prevailing medical knowledge, who eked out a miserable living through medicine or practiced on a part-time basis to supplement their income as farmers, planters, or merchants.

The lowest group in terms of training and skill were the folk practitioners and the quacks. In isolated areas particularly, any individual willing to give medicine a try could, with a little luck, set himself up in practice. If he or she possessed any knowledge of simples or herbal remedies and had learned a smattering of folk medicine, all that was needed for success was a number of patients with self-limiting medical disorders. A traveler in Connecticut encountered a former cobbler who, having chanced to "cure an old woman of a pestilent disease" and finding medicine more profitable than shoe repairing, "fell to cobling of human bodies." As the colonies increased in wealth and population, they began to attract quacks from abroad and to develop a few native ones. William Smith in his history of New York published in 1758 wrote: "Quacks abound like locusts in Egypt, and too many have recommended themselves to a full and profitable practice and subsistence."[9] Since medicine in the eighteenth century could neither prevent, cure, nor alleviate many of the disorders troubling patients, it is not to be wondered at that the public in Europe and the colonies frequently turned to anyone who promised relief. Moreover, the regulars within the profession frequently could not agree with each other, so that even intelligent laymen often did not know which way to turn.

Following the English example, where a Mrs. Joanna Stevens was awarded a grant of £5,000 by the British Parliament for discovering a lithontriptic, a medicine to dissolve urinary calculi, the colonial legislatures on several occasions rewarded individuals who claimed to have found some efficacious treatment. The Virginia House of Burgesses, for example, gave £100 to one Mary Johnson for discovering a cure for cancer and another £250 to Richard Bryan for his remedy for the "dry gripes," a name given to plumbism or lead poisoning. The Massachusetts General Court expressed a willingness to give Palmer Goulding a grant of land if he could successfully demonstrate his snake bite cure.[10] One of the more successful quacks in the late eighteenth century was Elisha Perkins of Connecticut with his magnetic tractors. Capitalizing on the interest in animal magnetism and electricity aroused by Franz Anton Mesmer and Benjamin Franklin, Perkins was one of the first of a long line of American entrepreneurs who cashed in on the latest scientific discoveries. As one might expect, the twentieth century with its radio waves, electronic devices, and atomic energy has also proved a gold mine for the unscrupulous.

MINISTER-PHYSICIANS

Last, but certainly not least, of the medical practitioners were the omnipresent preacher-physicians. Despite the growing number of professional and lay practitioners, ministers, in some cases out of necessity and others by choice, continued to provide medical services to members of their congregations and to the public at large. Anglican missionaries sent to the colonies in the late eighteenth century by the English Society for the Propagation of the Gospel often found their knowledge of medicine to be an effective way of reaching potential church members. In 1716 the Reverend Mr. Henry Lucas reported to the Society from New England that his "little knowledge in Physick" had given him "a great Opportunity for conversing with Men by whc. I have done that, wch. by preaching I could not have done."[11] Ministers in isolated areas often found that, as the best-educated man in a community without a physician, they were called upon for help. Many others discovered that medicine was an effective means of supplementing their income. The role of minister-physician elicited a mixed reaction from congregations. In some cases the congregation was glad to be relieved of providing full support for their minister and was happy to secure medical assistance. A few congregations, however, objected to receiving medical bills from their ministers, feeling that healing the sick was a normal responsibility for one whose life was presumably dedicated to the great Healer.

As educated and well-read individuals, it is not surprising that the ministerial profession provided a major share of the best medical writers in the colonial era. Thacher's broadside on small-pox in the seventeenth century was the first of a series of articles and pamphlets written by ministers on medical topics. Following a measles epidemic which killed five members of his household in 1713, Cotton Mather published an essay in which he provided a first-rate clinical description of the disorder and recommended a course of treatment which could scarcely have been improved upon. Familiar with the drastic therapy of his day, he began by warning against excesses in treatment: "Before we go any farther, let this Advice for the Sick, be principally attended to: *Don't kill 'em*! That is to say, With mischievous Kindness." "Indeed," he went on, "if we stopt here, and said no more, this were enough to save more *Lives* than our *Wars* have destroyed." He stressed the need for complete rest even when the patient suffered only a mild case, and he pointed out that "*a Fever*, (perhaps that which they call, the *Pleuritick*) too often follows the Measles." His final advice to the family of the patient reads: "Let him not be *well too soon*, and throw himself into a *Fever*, and throw away his *Life*, as many have inconsiderately and presumptiously done."[12] Cotton Mather's will-ingness to go counter to the active drugging and bloodletting of his day and his sharp observation that the sequela of measles is more dangerous than the disease itself show his forceful character and original mind.

Mather's chief claim to fame in the medical area lies in his sponsorship of inoculation or variolation in the colonies. Smallpox, as has been shown, was a dreadful disease and one that inflicted particular hardship upon American colonials. Sometime in antiquity, it was discovered that taking pus from the pustules of an active smallpox case and inserting it under the skin of a healthy individual would cause him to develop a relatively mild case of smallpox and henceforth be immune to the disease. The procedure is known as variolation, from the technical name for smallpox, *variola*, to differentiate it from the safer technique of vaccination. Inoculation was practiced in isolated rural areas of Great Britain and the Continent at least as early as the seventeenth century, but it was not until the years from 1714 to 1716 when a series of letters addressed to the Royal Society from Constantinople reported in detail on the procedure that interest became widespread.

Cotton Mather, who had an active interest in science and kept abreast of the latest developments, read the various accounts in the Royal Society's *Transactions*. He was particularly intrigued, since he had already heard of inoculation from his black slave, Anesimus. The latter claimed to have undergone the procedure, which he said was a common practice in his tribe. Mather decided in 1716 that, if smallpox again struck Boston, he would urge inoculation on the town physicians. In April 1721 several ships from the West Indies brought smallpox to the city, and Mather circulated a letter among the local physicians describing the practice and urging them to consider it. When the physicians did not deign to reply, Mather wrote a personal letter to Dr. Zabdiel Boylston, one of Boston's leading physicians. Two days after receiving Mather's letter, Boylston inoculated his six-year old son and two of his black slaves. When all three showed only the mildest of symptoms, Boylston inoculated several others.

Almost immediately the townspeople became outraged, or, as Mather recorded, a "horrid clamour" arose. He complained in his diary over "the vile Abuse which I do myself particularly suffer . . . for nothing but my instructing our base Physicians, how to save many precious Lives." Dr. William Douglass, the only one of Boston's ten physicians with a medical degree, bitterly criticized Boylston for mischievously "propagating the Infection" and called upon Mather and the advocates of variolation to put their reliance in "the *all-wise Providence* of God Almighty." Surprisingly, the town's ministers tended to support the innovation while most of the doctors opposed it. In 1722 Douglass wrote that his arguments with the clergy had "occasioned great Heats," and then added a little bitterly, "you may perhaps admire how they reconcile this with their doctrine of predestination." Not all clergy were convinced; one of them sermonized in 1722 that it was "an unjustifiable act, an affliction of an evil, and a distrust of God's overruling care. . . ." Another was apprehensive that inoculation, by freeing people from the fear of smallpox, would tend to promote "Vice and Immorality."

Although there were exceptions, the clergy throughout the colonies generally supported inoculation, and they deserve some credit for its widening use. As late as 1759 an Anglican missionary in New Jersey inoculated his own children, thus, he wrote, removing the prejudices and scruples of many of his congregation.[13]

As John Blake has pointed out, the clash between Mather and Douglass represented a conflict between the theocratic ideas of the old school New England clergy and the emerging professionalism of the physicians. Mather firmly believed in the right of the clergy to control the life of the community, and Douglass, speaking as a physician, was objecting to interference into professional matters by laymen. From Douglass's standpoint, smallpox was too dangerous a disorder to experiment with and too many questions about inoculation were unanswered. As it turned out, those undergoing inoculation, while suffering only a mild case themselves, were capable of passing a virulent and fatal disorder on to others.[14] Later events would show that smallpox inoculators not infrequently were responsible for serious epidemic outbreaks of the disease. Douglass correctly based his chief opposition upon the fact that not enough was known about variolation for it to be tried on a wholesale basis.

The major doubts about the efficacy of inoculation were laid to rest when the Selectmen of Boston compiled statistics on smallpox at the end of the 1721 epidemic. During the course of the outbreak almost 6,000 persons were infected with smallpox and approximately 300 were inoculated with it. The case fatality rate for those taking the disease naturally was about 14 percent against only 2 percent for those inoculated. Even Dr. Douglass conceded that variolation appeared to have promise, but he urged further experimental work by qualified physicians. In the succeeding years the use of inoculation gradually spread throughout the colonies.

As indicated earlier, many inoculators made little effort to isolate their patients and their careless techniques were often responsible for broadcasting the seeds of this deadly pestilence. It was not unusual for an inoculated patient "to do all Things, as at other times." If the patient was compelled to go to bed, the illness was, according to one account, only a minor inconvenience: "Ordinarily the Patient sits up every Day, and entertains his Friends, yea ventures upon a Glass of Wine with them."[15] The thought of a person with a mild case of smallpox going about his normal affairs or entertaining his friends is a frightening one, and it is small wonder that colony after colony passed laws forbidding inoculation. Whenever smallpox threatened or gained a foothold, however, these laws were usually held in abeyance. As the benefits of variolation were widely recognized, the tendency was to regulate the practice rather than to prohibit it. By 1760 the laws were rewritten so as to define the conditions under which inoculation could be performed and to set a minimum quarantine period for patients. At the outbreak of the Revolution, inoculation was widely practiced in the middle and southern colonies under reasonable legal safeguards. Massachusetts, the first colony to establish an effective quarantine system, continued to ban inoculation except when smallpox was present, but the repeated introduction of smallpox during the Revolutionary War convinced most residents of the Bay State of the need for inoculation.

The essential difference between the American and European experience with variolation was the extent of its application. In Britain and on the Continent inoculation was restricted largely to the upper class until the end of the century, whereas in the colonies it was applied on a large scale. For example, when the Revolution began, on the recommendation of his Physician-in-Chief, Dr. John Morgan, Washington ordered a general inoculation of all American forces.

There is little question that variolation proved a great boon to the American colonists. While it did play a role in spreading smallpox, the disease could not have been avoided, since American involvement in European wars and the growing commercial contacts made its repeated introduction almost inevitable. Smallpox was endemic in Europe, and it was only a matter of time before the same would become true of North America. In the colonies the wider use of inoculation led to improved techniques and a corresponding lower case fatality rate. It meant, too, that the great smallpox epidemics of earlier years no longer terrorized the population. True, the number of outbreaks increased, but they lacked the intensity and virulence of the earlier ones. The limited statistical information available shows that the case fatality rate for naturally acquired smallpox appears to have fallen as the eighteenth century advanced. Whether the wider use of variolation was responsible for this or whether it resulted from a century or more of natural selection—those with the greatest natural immunity tending to survive—is difficult to say. Variolation, however, did offer an alternative, and it helped to alleviate the psychological impact of this terrible disorder. Probably more important for both Europeans and Americans was that their familiarity with inoculation paved the way for the immediate acceptance of Edward Jenner's discovery of vaccination at the end of the century. The credit for introducing variolation into America rightfully belongs to Cotton Mather and Dr. Zabdiel Boylston. Even without their initiative it would have come, but they were the first to recognize its value and they hastened its advent. They provided the first relatively large-scale test, and the statistical evidence which they collected guaranteed that the practice would receive a fair trial.

Even more significant than Cotton Mather's role in introducing smallpox inoculation was his rationale for so doing. The development of microscopy in the seventeenth century had led Athanasius Kirchner (1602–1680), on the basis of the little "worms" he saw in the blood under his low-power microscope, to postulate the thesis that these tiny animals were the cause of infectious disease. His idea, known as the animalculaer theory, received only limited attention, but it persisted until the work of Pasteur and Koch demonstrated its essential validity. Alone among his fellow colonists, Cotton Mather was not only familiar with the thesis, but he himself espoused it. Upon first reading about inoculation, he indicated his belief that smallpox was a disease caused by these pathogenic animalculae, and when he began writing his major medical work in the 1720s, *The Angel of Bethesda*, he set forth his views in considerable detail. He described how swarms of these minute animals had been seen by microscopes, and he suggested that once in the body they "multiply prodigiously," corrupting the blood and injuring tender vessels. He even suggested that there was a specificity about the animalculae. In the case of "Itch" and syphilis, Mather described how the organisms could be transmitted from person to person by means of towels or direct contact. He also recognized that the invasions of these animalculae did not always cause disease, and he explained this fact on the grounds that, when bodily secretions and evacuations are normal, the body casts out the invaders. While based on the research and ideas of his predecessors, Mather's exposition of what we now term the germ theory is remarkable for its clarity and lucidity. It shows, too, his receptivity to new ideas.[16]

Mather's originality is shown by the way in which he applied the animalculae theory to explain why inoculation produced only a mild form of smallpox. In a pamphlet written in 1722, Mather asserted that the animalculae ordinarily entered the body through the respiratory passages and were quickly spread by the blood directly to the vital organs. In the case of inoculation, the contagion was introduced only at the periphery, which gave the body time to mobilize its defenses and resist the invader. The intriguing thing about Mather was his intellectual curiosity. He was not only receptive to new ideas, as shown by his willingness to test variolation, but, when they worked, he wanted to know why. Dr. William Douglass, during the heated debate over variolation, dismissed Mather as a credulous layman. In point of fact, Mather was probably the most original medical thinker of the colonial period.

The minister-physicians played a particularly important role during the great "throat distemper" epidemic of the 1730s, and at least two of them made significant contributions to medical knowledge. The Reverend Mr. Jabez Fitch collected and published an excellent statistical account of the disease in New Hampshire. On the basis of his careful observations, we can be reasonably sure today that diphtheria was not the new disease it was thought to be in Fitch's time. The second minister-physician, the Reverend Mr. Jonathan Dickinson, wrote one of the best medical treatises on the disease. In the characteristic fashion of his day, he described a bewildering array of symptoms and an equally wide variety of medicines, ranging from Virginia snakeroot to laudanum and calomel.

Preacher-physicians were particularly active in New Jersey. The Reverend Mr. Robert McKean of Perth Amboy, another Society for the Propagation of the Gospel missionary, in 1766 was chosen as the first president of the New Jersey Medical Society, and during the first ten years of this Society's existence, six of its thirty-six members were pastor-physicians. The German ministers who came to Pennsylvania also found their congregations asking for more than spiritual consolation. The Reverend Mr. Henry Melchior Muhlenberg in a bitter moment likened himself to a "privy to which all those with loose bowels came running from all directions to relieve themselves." Fortunately he was well prepared to handle complaints of the spirit and the bowels, since he had been trained in medicine in Halle. Although his main objective in coming to America was to organize Lutheran churches, he spent a good deal of his time practicing medicine.[17]

One can scarcely leave the minister-physician without a mention of John Wesley's *Primitive Physick*. This classic do-it-yourself medical book went through thirty-two English and seven American editions between 1747 and 1829. Although it included many of the esoteric remedies of the eighteenth century, Wesley counseled his readers to beware of excessive bloodletting and strong drugs, a factor which no doubt helped its sale. Another reason for its widespread distribution was that it enabled the patient to save medical fees. This latter may have been a source of the occasional clashes between doctors and ministers. Wesley himself was dubious of the medical profession and advised his followers to consult only godly doctors. The doctors in turn accused the ministers of dabbling in medicine far more than physicians meddled in theology; thus, the doctors asserted, ministers were more inclined to quackery than doctors to heresy.[18]

LEADING PHYSICIANS

Although the number of able physicians in the colonies was quite high, none of them rank with Cotton Mather as an original contributor to medicine. Dr. William Douglass, whose opposition to Mather in the inoculation controversy has already been discussed, was a dogmatic and assertive Scotsman with a medical degree from Leyden. Despite a personality problem, Douglass was an able individual, and he wrote an excellent clinical account of a scarlet fever outbreak in Boston. Entitled *The Practical History of a New Epidemical Eruptive Military Fever, with an Angina Ulcusculosa Which Prevailed in Boston New-England in the Years 1735 and 1736*, this clear depiction of scarlet fever was published twelve years before Dr. John Fothergill, the famous English physician, issued his classic account. Douglass also had an active interest in natural history and collected several hundred botanical and mineral specimens in and around Boston.

During the colonial period literally nothing was known about the causes of the great epidemic disorders, and in desperation every possible lead was followed. Since scientifically inclined individuals were beginning to turn to observation and to the collection of statistical data, one blind alley they pursued in quest of an explanation for epidemics was meteorology. They sought to keep exact records of the daily changes in temperature, humidity, and so forth and to correlate these records with the rise and fall of particular epidemics. The idea dates back to one of the books of Hippocrates, *Airs, Waters, and Places,* which stressed the role of environment in disease causation. Sydenham's "epidemic constitution"—a peculiar combination of meteorological phenomena and other factors which presumably turned normal summer or winter fevers into serious epidemic diseases—was a variation of the Hippocratic idea. Douglass was one of the first colonial physicians to begin gathering this information. He was, however, too preoccupied with the inoculation controversy and maintaining his position as the informal leader of the Boston physicians to make any important contributions in natural history and related sciences.

Douglass was only one of four colonial physicians whose work contributed to and was recognized by the international natural history circle.[19] Interestingly, three of them were Scotsmen and the fourth had received much of his education at the University of Edinburgh. The second of this group was Cadwallader Colden. Colden took his M.A. degree at Edinburgh before the University offered training in medicine and then headed south to London for his medical education. He subsequently emigrated to America, first to Philadelphia and then in 1718 to New York where he began investigating American plants (botanical remedies still constituted a major part of the materia medica, and it was natural that any physician with intellectual curiosity would be interested in herbals). Subsequently Colden encountered a copy of Linnaeus's *Genera Plantarum* and quickly mastered the Linnaean system of plant classification—an accomplishment which placed him among a select group of Britishers at that time. Colden's interest in botany came to the attention of Peter Collinson, an English Quaker who stimulated and encouraged much of the work by colonial naturalists. Through Collinson, Colden became known to the two leading European naturalists, Linnaeus and Gronovius, both of whom had praise for his description and classification of the plants he discovered in New York.

Although he practiced medicine only briefly, Colden was acutely conscious of the need to raise the status of the medical profession, and he constantly urged government support for medical education and research. In 1720 he published his first medical article, *Account of the Climate and Diseases of New York*. Colden's study on climate and disease antedates that of Douglass and, in addition, is much more thorough. In it Colden attributed the relatively small amount of consumption (pulmonary tuberculosis) in New York, when compared with England, to the pure air. Colden's second and most important medical work was his essay entitled *The Fever Which Prevailed in the City of New York in 1741–42*. Yellow fever appeared widely in the American colonies in 1741, and, although New York City suffered only lightly, the disease aroused considerable apprehension. In his essay, Colden reviewed the history of yellow fever and then turned to the conditions in New York City which he felt provided a potential breeding ground for the fever. He noted that the disorder invariably appeared in the vicinity of the docks—where dirt and filth tended to accumulate—and ships in those low-lying areas of the city which had been built upon swampy ground. He questioned the traditional belief that the high morbidity and mortality among infants and children during the summer was due to eating fresh fruit, pointing out that country children, who had far greater access to fruit, did not die in such numbers from these summer complaints. The real cause, he wrote, was the deleterious atmosphere and the unsanitary condition of the city.

Having stated what he believed were the conditions predisposing to epidemic fevers, Colden then made a series of specific recommendations to the city officials. The city must make arrangements to drain all low-lying damp grounds and see to it that "all the filth and nastiness of the town be emptied into the stream of the river. . . ." The deplorable sanitary and drainage conditions, he said, resulted from leaving the responsibility for drainage in the hands of private individuals. The solution was to make the city responsible, "then every one, since it would cost him no more, would be desirous and careful to have his cellar clean and dry, and his nostrils freed from an offensive stench." He stressed the need for conscientious officials, "men of Known industry, and zeal for the welfare of the town. . . ." The force of Colden's logic and his prestige as a colonial official gave his recommendations real meaning. In May 1744 the Provincial Assembly enacted "A Law to Remove and Prevent Nusances within the City of New York." On the basis of this law, the Common Council of New York City promulgated a sweeping sanitary ordinance and followed up by appropriating funds for cleaning the city. The preamble to the city ordinance stated the principle which was to dominate public health for the next 150 years: ". . . the health of the Inhabitants of any City Does in a Great Measure Depend upon the Purity of the Air of that City and that when the Air of a City is by Noisome Smells Corrupted, Distempers of many Kinds are thereby Occasioned. . . ."[20] The law established a table of fines for each offense against the sanitary code and divided the revenues between the individual responsible for prosecution and the church wardens. The system worked well up to the time of the Revolution, although its success was more likely due to the tradition of cleanliness among the town's inhabitants.

Colden's thesis was scarcely an original one. A good part of it was borrowed from a classic work by the Italian clinician and epidemiologist, Giovanni Maria Lancisi, *De nosiis paludum effluviis,* published in 1717. Yet Colden obviously kept abreast of the current medical literature, he was receptive to new concepts, and he succeeded in applying his sanitation ideas on a large scale. His essay on fever is not only the first significant writing on sanitation in the American colonies but, more important, it bore fruit.

The third of this group of Scottish physicians to make a name for himself in botany was Dr. Alexander Garden of Charleston. Garden, however, was a naturalist first and a physician second, and all his major contributions relate to botany and zoology. The fourth of these botanist-physicians was Dr. John Mitchell of Urbana, Virginia. Mitchell's background is uncertain, but after receiving an education at Edinburgh and Leyden he settled in Virginia. He, too, came under the influence of Peter Collinson and was introduced into the European natural history circle. Ill health forced Mitchell to return to England in 1746, but before he did so he had written several papers on botanical subjects and had discovered some twenty-five genera, at least ten of which had not been described previously. In England he published three books and achieved a measure of fame for his *Map of the British and French Dominions in North America.* This map, which remained the standard work for many years, was used in settling British and French claims in the peace treaty ending the American Revolutionary War.

Mitchell's medical contribution, although indirect, was to have a strong impact upon nineteenth-century medical practice. Following the outbreaks of yellow fever in Virginia in 1737 and 1741, Mitchell wrote an essay on yellow fever which he sent to Benjamin Franklin for presentation to the Society for the Promotion of Useful Knowledge. Some years later this manuscript came to the attention of Dr. Benjamin Rush, who used it in preparing his lectures on medicine. During the 1793 Philadelphia yellow fever epidemic, Rush reread the manuscript and became convinced on the basis of Mitchell's experience that his own therapy had been too mild. The result, as will be seen later, was to be of major consequence to thousands of American practitioners and their patients.

Another Scot interested in botany but who was primarily a physician was Dr. John Lining of Charleston. Lining's best-known work is a description of the yellow fever outbreak in Charleston in 1748, a careful and precise clinical account in which he sought to correlate weather conditions with disease. Lining also deserves some credit for his efforts, even if they were not successful, to investigate physiology. During the summer of 1740, he wrote, "as opportunity served, I weighed myself every hour, second or third hour, through the day, to investigate the difference of the urine and perspiration in the different hours of the day, under different circumstances. . . ."[21] However admirable Lining's intent, the answers to his research would have to await a vastly improved technology and a fundamental breakthrough in science.

There were other physicians, too, who dabbled in botany—and other botanists who dabbled in medicine. John Bartram, for example, made his name in natural history, but to support himself he had to farm and occasionally practice medicine. Among the physicians who concentrated their intellectual energy primarily upon medicine was Dr. John Bard, the outstanding practitioner in New York City prior to the Revolution. Born in Burlington, New Jersey, Bard received a private education and was then apprenticed to Dr. John Kearsley, an irascible English surgeon in Philadelphia. After practicing in that city for some years, Bard was persuaded by his friend Benjamin Franklin to move to New York. Here he quickly established an excellent reputation. During his long career, he wrote several excellent papers on medical topics. In 1759, Bard and Dr. Peter Middleton performed the first dissection for teaching purposes in America, using the body of an executed murderer. In recognition of his long and active career in medicine, when the Medical Society of the State of New York was organized in 1788, Bard was elected its first president.[22]

John Bard's son, Samuel, continued his father's tradition. Following graduation from King's College, in 1760 he was sent abroad for study, and immediately encountered one of the hazards facing all colonists who ventured across the Atlantic. His ship was captured by a French privateer, and young Bard spent five months in a French prison until he was released through the efforts of Benjamin Franklin. Undeterred by this experience, Bard began studying medicine in London and Edinburgh, taking an M.D. degree in the latter institution, and returned to join his father in medical practice. Prior to the Revolution Bard published an article entitled the "Angina Suffocativa, or Sore Throat Distemper" in New York. Although only one of many articles published on diphtheria during these years, it is an excellent clinical description of the disease.

The city of Philadelphia produced several excellent physicians, at least two of whom rank with the best in the colonies. One of the first was John Redman (1722–1808), who was educated in Philadelphia, served an apprenticeship under Dr. John Kearsley, later attended Edinburgh University, and took a medical degree at Leyden. He was an able physician, a strong supporter of inoculation, and best known for the able young physicians who studied under him, men such as John Morgan, Benjamin Rush, and Caspar Wistar. John Morgan (1735–1789), one of the first of these apprentices, far outshone his preceptor Redman. Morgan was educated at a private academy and then apprenticed for six years to Dr. Redman. While serving this apprenticeship, he enrolled in the College of Philadelphia (University of Pennsylvania). On completing both his apprenticeship and his college degree in 1756, he joined the Pennsylvania Provincial forces and served as a surgeon during the French and Indian War until the end of hostilities.

Recognizing the need for additional medical study, Morgan decided to further his medical education in Europe. As was true of so many young colonists going abroad, he left Philadelphia in 1760 armed with letters from Benjamin Franklin. Morgan spent a year in London studying under John and William Hunter and came under the influences of Dr. John Fothergill. The latter was an English Quaker physician and naturalist who counseled and encouraged many of the young colonists who came to London to further their medical education. He was a friend of Franklin's and enjoyed a wide range of contacts in the London intellectual world.

From London Morgan moved on to spend two years taking an M.D. degree at the University of Edinburgh. Next he embarked on a grand tour of Europe, stopping off in Paris for three months to study medicine before going to Italy where he made a courtesy visit to Giovanni Morgagni in Padua. Before returning to America in 1765, Morgan had gained membership in several leading medical and intellectual societies in London, Edinburgh, Paris, and Rome. From the standpoint of his American contemporaries, his most signal honor was membership in the Royal Society. While in London Morgan was already planning to establish a medical school and to organize a medical society on his return to Philadelphia. As will be seen, he succeeded in both enterprises and subsequently played a significant role in the American Revolution.[23]

Along with John Morgan, the other outstanding Philadelphia physician was William Shippen (1736–1808). Shippen graduated from the College of New Jersey (Princeton) in 1754 and began an apprenticeship in medicine under his father, William Shippen, Sr., a prominent medical man in his own right. In 1757 the younger Shippen sailed for Great Britain, where he spent three years in London working with the celebrated English obstetrician William Hunter. Shippen was also fortunate enough to enter the circle of Dr. John Fothergill, joining in the breakfast sessions which the busy Fothergill devoted to his younger protégés. Following his London studies, Shippen moved to Edinburgh where he acquired an M.D. degree and spent some time in Paris and Montpelier.

Shippen was interested in offering private courses in midwifery and anatomy, and he was encouraged in the project by Fothergill, who gave him a number of anatomical drawings and casts. In November of 1762 he began teaching the first formal course of anatomy in the colonies. Although he used materials donated by Fothergill, he relied largely upon the dissection of human subjects—a practice which caused considerable popular resentment and on several occasions led to his dissecting rooms being mobbed. Nonetheless, the course proved successful, and the number of students grew rapidly. Shippen next added a course in midwifery for medical students and prospective midwives. When Morgan returned in 1765 and a medical school was established, Shippen and Morgan became embroiled in a personal controversy which peaked during the Revolutionary War and which was to plague them for the rest of their lives.

One can scarcely leave Philadelphia without some mention of Dr. Thomas Bond (1712–1784). A native of Maryland, Bond served an apprenticeship with Dr. Alexander Hamilton of Annapolis and then crossed the Atlantic to study medicine on the Continent. He began practicing in Philadelphia around 1734 and gained a fine reputation as a physician and surgeon. During his lifetime he published two first-rate clinical papers, but his chief claim to medical fame comes from his role as the prime mover in promoting the Pennsylvania Hospital and his long association with that institution. In 1766 he began giving lectures on clinical medicine at the Hospital. Although he was not on the faculty of the newly organized Medical School, the students were advised to attend Bond's lectures. Aside from his contributions in medicine, Bond is equally well known for his leadership in founding the American Philosophical Society in 1768. These brief biographical sketches do not exhaust the list of worthy practitioners, but colonial physicians collectively contributed little to advancing medical knowledge. The chief significance of those discussed was that they helped lay the basis for an effective American medical profession by keeping in touch with European developments and by promoting medical education, hospitals, and professional societies in the colonies.

THE MEDICAL SIDE OF BENJAMIN FRANKLIN

Ironically, the two Americans in the colonial period who made the most original contributions to medicine were both laymen. The first was, as we have seen, the Reverend Cotton Mather and the second was Benjamin Franklin—the one man whose interests encompassed nearly all areas of American thought and action. While apprenticed to his brother James, young Ben became involved, if only slightly, in the inoculation controversy. Although James Franklin's paper, the *New England Courant,* had bitterly attacked Cotton Mather in 1721–22, Ben Franklin soon became a staunch advocate of inoculation, and later in his own newspaper, the Pennsylvania *Gazette*, he strongly supported the practice. Despite the vitriolic clash between his older brother and Cotton Mather, Ben realized Mather's ability and on a return trip to Boston reestablished good relations. He relates that on leaving Mather's house the old minister suddenly said, "Stoop, stoop!" Before Franklin realized what was meant, he hit his head on a low beam. Mather, who never missed an opportunity to moralize, told Franklin to "stoop as you go through [the world], and you will miss many hard thumps."[24]

Franklin's experiments with electricity are common knowledge. What is not so well known is that he tried to use electricity to stimulate muscular action in patients suffering from various forms of paralysis. He experimented on several patients in 1757 and discovered that although they showed an immediate improvement for two or three days, by the fifth day they became discouraged and discontinued the treatment. Unlike so many discoverers of purported medical cures, Franklin was not carried away with enthusiasm. He reported that while he felt that electrical treatments might have value in the hands of a skilled physician, he had serious doubts about their usefulness. His own medical problems led him to devise two useful medical aids. One of these was his invention in 1784 of bifocals so as to avoid having to carry two pair of glasses around. The second arose from his bouts with urinary calculi or bladder s ones. Probably as a result of his own painful experiences, he devised a flexible silver catheter, personally directing the silver-smith in the work.[25]

A brief mention was made earlier of Franz Anton Mesmer, a Frenchman who claimed to have discovered a rather mysterious substance he called animal magnetism. He won a good deal of popular support, although the European medical profession was quite skeptical. In Paris a special commission was appointed to investigate Mesmer's claims. Franklin, one of the five judging academicians, shrewdly pointed out that the successes attributed to Mesmer were largely due to the imagination of the patients. From his own knowledge of medicine and his experiments with electricity, Franklin had come to some understanding of what we today term psychosomatic medicine. Although the commission dismissed

Mesmer's claims, the concept of animal magnetism continued to have considerable public appeal.

Throughout his career Franklin was asked for—and gave—medical advice. His approach to medicine was that of a keen observer and a sensible practical individual. In 1744 he warned his parents that the lithontriptic of Joanna Stephens, the medicine supposed to dissolve urinary calculi, was not really effective. A few years later he advised one of his friends "not" to stop taking cinchona bark for fever and ague for at least two or three weeks after the last bout with the fever. Since even today the treatment to eliminate malarial parasites is a long-term one, Franklin's advice was sound. He was a constant advocate of "fresh air and exercise" which he thought were invaluable in preventing disease. It was particularly important, he said, to prevent diseases, "since the cure of them by physic is so very precarious." In 1773 he wrote to Dr. Benjamin Rush: "I hope that after having discovered the benefit of fresh and cool air applied to the sick, people will begin to suspect that possibly it might do no harm to the well." In this same letter he also suggested that colds and influenza were spread in close, ill-ventilated places. In the eighteenth century gout was associated with excessive eating, drinking, and sexual activities. When Franklin fell prey to this painful metabolic disease, an old friend, Madame Brillon, wrote teasingly to him in 1780 that it was not his indolence or greed but his amorousness which had brought on the disease. Franklin replied that he was sure excessive sexual indulgence had not brought on his disorder since it had not bothered him when he was young![26]

During the course of a long career, Franklin observed and commented upon a wide range of medical topics. In addition to those already mentioned, he wrote on the heat of the blood, deafness, infant mortality, and medical education. Franklin was a shrewd promoter, and this ability proved useful in the case of the Pennsylvania Hospital, the oldest hospital still in operation in the original American colonies. Dr. Thomas Bond had been trying unsuccessfully to raise funds by popular subscription when he was advised to see Franklin. Franklin was quite enthusiastic and immediately began publicizing the project. Realizing that government money was needed, he approached some of the legislators, suggesting that they match the money raised by private subscription. On receiving some encouragement, he drew up a bill which stated that the provincial appropriation was conditioned on the raising of £2,000 from private individuals. As Franklin later wrote, the legislators agreed to support the measure since they thought that so large a sum could not be raised privately. When the bill did pass, Franklin then used the promise of government money to persuade private donors to contribute their share.[27] The hospital might have been organized without Franklin, but his support hastened the process and guaranteed firm backing for the institution.

Unlike Cotton Mather, whose preoccupation with theology necessarily limited the scope of his activities, Franklin ranged over and dabbled in almost every type of intellectual, political, economic, and social activity. Both men had first-rate minds, and they seldom mistook trees for woods. It may be symbolic of the state of American medicine that the two men who contributed the most original work in medicine were laymen.

THE PUBLIC IMAGE OF THE COLONIAL PHYSICIAN

The nature of medical work and the close relationship of the profession with its clientele make it difficult to ascertain precisely what the public thinks of physicians at any given time. A great deal of ambivalence always exists in the public reaction to doctors. The same individuals who may denounce the profession collectively will, in the next breath, swear by their own physicians. Public opinion in the colonial period showed some of this ambivalence, but there was a far greater suspicion of medicine than holds true today. Understandably intelligent and articulate men, supported by the more able physicians, generally denounced the increasing number of ignorant empirics, quacks, and charlatans as the eighteenth century advanced. More serious than this, however, was a widespread skepticism of medical theories and of the harsh and drastic measures employed by even the best-trained practitioners.

In an age when medicine was taught largely by lectures and reading, any educated individual could emulate the physician in "reading" medicine and was thus in a position to pass judgment upon the rationale of his physician's practice. While the more intelligent of the university-trained physicians learned from experience and used discretion in applying the various forms of therapy, too many others zealously followed the medical theory of their preceptors or rigorously applied traditional therapeutics regardless of the consequences to the patients. To compound the situation, public disagreements among even the better physicians over the cause, nature, and treatment of diseases were common and served only to increase public skepticism.

As mentioned earlier, historians generally agree that the caliber of medical practitioners was reasonably high during the early years of settlement, and, as it became clear that British North America offered no royal road to wealth, the quality of physicians and surgeons declined. Hence it is no accident that the first complaints about the medical profession were not recorded until well into the colonial period. The celebrated Virginian William Byrd, whose diaries tell us so much about colonial life, was one of those who regarded the medical profession—and other professions, too—with more than skepticism. He once referred to New Jersey as "a Place free from those 3 great Scourges of Mankind, Priests, Lawyers, and Physicians. . . ." Speaking of Virginia in 1706, he wrote that the colony had men who claimed to be doctors, "but they are generally discarded Surgeons of Ships" who "know nothing above very common Remedys." Dr. William Douglass of Boston had nothing but contempt for most of his fellow practitioners, an attitude scarcely conducive to instilling public confidence in his profession. So many quacks and poorly trained doctors abounded, he wrote, there was often "more danger from the physician than from the distemper."[28]

Colonial records show many instances where patients did fall victims to medical treatment, a few of which have been alluded to earlier. Occasional newspaper editorials decried cases where individuals who sought medical help for a minor illness were promptly purged, bled, and blistered to death. John Oldmixon, an early historian, summarized what may well have been a general attitude when he wrote that the Virginians "have but few Doctors among them, and they reckon it among their Blessings, fancying the Number of their Diseases would increase with that of their Physicians." In 1763 a young British physician asked John Watts for assistance in establishing a practice in New York. Watts wrote that he would welcome him even "tho' a Professor of that black Art, in hopes that he may be an exception to the general Rule. . . ." He warned that the doctor would not have an easy time, adding cryptically, "but for the [medical] faculty, it is a healthy Climate. . . ." The following year he replied to a request about the possibility for a medical lectureship in anatomy by declaring there was little hope, explaining, "we have so many of the Faculty allready destroying his Majestys good Subjects, that in the humor people are, they had rather one half were hanged that are allready practicing, than breed up a New Swarm."[29]

Most of the complaints about doctors in these years related to the excessive number of untrained practitioners and charlatans. The preface to the 1760 medical licensure law in New York begins: "Whereas many ignorant and unskilful persons in Physic and Surgery . . . do take upon themselves to administer physick, and practice surgery . . . to the endangering of the lives and limbs of their patients. . . ." A few years later Dr. Peter Middleton of New York City deplored the fact that competition from quacks and empirics had forced even respectable physicians to prescribe popular nostrums and secret remedies. "Such being the state of physic here," he asserted, "what wonder is it that this city should be pestered in so remarkable a manner with the needy outcasts of other places, in the character of doctors; or that this profession of all others should be the receptacle and resource for the refuse of every other trade and employment."[30]

Despite strong competition, once a physician had established a sound middle- or upper-class practice, his financial position was quite good—but, unless a young physician belonged to a well-to-do family or had medical connections, this was not easy to do. Precisely because the practice of medicine was accessible to anyone, the ratio of practitioners to population was always high, resulting in a low income for the average doctor. A young Philadelphian sent abroad for his medical training informed his father that he had no desire to return home. The prospect of practicing in Philadelphia held little appeal for him. Fees were so low, he wrote, that it "is a severe piece of Drudgery" for a physician to "maintain his family Genteelly."[31] The economics of medicine were undoubtedly one of the factors which drove many physicians into becoming planters, merchants, government officials, and, occasionally, ministers.

Aside from the limited economic opportunities in medicine, it did not have the prestige of either the ministry or law. One could become an apprentice-physician with minimal education—and many of the empirics were virtually illiterate. Under these circumstances, educated practitioners who left the profession for more lucrative fields, such as administration, business, or planting, seldom returned to the practice of medicine.[32]

Quite a few men with training in medicine held positions in the provincial governments, which, as Whitfield Bell noted some time ago, raises an interesting point. Why was it that with a few exceptions, most notably Cadwallader Colden in New York, these former physicians took so little interest in public health or made so few efforts to secure medical licensure laws?[33] We can assume, however, that those who left the profession were scarcely dedicated physicians, but rather were men who in most instances had taken up medicine as a means of making a living. In addition, the climate of opinion in the colonies was scarcely receptive to any form of government regulation except in emergency situations. Quarantine and isolation measures were accepted when epidemics threatened, but, in normal times, they and other public health measures received short shrift. And with a good part of the public dubious of all professions and holding the medical profession in particular distaste, there was little chance for a medical society or any other professional group to receive the right to regulate its practitioners.

The relationship of physicians to their female patients is always a delicate one, and the charges and countercharges in court records show that colonial physicians had at least their share of moral problems. In North Carolina a Dr. Boyd, a medical graduate of Edinburgh and an ordained minister, was rumored to have "poysoned a man [in order] to lye with his wife." He brought suit for character defamation, and, since he continued to practice medicine, the suit must have been successful. Another Carolina doctor was not so fortunate. In 1736 a widow sued a neighbor for saying she "had often lain & coppulated with" her physician, Dr. Thomas Hall of Brunswick. The disposition of the case is not clear, but, significantly, Dr. Hall's name does not appear again in the local records. Another Carolina doctor, Josiah Hart, who later became a pioneer Baptist minister, sued a libeler who had accused him of having impregnated a black slave belonging to a Mr. Burgess. If for nothing else, the libeler deserved to be punished for his perverted sense of humor; he was specifically accused of having said that Mr. Burgess employed Dr. Hart "to cure his Negro wench's sore Eyes and he . . . began at the wrong End."[34] With a relatively low educational level, virtually no code of ethics, and many quacks and charlatans in the medical profession, the fact that even this many cases of this kind finding their way into court probably means they represent only a small percentage of the actual number. The nature of these offenses, however, leaves little historical evidence. One can only assume that medical practitioners then as now reflected the general level of morality.

One last point with respect to colonial doctors. For most of them medicine was a way of making a living, far more of a trade than a profession. As such, they felt little obligation to provide free medical care for the poor. No dispensaries or clinics existed, and, while individual physicians undoubtedly provided some charity work, it was not the general rule. The deserving poor who received medical care did so at the expense of the township or community. The occasional testimonies in newspapers and other colonial records to the fact that a deceased physician had rendered help to the poor implies that this conduct was not typical, and the same implication can be seen in the constant advice to medical students to treat the sick regardless of their financial condition.

In summary, many physicians were respected and affluent members of their community, but this respect arose from their personal qualities rather than their status as physicians. The majority of doctors were ill-prepared and poorly paid. They had little professional consciousness and held only a very limited concept of professional ethics or responsibilities. By the time of the Revolution the situation was beginning to change, but the road ahead was still a long one. The public in the eighteenth century accepted the physicians on these terms; they liked and respected individual practitioners, but they were dubious of medical theories and had serious reservations about the profession as a whole.

COLONIAL HOSPITALS

The first hospital built in the British American colonies was constructed in 1612 in Virginia near the falls of the James River. A contemporary account describes it as a "Hospitall with fourescore lodging . . . for the sicke and lame, with keepers to attend them for their comfort and recoverie." Nothing further is heard of this institution, and in all probability it was burned during the Indian uprising of 1622. The early proprietors of the colony also sought to build "guest-houses" for the sick; but, once Virginia became a Royal colony in 1624, the Royal government took no interest in the matter. Probably the next hospital in the colonies was a small military hospital erected in New Amsterdam in 1658 and placed under the charge of Matron Hilletje Wilburch.[35] For the next one hundred years the history of hospitals in the English colonies is vague, and the claims for priority in the founding of hospitals depend largely upon how one defines a hospital.

Until well into the nineteenth century the line between hospitals and almshouses was never sharply defined. Even those institutions designed to provide care and treatment for the sick often became filled with the aged poor and chronically ill. Local authorities in all the colonies were compelled to make some provision for those who could not afford medical care. The standard practice was to designate one physician to attend those in necessity or else employ a doctor as the occasion arose. Since sick strangers and other impoverished individuals often had no place of residence, it was also necessary to rent or buy a house in which to treat them. By the eighteenth century the larger towns had established almshouses and had appointed physicians to attend to the residents. In describing these institutions, the terms almshouse and hospital were used interchangeably, leading to much of the present confusion.

Whether these establishments can be classified as hospitals or poorhouses lies at the crux of the dispute as to priority between Charity Hospital of New Orleans and the Pennsylvania Hospital. Both claim to be the oldest hospital in the present United States. While Charity was founded in 1736, some sixteen years before the Pennsylvania Hospital, the supporters of the latter claim that Charity was merely a poorhouse during the eighteenth century. Before taking up this question, it will help to look at the history of hospitals in Louisiana. The French began settling the Louisiana Territory along the Gulf Coast around 1699 and established several excellent military hospitals. The Company of the Indies, the French equivalent of the Virginia Company, was quite paternalistic, sending surgeons, apothecaries, midwives, and ample medical supplies to its colony in Louisiana. In 1722 a large military hospital was built in New Orleans following a hurricane which destroyed the existing one. We do not know the number of patients for which it was designed, but during the sickly autumn of 1723 over 800 patients were jammed into it. In 1726 the Ursuline Sisters of Rouen were invited to take charge of the hospital, which was called the Royal Hospital. An agreement was worked out by which the Company of the Indies would provide transportation and support for a group of six nuns, including the Mother Superior, and four servants. This small group of Ursulines arrived in 1727 and the Ursuline Order continued to administer the Royal Hospital until 1770. During these years and for the rest of the eighteenth century the Royal Hospital continued to receive government support from both the French and Spanish regimes, and the institution did not close until the American occupation of Louisiana in 1804.[36]

As the expenses of the Louisiana colony mounted during the early years, the French government began objecting to civilian use of the Royal Hospital, since it was intended for military purposes. In response to these objections, Jean Louis, a sailor and boat-builder, willed his entire estate worth 10,000 livres, a relatively large sum, "to serve in perpetuity to the founding of a hospital for the sick of the City of New Orleans." In 1736 a small temporary hospital was established and plans were made for a new brick building, which opened in 1737. During its early days the hospital was variously named. It was at all times a "charity" hospital and eventually the name Charity Hospital became official. During the ensuing years, the Hospital was rebuilt several times, and eventually became the first state-operated hospital in the United States.[37]

To dispense with Charity's claim to being the oldest hospital in the United States on the grounds that it was more of an almshouse than a hospital implies that the Pennsylvania Hospital never served in this capacity. The truth is that all hospitals in the eighteenth century were eleemosynary institutions, designed to take care of sick strangers and the sick poor. While it is true that Charity at times held many chronically sick, it always provided medical care for those who could not be treated in their homes. It should be remembered that even as late as 1900 most so-called decent, respectable people expected to be treated at home and, when the time came, to die in their own beds.

It should also be mentioned that one of the aims of the

almshouses was always to provide care for the sick poor. For example, the Philadelphia Almshouse, which was founded in 1729, ultimately became the Philadelphia Hospital, the forerunner of the Philadelphia General Hospital (Blockley Division) of today. Dr. Robert J. Hunter, the historian of the Philadelphia General Hospital, declares that the Almshouse was "a hospital in every sense . . . an institution where people with many kinds of illness were receiving medical care. . . ."[38] In 1736 New York City opened a similar institution, called the Alms House. One room with six beds was set aside as an infirmary, providing the city with its only "hospital" facility for many years. This same year witnessed the establishment of St. Philips, a combined workhouse and hospital, in Charleston. These almshouses, however, were designed primarily as welfare institutions and, while they provided some medical care, it was only incidental to their main purpose.[39]

In addition to the almshouse, another precursor of the modern hospital was the pesthouse, lazar house, or lazaretto. These institutions, which date back to the early eighteenth century, were designed to protect the public and not to help the patient. Their main purpose was to isolate patients with infectious or communicable diseases.

Boston was probably the first town to set aside a hospital or pesthouse for those sick with pestilential diseases. As early as 1702, and possibly well before this, smallpox victims were removed from town. In 1717 the General Court of Massachusetts built one on Spectacle Island to isolate "infectious persons" arriving by sea. Bedloe's Island in New York Harbor was first designated as the location for the city's pesthouse in 1738. Some years later the City Council, leaving no doubt that patients sent to the pesthouse would receive no more than custodial care, appointed John Brown, a "city Labourer," as "Overseer and Manager of Bedloe's Island. . . ."[40] Philadelphia built its first pesthouse on Province Island in 1743, and by this time almost every major port city had some type of isolation center.

As already noted, the oldest institution in the thirteen original British colonies still in existence today is the Philadelphia Hospital. The idea for the hospital was first conceived by Dr. Thomas Bond and, as mentioned earlier, was brought to fruition in 1752 with the aid of Benjamin Franklin. Unlike the almshouses which were open to what were considered the "deserving" poor regardless of circumstances, the first regulation of the Pennsylvania Hospital specified that "no Patients shall be admitted whose Cases are judg'd incurable, Lunaticks excepted; nor any whose Cases do not require the particular Conveniences of an Hospital"; the second rule forbade the admission of persons with "the Small-pox, Itch, or other infectious Distempers," unless special apartments were prepared for their "Reception." A third rule stated that women with children would not be admitted unless provision was made for the care of the children elsewhere, "that the Hospital may not be burthen'd with the Maintenance of such Children, nor the Patients disturbed with their Noise." After specifying what procedures the poor needed to follow in order to gain admittance, the regulations stated that "if there shall be Room in the Hospital to spare, after as many poor Patients are accommodated as the Interest of the Capital Stock can support, the Managers shall have the Liberty of taking in other Patients, at such reasonable Rates as they can agree for." While caring for private patients was purely secondary to the main purpose of the Hospital, this is the first instance in the colonies where provision was made to receive paying patients. Another regulation—which makes it clear that the founders were creating a hospital rather than an almshouse—stated that all patients must be discharged as soon as they were cured or "after a reasonable Time of Trial are judg'd incurable."[41]

Some of the other regulations are of interest since they throw light on early hospital conditions. Patients were forbidden to "swear, curse, get drunk, behave rudely or indecently, on Pain of Expulsion after the first Admonition." They were also enjoined from playing cards, dice, or any other games within the hospital and from begging anywhere within the city of Philadelphia. The last of the hospital rules required all patients "as are able [to] assist in nursing others, washing and ironing the Linen, washing and cleaning the Rooms, and such other Services as the Matron shall require."[42]

As one of the inducements to encourage the Legislature to appropriate funds for the Hospital, Franklin had persuaded three physicians, Drs. Lloyd Zachary, Thomas Bond, and Phineas Bond, to offer their services free of charge for three years. Once the precedent of free service to the Hospital was established, the practice continued. The six practitioners who were selected to serve in the Hospital in May 1752 not only attended the patients gratis, but they also provided free medicines until December 1752 when the directors opened an Apothecary's Shop in the Hospital. Aside from a measure of prestige, the Hospital physicians were allowed to bring apprentices or students into the Hospital for clinical training at a charge of one English guinea per year.[43]

During the first fourteen months of existence, the Hospital admitted 64 patients, of whom 32 were cured, 5 discharged as incurable, 4 were considered to have been helped, 1 discharged because of "irregular Behavior," 6 were "taken away by their Friends," 2 simply left on their own, and 5 died. The largest category of patients admitted during the first two years or so were those listed as suffering from "Ulcers, with Caries, &c." A total of 37 were admitted under this heading, of whom 21 were cured, 4 relieved, and 3 died. The next largest group was the "Lunatics," of whom 18 were admitted. Only 2 were reported cured and another 3 relieved. Tying for third place, each with 9 admittances, were "Dropsies" and "Scorbutick [scurvy or scurvous] and scrophulous Diseases." Of the latter category, 6 were cured and 1 relieved. Of the 9 patients with "Dropsies," only 4 were cured and 1 helped. The Hospital appears to have had some success in dealing with "Rheumatism and Sciatica," but both of these complaints tend to be self-limiting. Of the six individuals admitted in this category, four were cured and two were still under treatment at the end of the period. Three patients were admitted with ague, all of whom were cured, and three each with cancer, "Falling Sickness," and "Fistula in *Ano*." Two of the patients with "Falling Sickness" died, but the other was cured. The physicians claimed more success with cancer and the "Fistulas," since they discharged two out of the three cases each as cured. Rather surprisingly in view of the usual complaints in the eighteenth century, only two individuals were admitted with "fevers," both of whom were cured, and only one each with consumption and flux. The flux victim died and the consumption patient (probably a case of pulmonary tuberculosis) was reported to have been taken away by friends.[44]

The success of the Pennsylvania Hospital encouraged the local medical society in New York City to attempt to establish a comparable institution. New York had a workhouse or almshouse, but it had no place specifically designed to care for the sick. Moreover, the better physicians recognized the value of a hospital in providing clinical training. With the founding of King's College Medical School, the need for a hospital became more evident. As already noted, in his address at the first graduation of the Medical School in 1769 Samuel Bard appealed for the establishment of a hospital on grounds of humanity and upon the role of the hospital in providing an essential part of the physician's training. Led by Samuel Bard, Peter Middleton, and John Jones, and with strong support from Cadwallader Colden, the Society of the Hospital in the City of New-York in America was chartered by the provincial government. The Society soon raised £800 by private subscription, secured a plot of land from the city as a building site (which was subsequently exchanged for £1,000), and persuaded the provincial legislature to grant an annual allowance of £800 per year for twenty years. Construction began in 1773, but as the building was nearing completion it was virtually destroyed by fire. The legislature quickly appropriated an additional £4,000 and construction began anew. The time was scarcely propitious, and the war intervened before the building was finished. The fire and the war were only two of the problems besetting the institution, and it was 1791 before the New York Hospital officially opened.[45]

Before leaving the subjct, brief mention should be made of the inoculation hospitals. These, in effect, were much improved versions of the pesthouses, and arose from a recognition that persons urdergoing variolation needed close medical attention— and, more important, were a potential threat to the community. A number of these hospitals were opened by private physicians or "inoculators" who used their own homes or some other building. During a smallpox epidemic in the winter of 1764 the Province of Massachusetts opened two large inoculation hospitals, one at Point Shirley and another at Castle William. By the time of the Revolution, inoculation hospitals of various sorts were scattered throughout the colonies. Their purpose, as indicated, was primarily to isolate those undergoing smallpox inoculation, and they can scarcely be called true hospitals. Aside from pest houses, almshouses, and inoculation centers, at the end of the colonial period only two hospitals, the Pennsylvania Hospital and Charity Hospital in New Orleans, were in existence.

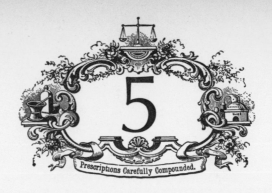

MEDICAL EDUCATION, LICENSING, AND SOCIETIES

EARLY in the eighteenth century, Britishers, at home or in the colonies, turned to the Continent for their medical education, with most of them going to Leyden. By the second half of the century, Edinburgh and Glasgow were emerging as centers for medical education and the London hospitals were providing first-rate clinical and surgical training. Since these hospitals could not offer degrees, the standard practice for young colonists was to spend one to three years in London and then move to Scotland for a year or so to acquire a medical degree. The University of Edinburgh was in the anomalous position of offering easy degrees to those who wished them but also providing sound training for those earnestly seeking an education. Benjamin Bell wrote in 1770 that medicine was taught in Edinburgh "in greater perfection than in any other part of Europe"—but that its surgery fell "greatly short of either Paris or London."

A medical degree carried prestige in the colonies, but, as

Whitfield Bell has pointed out, it was no guarantee of professional competence. Aside from those individuals who sought a degree rather than an education, not infrequently men who had spent a few months at Edinburgh or Leyden simply assumed a medical degree upon landing in the colonies. Moreover, even those with legitimate degrees often found themselves in an isolated town or rural area, with little intellectual contact and no professional support.

Long before any formal teaching of medicine in the colonies, at least two medical degrees were awarded. In 1663 the General Court of Rhode Island conferred a medical degree upon one John Cranston in the process of giving him a license to "administer physicke and practice chirurgery." One section of the act read that Cranston "is by this Court styled doctor of physick and chirurgery. . . ." Sixty years later, 1723, Yale bestowed a medical degree upon a Daniel Turner in return for a gift of books.[1] Happily today, degrees of this sort do not carry the right to practice medicine.

Two of the earliest steps toward providing formal medical training in the colonies have already been touched upon: the private course in anatomy offered by John Bard and Peter Middleton in 1750 and William Shippen's courses in anatomy and obstetrics. In addition, Dr. Thomas Wood in New Brunswick in 1752 and Dr. William Hunter in Newport, Rhode Island, in 1754 and 1756 offered private lectures in anatomy. The first formal course in anatomy associated with a regular educational institution was given by Dr. Samuel Clossy at King's College (Columbia) in New York in 1763, but another five years elapsed before this course became part of a medical curriculum.

In the meantime, Drs. William Shippen and John Morgan were pushing ahead with their respective plans to establish a medical school in Philadelphia. Both Shippen, who had preceded Morgan to Britain by several years, and Morgan had discussed their hopes with Dr. John Fothergill and other sympathetic British physicians and received strong encouragement. Shippen contemplated establishing an independent medical school with the power to grant degrees, and, when he returned to Philadelphia in 1762 and began his course in anatomy, it was generally assumed that this was the precursor to a full-scale medical curriculum. The formation of the school was to await the return of Morgan with a medical degree. Dr. Fothergill, who was fully aware of these plans, referred to Morgan on one occasion as Dr. Shippen's "able Assistant." Morgan, in the meantime, gradually pushed his own plan for a medical school associated with the College of Philadelphia and in the process simply ignored his old friend Shippen, a course of action which soon led to bitter enmity between the two men.

Immediately on his return to Philadelphia in the spring of 1765, Morgan approached several of the trustees of the College of Philadelphia with a design for a medical school and asked for an appointment as professor of medicine. On May 3 the trustees acted favorably upon his request and gave him permission to present the next commencement address. During the two-day commencement, May 30 and 31, Morgan delivered the *Discourse upon the Institution of Medical Schools in America* which was to mark the high point of his career. In it he first pointed to the defects and narrowness of the apprentice system for training physicians and excoriated the majority of American physicians who, he declared, by their ignorance were slaughtering their patients "and laying whole families desolate." He then turned to the advantages offered by Philadelphia: the presence of a number of well-trained physicians, the existence of a hospital and a college, and the city's central location with respect to the other colonies. He stressed the need to provide prospective physicians first with a general education and second with a sound scientific training, for he said, "there is no art yet known which may not contribute somewhat to the improvement of Medicine. . . ." Reflecting the new European ideas, he emphasized the need for clinical observation and physical experiments and insisted that medicine was a science. Flying in the face of accepted American practice, which required physicians to combine medicine, surgery, and the compounding of drugs, Morgan asserted that each of these was a separate profession. It was common sense, he declared, that no man could be an expert in more than one of these fields. Morgan's appeal for a medical school was successful, but his call for the separation of medicine, surgery, and pharmacy had virtually no effect.[2]

As already noted, Morgan scarcely mentioned Shippen in connection with his proposed medical school and appears to have made no effort to keep him informed. He took full credit for the proposal and only casually and patronizingly suggested that Shippen would be a logical choice for the professorship in anatomy. Aside from antagonizing Shippen and his friends, Morgan's attempt to deprive Shippen of all credit ultimately hurt his own reputation. Whatever the consequences of this action, the school was organized in 1766 with Morgan as professor of botany and practice of medicine, Shippen as professor of anatomy, and William Smith, the Provost of the College, giving a course in natural and experimental philosophy. In 1768 Adam Kuhn was appointed professor of botany and materia medica, and the following year, on his return from Edinburgh, Benjamin Rush joined the faculty as professor of chemistry. Dr. Thomas Bond, although not officially a member of the faculty, taught clinical medicine. The school opened its doors in 1766 and graduated its first class in 1768. By this date the enrollment was close to forty students. The quality of the teaching was probably not too high. For example, the first chemistry course at the College consisted of the instructor reading back the notes which he had taken in Cullen's classes at the University of Edinburgh. Yet this form of pedagogy characterized most teaching institutions during the eighteenth and nineteenth centuries.[3]

The example of Philadelphia stirred physicians in New York City into action. The two Bards, John and Samuel, both recognized the need for formal medical training in the colonies, but they had some reservations about New York City as a possible site for a medical college. The father, John Bard, thought the city's lack of a hospital was a serious handicap, while his son Samuel noted that there was no medical library and that New York was too close to Philadelphia where a medical school had already made a good start. Nonetheless, a group of able New York physicians had already organized a medical society and in 1767 several of the members urged the trustees of King's College to follow the example of the College of Philadelphia. In response, the board of trustees established a full medical training program by appointing six professors: Samuel Clossy, professor of anatomy; John Jones, professor of surgery; Peter Middleton, professor of physiology and pathology; James Smith, professor of chemistry and materia medica; John V. B. Tennant, professor of midwifery; and Samuel Bard, professor of theory and practice of physic. The faculty came from varied backgrounds: Clossy was an Irishman and Peter Middleton a Scot, while the others were colonial born. All of them received at least part of their medical education in Europe, and each one achieved some measure of distinction. For example, Samuel Bard wrote a classic account of diphtheria, Jones served in the Revolutionary War and wrote the first American work on surgery, and Tennant, who was from New Jersey, was a member of the Royal Society.[4]

In his inaugural address, Dr. Peter Middleton cursorily surveyed the history of medicine and rejoiced that by the opening of the college "we may in a great measure prevent the future necessity of long and perilous voyages to Europe; as well as large Remittances of money, which never more returns!" When the first graduating ceremonies were held on May 16, 1769, Dr. Bard spoke at length on the duties of a physician. This discourse, which was subsequently published, is the first American tract on medical ethics. It is probably more significant because of Bard's eloquent plea for the establishment of a public infirmary or hospital. He pleaded his cause so well that the provincial governor, Sir Henry Moore, promptly subscribed £200 toward the project. The graduates at this commencement received bachelor of medicine degrees. The following year, 1770, the school awarded to Robert Tucker the first doctorate in medicine conferred in America.[5]

Despite the troublesome times foreshadowing the approaching revolution, both schools prospered. Graduates of the two schools ordinarily received an M.B. degree, which was given following two courses of lectures. The two courses of lectures, however, were identical but the students were expected to have served a preceptorship or apprenticeship with a practicing physician for at least two years. The doctorate in medicine required a minimum of seven years of medical practice and the completion of a satisfactory thesis. Between 1768 and 1774 the College of Philadelphia awarded twenty-nine M.B. degrees and five M.D. degrees. King's College in this same period conferred twelve M.B.'s and two M.D.'s.[6] The outbreak of the Revolutionary War interrupted formal medical education for some years, but both these institutions eventually reopened.

MEDICAL LICENSING

The principle of regulating or controlling the practice of medicine is an old one, dating at least as far back as the Code of

Hammurabi, two millennia before Christ. In late medieval England, since education was in the hands of the church, the licensing of physicians was under the jurisdiction of the ecclesiastical authorities. During the Renaissance, the regulation of medical practitioners gradually shifted to the universities and to the early professional guilds—the Royal College of Physicians and the various "Companies" of surgeons and apothecaries. American colonists, then, were familiar with the concept of licensing medical practitioners, but it was not until the eighteenth century, when colonial America began to mirror the urban culture of England and when the educational qualifications of physicians began to rise, that the first call for the licensing of medical practitioners was heard. As noted, a few tentative steps were taken in Massachusetts and New York in the seventeenth century, but there is no evidence that any of the early measures were enforced.

The American emphasis upon practicality has led many American historians to assume that common sense and sound practical experience provided a better basis for learning medicine in the eighteenth century than years of formal academic study and reading—particularly when university-trained physicians seemed better versed in the subtle philosophical distinctions between the various medical theories than in clinical medicine. There is some truth in this assumption, and certainly many colonials, laymen and medical practitioners alike, believed it. The essential factor is what might be called practical intelligence. An intelligent and conscientious individual trained under an able physician was more likely to make a good doctor than a mediocre person with the most advanced medical schooling, or possibly even a university product whose mind tended to revel in philosophical abstractions. All one can conclude is that the intelligent man will always do well, but the better his training, the greater will be his knowledge and understanding.

The assumption that apprentice-trained American practitioners were at least as good as their university-educated colleagues was strengthened by the fact that the eighteenth century was preeminently an age of medical theories, and too many physicians were guilty of practicing theoretical medicine regardless of its consequences to their patients. Fortunately only a few were like the eighteenth-century Scottish physician reputed to have said that he was not going to practice unphilosophical medicine merely because his patients died. One might also ask whether the best of the university products emigrated to the colonies. Some of them, as we have seen, were able men, but it is likely that the best graduates were inclined to stay in Britain and the Continent, in close proximity to the centers of medical learning.

One of the wisest of American medical historians, Richard H. Shryock, was the first to raise the question as to the medical skill of colonial physicians whose knowledge rested solely on an apprenticeship. Just what the colonists themselves thought is not clear, since medical practitioners of all backgrounds were subject to satirical and often caustic criticism. The important question which Shryock asked was why, if practical training was so effective, were so many of the better practitioners calling for the regulation of medical practice and urging the establishment of medical schools?[7] Physicians who had studied abroad and were in a position to make a comparative judgment of colonial practice were usually the harshest in their criticism of colonial doctors. Men such as William Douglass, John Morgan, Peter Middleton, and John Bard without exception favored raising educational qualifications and licensing medical practitioners.

The first eighteenth-century law relating to physicians was more concerned with protecting patients from exorbitant fees than with raising the caliber of medical care. This law, passed by the Virginia legislature in 1736, specified what fees and charges doctors could collect. A standard fee was set for visits in town and the other fees were based largely on the distance traveled. Rather significantly, in the light of the earlier discussion, the law stated that university-trained physicians could charge a fee double that of those with merely an apprenticeship in medicine. We might also call this Virginia measure the first "truth in advertising law." Practitioners were required to specify the drugs used in their prescriptions, and any physician or apothecary failing to do so could be subject to legal action. At the end of two years the law was allowed to lapse, and although at least three more bills to regulate medical fees were introduced during the colonial period none of them passed.[8]

Before attempting to deal with its physicians, in 1738 New York City sought to establish some control over midwives. A law to regulate midwives required all applicants to "take the Oath of a Midwife" which specified precisely how the midwives should conduct themselves. No provision was made for examining candidates, and the law was obviously concerned more with ethical conduct than with medical qualifications. A section of the law showed that obstetrics was still clearly in the woman's domain, since the oath included a vow not to "open any mystery appertaining to your Office, in the presence of any Man, unless Necessity . . . constrain you to do so."[9]

Agitation to license physicians first began in New York in the 1750s. A letter to a newspaper editor in 1753 pointed out that some type of regulation was necessary to prevent "the dismal havock made by quacks and pretenders." With strong support from prominent physicians and the help of Cadwallader Colden, at that time a member of the Governor's Council, in 1760 the Provincial Assembly passed the first colonial medical licensure law.[10] The law was a good one, since it provided for the examination of physicians by government officials who were authorized to seek the assistance of reputable physicians. Enacting laws, however sound, is meaningless without enforcement, and, other than establishing the principle that medical practice was a matter of public concern, the law proved useless. Quacks and charlatans continued to practice in the city, and there is no record of any conviction for failing to secure a license.

Twelve years later, in 1772, the New Jersey Medical Society secured the enactment of a similar law on a province-wide basis for New Jersey. The provisions of the law closely followed those of the 1760 New York City measure, and it is quite likely that the end results were the same. As was the case in the New York law, there is no evidence to show that the New Jersey measure was enforced. Aside from one or two other abortive attempts to secure medical regulation (for example, a licensing bill was defeated in South Carolina in 1765), nothing further was accomplished in the colonial period, and the advent of the Revolution meant that medical licensing would have to await more orderly times.

MEDICAL SOCIETIES

One of the first signs of an emerging professional consciousness is the development of professional organizations. As already indicated, among colonial physicians this came around the midcentury. Other than that they existed, we know little about the early medical societies. The first for which we have any evidence was the Medical Society of Boston which, according to a letter written by Dr. William Douglass, was organized early in 1736. In February of that year Douglass informed Dr. Colden of New York that the Society proposed publishing a series of *Medical Memoirs*, but apparently the project fell through. In the succeeding years there are only a few scattered references to the Society in the Boston *Weekly News-Letter*.

The second medical society may have come into existence in New York City around 1749, although the evidence is scant. A manuscript notebook of Dr. John Bard dated this year contains an essay on pleurisy with a notation stating that it was delivered before the Weekly Society of Gentlemen of New York. No evidence corroborating Bard's statement has been found, however. Dr. James J. Walsh, medical historian of New York, mentions the existence of a group known as the "Physical Society," which appears to have been comprised largely of physicians. Since medical schools offered the only formal training in science, physicians invariably constituted a good share of the membership of eighteenth-century scientific societies, and the "Physical Society" was probably a small group of scientifically inclined individuals.[11]

In June 1755 the physicians in Charleston, South Carolina, met under the leadership of Dr. John Moultrie in order to promote "the better Support of the Dignity, the Privileges, and Emoluments of their Humane Art. . . ." In a statement published in the *South Carolina Gazette*, they asserted they were summoned to the homes of patients "under the greatest Inclemencies of the Weather," but they were "often slowly and seldom sufficiently paid." In a commentary upon the practice of medicine, the statement read that the physicians did not "think the Payment of an Apothecary's Bill a sufficient Reward to him who acts in the three distinct Offices of Physic, Surgery, and Pharmacy." In view of the foregoing, the physicians had resolved to make no further visits unless they received a reasonable fee, payable on each attendance upon the patient.

The only result of this bold proclamation was a series of letters to the newspapers, some satirical and others highly derogatory of the profession. The storm of outrage which greeted the physicians' statement apparently had its effect, for nothing further was heard of either the Charleston medical organization or the proposal about fees.[12] The complaints of the physicians were undoubtedly justified, but much of the problem lay in the excessive number of practitioners in Charleston. When Benjamin Rush sounded out Dr. Lionel Chalmers about coming to Charleston to practice medicine in 1772, Chalmers discouraged him. "In this town," he wrote, "there may be 11,000 to 12,000 persons of all complexions and we have between 30 and 40 persons who practice Physick, most of whom, tis true, have not much to do. . . ."[13]

Philadelphia, which was the scientific center in the later colonial period and the home of the first medical school, never had a significant medical association in the colonial period. The only medical society was a small short-lived group organized largely on the initiative of Dr. John Morgan in 1767. By this date Morgan had already antagonized many of the older physicians by his brashness and the manner in which he had promoted the medical school. He compounded his error by organizing a group of young physicians into a society and then inviting the more established physicians to join. To make matters worse, he did not extend an invitation to the two Shippens to join, an action which led Dr. Thomas Bond, one of the leading physicians, and his brother Phineas to turn down membership. The Medical Society of Philadelphia survived less than two years. In November 1768 its entire membership of twelve physicians merged with the American Society, one of Philadelphia's two scientific organizations, and became the American Society's medical committee.[14]

The more able and intelligent Philadelphia physicians, who in any other colonial city would have been organizing medical societies, were too active in general scientific pursuits to concentrate upon medicine. By 1768 the American Society and the American Philosophical Society were vying for leadership among Philadelphia intellectuals, a surprisingly high percentage of whom were physicians. For example, Dr. Thomas Bond was the leading spirit in the American Philosophical Society. Thus it was that the very activity and keen interest in the scientific area in the city mitigated against the development in these years of a strong medical organization.

The most effective medical organization in the colonial period was the New Jersey Medical Society, founded in New Brunswick in 1766. It holds the distinction of being the only colonial society to survive the Revolution. In 1790 it was incorporated as the Medical Society of New Jersey, a name which it holds today. The founders spoke of the "low State of Medicine in New Jersey" and dedicated themselves to discouraging "quacks, mountebanks, imposters or other ignorant pretenders of medicine. . . ." The major complaint of colonial physicians arose from the relatively low fees they could charge and from their inability to collect even these. The ease with which one could take up the practice of medicine and competition from quacks and irregular practitioners led to fierce competition, a competition which worked to the disadvantage of well-trained doctors. Hence the first action of the fourteen founding members of the New Jersey Medical Society was to draw up "A Table of Fees and Rates."[15]

This fee bill, like the earlier one in Charleston, brought outraged protests, and four months later the Society rescinded the requirement that its members adhere to it. While doing little to improve the financial status of New Jersey physicians, the fee bill does tell us a great deal about their medical practice. The doctors set no fee for one or two visits in town, charging, like the English apothecaries, only for the medicines. Where daily visits were required for long periods, the fee was ten shillings per week. For out-of-town services, the fee depended upon the distance to be traveled. It is also clear, as David Cowen notes, that most of the physicians' work was done at the bedside of the patient. This same medical society, it will be recalled, elected a minister-physician as its first president and included a goodly number of ministers among its membership. A second major aim of the Society was to raise professional standards by securing some method of licensing practitioners. To this end, it successfully promoted a medical licensure bill.[16]

In Connecticut two local societies were organized in the 1760s. A small group of physicians in Norwich debated in 1763 whether or not to apply for licensing powers, and, deciding the time was not ripe, voted against seeking them. The physicians in Litchfield County were more adventurous. Some thirty of them organized in Sharon in 1767 and in 1769 unsuccessfully petitioned the provincial legislature for the authority to examine and license practitioners. Once again the newspapers and public arose in opposition and the cry of monopoly was raised. Following this unsuccessful attempt, the next year the Society appealed to the public. Although the appeal proved fruitless, it is of interest since the Society mentioned that its membership now included doctors from the neighboring provinces. Sharon lies close to the boundaries of New York and Massachusetts, and the Sharon Medical Society had the distinction of being the only interprovincial medical association.[17]

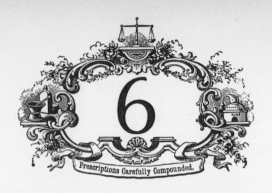

Prescriptions Carefully Compounded.

MEDICAL ASPECTS
OF THE
REVOLUTIONARY WAR

THE panoply and accounterments of war—brilliant uniforms, colorful flags, bands, and marching men—and the courageous action of individuals or armies have always made wars a subject of fascination to readers. The words glory, valor, and victory carry a far more heroic connotation than disease, casualties, and death—which explains why, for the millions of words written about wars, scarce thousands have been devoted to describing the medical and health aspects of soldiering. The American Revolution is no exception. Of all the many journals kept by participants in this struggle, not one of them deals more than cursorily with military medicine. Ironically, even the physicians and surgeons who record-ed their experiences were more intrigued with marching and battles than with their aftermath. The most complete journal written by a physician was that of Dr. James Thacher of Massachusetts—but Thacher, too, wrote primarily of his military experiences and only incidentally on medical subjects. Of the four men who served successively as Medical Director of the Continental forces, only Dr. John Morgan, who sought to vindicate himself from the charges which had led to his dismissal, wrote anything about his medical work. Fortunately, despite the paucity of medical writings and the lack of medical journals, we can glean enough from the wide variety of historical sources relating to the Revolution to draw a reasonably accurate picture.

Altogether approximately 1,400 physicians and surgeons enrolled in the Continental Armies during the Revolution, although many served in a purely military capacity. Quite a few of these individuals had also been active in the events leading to the War. The first Provincial Congress of Massachusetts, for example, included no less than twenty-one doctors. One of them, Dr. Joseph Warren, helped spread the alarm to Lexington and Concord and another, Dr. Benjamin Church, was appointed the first Medical Director of the Continental Army. Six physicians, two each from Massachusetts and Connecticut, and one each from Pennsylvania and New Jersey, were among the signers of the Declaration of Independence. Several others achieved high military rank, including Arthur St. Clair and James Wilkerson, both of whom subsequently served as Commander-in-Chief of the Army, and Dr. John Thomas, Major General and Commander of the Northern Army of 1777. As might be expected in a time of divided loyalties, a good number of physicians remained loyal to Great Britain and still others sought to maintain a measure of neutrality.

The overall picture of military medicine is a rather confused one, since the colonials had neither an effective central government nor a national army at the outset of hostilities. At first the provincial governments provided some elementary medical services in conjunction with their military forces. Subsequently the Continental Congress created its own army and medical department and began to superimpose a central authority over the provincial forces. This latter proved difficult, and it was not until 1781 that the Continental Medical Department was able to extend its medical jurisdiction over the southern colonies. To complicate matters, a sharp conflict immediately developed between the Medical Department of the Continental Army and the regimental surgeons. The armies commanded by Washington and his officers consisted of the Continentals, or regulars, and the colonial militia, the latter usually drawn from the general area of conflict. For example, during the first years the war was fought largely in New England and the middle colonies and during the later years in the South. The militia regiments had their own surgeons, many of whom were political appointees, a situation which compounded their medical incompetence.

The health, medical care, and welfare of any given body of troops depended upon a number of factors: the ability of the commanding officer, the quality of the regimental surgeons and the general hospitals, the availability of food, clothing, and medical supplies, and the willingness of Congress or the provincial legislatures to provide adequate appropriations. A weakness in any one of these areas could and did cause a great deal of unnecessary suffering and death. For example, the rations prescribed for the soldiers were fairly generous and were comparable to those given to the British troops. The Massachusetts forces were supposed to receive a daily allotment of $1/2$ pound of salt beef, $1/2$ pound of pork, 1 pound of bread, and 1 gill of rice, peas, or other "equivalent." An additional weekly allowance of 6 ounces of butter, $1/2$ pint of vinegar, and $1/6$ pound of soap was also provided. When it was available, this ration could be replaced with a weekly ration of 7 pounds of fresh beef and 7 pounds of flour. A similar ration was subsequently prescribed for the Continental Army. Unfortunately, the lack of trained cooks and the unsanitary conditions under which the food was prepared negated much of the value of this diet. Furthermore, rising prices, inadequate appropriations, and other factors often drastically reduced the available food supply.[1] For example, the rapid movement of troops as the balance of war shifted placed enormous strains on the local economy, and inadequate transportation compounded the problem. Hospitals were especially affected by transportation difficulties, since a hospital might be desperately short while ample supplies were available 50 or 100 miles away. Repeatedly hospitals, both permanent and makeshift, had to be evacuated as the battle lines surged back and forth, adding to the confusion and further complicating the supply problems.

As might be expected, the quality of medical care varied widely from region to region. The multiplicity of forces in the field, the short-term enlistments, and the amorphous medical organization makes it almost impossible to know the exact number of sick, wounded, and dead. For example, throughout the war years thousands of soldiers furloughed because of sickness or injuries never returned. How many of these subsequently died will never be known. The vicissitudes of battles and campaigns also add to the difficulties of ascertaining exact figures. Disastrous defeats so scattered some forces that one can only estimate the number of dead, wounded, and deserted.

Notwithstanding all these difficulties, it is possible to come up with the casualty rates. Military historian Louis C. Duncan estimated that during 1776 the American forces consisted of 47,000 Continental troops, whose enlistment period was for one year, and 27,000 militia who had volunteered for terms ranging from a few days to several months or more. Of this total, about 1,000 were killed in battle or died from their injuries, 1,200 suffered wounds, 6,000 were taken prisoner, 10,000 died of disease, and several thousand either deserted or simply disappeared. The following year, while maneuvering around Philadelphia, army records in August show that about 26 percent of Washington's forces were sick. Dr. James Thacher, who participated in the fighting from Breed's Hill to Yorktown, estimated the total American deaths during the entire war at 70,000, roughly 10,000 per year for the seven years of military activities, 1775–81. Duncan considers this figure reasonable, but he doubts that it includes the thousands of sick who simply went home and for whom we have no records. Nearly every observer agrees that the ratio of sick to battle casualties was very high. Dr. James Tilton, a Delaware physician who later became Surgeon General of the Army, declared that "we lost not less than from ten to twenty of camp diseases for one by weapons of the enemy."[2] Most other contemporary estimates place the figure at closer to nine to one—approximately nine deaths from sickness for each one resulting from battle action. American casualties were much higher than those for the British. The British troops, however, were veterans whose enlistment period was twenty years. Most of them had already encountered and survived the main camp diseases. They were also better disciplined and backed by a more effective medical department.

The major diseases affecting the American forces were small-pox, which was a problem primarily in the first two years, dysentery, respiratory complaints, malaria, and the so-called camp fevers, probably typhus and typhoid. Smallpox always had been a serious threat in the colonies, but the long years of war at the midcentury and the more general use of smallpox inoculation tended to make it both more familiar and less dangerous. Even so, the Revolution mobilized thousands of young men, many from relatively isolated areas, leading to widespread outbreaks of smallpox and other diseases. In June of 1776 John Adams wrote from Philadelphia almost in despair: "The small pox! the small pox! What shall we do with it? I could almost wish that an inoculating hospital was opened in every town in New-England." Reflecting a typical colonial viewpoint, he added: "It is some small consolation that the scoundrel savages have taken a large dose of it." The disease was a constant factor in the early military actions and may well have been decisive in the unsuccessful attempt to capture Quebec in the winter and spring of 1776–77. When the American forces were attempting to regroup in June of 1776, General John Sullivan reported to General Washington: "There are some regiments all down with the small-pox—not a single man fit for duty," and a day later Benedict Arnold reported that half of his forces were sick, "mostly with the smallpox." The American forces converging on Quebec were forced to make long hard marches through the wilderness on limited rations and in bitter weather. These difficulties might have been surmounted, but the widespread dysentery and smallpox virtually precluded any chance of victory.[3] Fortunately, by the end of the first two years of fighting, most of the troops had either survived smallpox or else had been inoculated. Henceforth, although flaring up on occasions, smallpox was no longer a serious problem.

When Washington was besieging Boston in the fall of 1775, the chief disorders in addition to smallpox were dysentery, respiratory diseases, rheumatic complaints, malaria, and what was probably typhoid. These same ailments plagued General Gates's forces before Ticonderoga in the summer of 1776. His men were reported as suffering from "bilious, remitting and intermitting fevers with some of the putrid kind; dysenteries, diarrhoeas, with rheumatick complaints." The remitting and intermitting fevers were malaria, and the bilious and putrid fevers were most likely typhoid and typhus. Typhus has never been a serious problem in the United States, but it was probably responsible for a good share of the "putrid" camp fevers. Typhoid, which arrived early in the colonies and exacted a steady toll from the American population until well into the twentieth century, is another likely suspect. Malaria troubled the troops in all sectors, but it was present in its most acute form in the southern colonies. Northern soldiers campaigning in the South were particularly susceptible, although the fever represented a hazard to all forces. As early as 1776 Congress ordered its medical committee to send 300 pounds of Peruvian bark (cinchona) to the Southern Department. During the siege of Yorktown, according to Thacher, the New England troops in particular suffered heavily from malaria.[4]

Dysentery has been a concomitant of every military campaign, and invariably its incidence has been highest at the outset of hostilities. The explanation for this is that the incidence of dysentery correlates closely with discipline and the effectiveness of sanitary regulations. The New England troops gathered around Boston in the first years of the war were notorious for urinating and defecating in the area surrounding their camps. Washington commented that he thought the New England troops would fight well, but that they were "an exceedingly dirty and nasty people."[5] The New Englanders were no worse than any other soldiers. Poorly disciplined troops neither build adequate latrines and sanitary facilities nor use the available ones, with the result that in short order they contaminate their water supply. The famous eighteenth-century English army surgeon Sir John Pringle, and others long before him, had stressed the necessity for providing proper sanitary facilities and for strictly enforcing the regulations about their use, but the lesson has had to be relearned in every war. Discipline was a major problem in the colonial armies, and few officers recognized the value of camp hygiene. The more able ones learned from bitter experience, but progress was slow. Although the incidence of enteric diseases dropped off somewhat as the fighting continued, the rapid turnover in the American forces brought about by short-term enlistments meant that diarrheas and dysenteries were a constant factor in reducing the effectiveness of colonial fighting forces.

The extent to which disease rather than battle wounds was a major source of casualties is clearly shown by the hospital reports. For example, during March 1780 a military hospital in South

Carolina reported 302 admissions. Of these patients, only 12 had gunshot wounds; the rest were admitted for a wide range of medical complaints, including many with diarrheas and dysenteries, 66 cases of continued fever (probably typhoid), 60 cases of intermittent fever (malaria), 44 with rheumatism, 34 with ulcers, and 20 suffering from venereal disease.[6] The constant shortage of supplies in the Continental Army meant that malnutrition and exposure were significant factors in the health of the troops. Inadequate diets undoubtedly account for much of the diarrheas, and lack of adequate clothing and shelter help to account for the relatively large number of rheumatic complaints.

The history of the organization of American medical services from the opening of hostilities to the end of the war is an equally interesting and confusing picture. The Province of Massachusetts was the first governing body to take firm and definite action to raise troops and to provide for their medical care. In February 1775 its Provincial Congress appointed Drs. Joseph Warren and Benjamin Church to study the medical needs of the Massachusetts militia. The following month the same Congress voted funds to buy medical supplies and to establish hospitals. In May, after it had become apparent that a number of the regimental surgeons were not qualified, the Massachusetts Committee on Public Safety appointed an eight-man medical committee to examine them.[7] This action provided no solution to the supply problems and other difficulties involving the regimental surgeons, but it did help to weed out the more inefficient and untrained ones. It may also help to account for the relatively good health enjoyed by the New England troops as compared to those from the middle and southern colonies.

In May 1775 the Second Continental Congress assumed charge of the colonial militia assembled to besiege the British force in Boston. One of its first acts was to create an Army Medical Department headed by a Director General and Chief Physician at a salary of $4 per day. In addition to the Director, the Department was to consist of 4 surgeons, 1 apothecary, 20 surgeon's mates, 1 clerk, 2 storekeepers, and 1 nurse for every 10 sick men. Since Massachusetts was the mainstay of the colonial forces, the choice of Director fell to Dr. Benjamin Church, a prominent Boston physician and active patriot. Dr. Church, and his next two successors, faced an impossible task. The Continental Army itself was made up of various provincial units and it was to take several years of fighting to create a unified army. Washington had considerable support from the Continental Congress in building an army, but both he and Congress underestimated the Army's medical needs. Hence Dr. Church's effort to build a medical division from the ground up was made immensely more difficult by the failure of the Continental Congress and the provincial legislatures to provide sufficient funds for personnel, equipment, and supplies. Even Washington did not fully realize the importance of a healthy army until the war was well along. As late as January 1777 he marched his army from Trenton to Princeton without taking along a single surgeon or telling his medical officers of the move.[8]

Dr. Church's first action was to take over the hospitals established around Boston by the Massachusetts government. These consisted of private homes and miscellaneous buildings which were now called the General Hospital. Church then ordered that regimental hospitals be closed and that all patients needing hospitalization be sent to the General Hospital. The regimental surgeons resented this infringement upon their authority and soon carried their complaints to Congress. In the meantime, Dr. Church was trying to build a competent staff, standardize procedures, provide a satisfactory system of records, and find the much-needed medical and hospital supplies. As criticism of his administration mounted, Washington ordered an investigation, but before the inquiry was completed, Dr. Church was discovered to have been in treasonable correspondence with a British officer. As the clash between the motherland and the colonies mounted, he apparently sought to hedge his bets by supplying the British Commander, General Gage, with information. A letter which he had asked his mistress to pass on to the British was accidentally intercepted and Church's career came to an abrupt end. Suffice it to say, he was dismissed from his post and placed in jail, but neither the Articles of the Continental Army nor the Continental Congress had provided for dealing with such cases. John Adams wrote in disgust that no one knew what to do with Church: "There is no law to try him, and no court to try him," adding that Church deserved far more punishment than he would receive. The problem was solved when Church's health failed, and he was permitted to sail for the West

Indies. In a tragic finale to his life, the ship was lost at sea with all hands.[9]

On October 16 Congress selected Dr. John Morgan, the distinguished founder of the Philadelphia Medical College, to fill Church's position. The choice was an excellent one for America, but an unfortunate one for Morgan. He was able, energetic, and well qualified, and, although he accomplished a great deal, his position was a hopeless one. On entering into his duties, he discovered that no records existed showing how many patients were hospitalized. He promptly ordered weekly returns of the sick and requested an inventory of supplies. He was horrified to discover only a handful of medicines, a few hundred bandages, virtually no surgical instruments, and scarcely any blankets. The limited funds appropriated by Congress were clearly insufficient for the needs of the General Hospital and the Medical Director's staff, and no appropriation had been made for equipping the regimental surgeons. When his urgent requests to the Continental Congress for additional supplies proved fruitless, Morgan began scouring the countryside, appealing to private citizens, local groups, and provincial governments for help. By these means he managed to accumulate a limited amount of medical stores and to equip his own surgeons and hospitals. He next turned his attention to the regimental surgeons. They, too, were clamoring for hospital and medical supplies, and they assumed that they had a claim to any available material. When Morgan sought to preserve his limited supplies for the use of his own staff, the regimental surgeons were outraged.[10]

At this point it might be well to explain that regiments usually were recruited in a single community or local area and the surgeons were appointed by the commanding officer. A few surgeons brought their own instruments and medicines, but many of them were told or assumed they would be supplied by the Army. The Continental Congress, however, simply created a small Medical Department and left the status of the regimental surgeons in a limbo. Unaware of this, and seeing Morgan with what seemed a great deal of supplies, understandably the regimental surgeons blamed him for their troubles.

Except in Massachusetts and one or two of the other New England states, little effort was made to insure that regimental surgeons were qualified. Morgan described many of them as "unlettered, ignorant, and rude to a degree scarcely to be imagined." Some of them, he added, had no training in physic and had never seen an operation. In light of the prevailing medical treatment, one might well wonder whether or not this was a handicap. Dr. Thacher, one of the better surgeons, was called upon with two other army doctors to deal with a soldier bitten by a rattlesnake. The three surgeons forced the patient to swallow repeated doses of olive oil until he had ingested a quart, and in the meantime kept rubbing the affected leg with mercurial ointment. Within two hours, Dr. Thacher reported, the crisis passed and the patient was saved. The knowledge that his physicians were doing everything possible to save him may have supplied the necessary psychological lift to enable the soldier to survive both the snake bite and the therapy. Dr. William Eustis of Massachusetts treated a patient shot through the lungs with repeated and liberal bloodletting. The patient's survival was attributed "to the free use of the lancet and such abstemious living as to reduce him to the greatest extremity."[11]

Despite the heroic tactics used by surgeons, there was a large and useful body of medical knowledge available to trained physicians, and Morgan was justified in seeking to improve the caliber of the regimental surgeons. His efforts to do so and to provide for an effective system of sick returns, however, merely added to their bitterness. In addition to his other difficulties, Morgan soon found himself in conflict with Dr. Samuel Stronger, the director of the Hospital in the Northern Department, who considered himself at least on an equal basis with Morgan. This problem was not completely resolved until Congress eventually dismissed both men.

By the time Washington had marched south to the defense of New York in 1776, Morgan, overcoming almost insuperable difficulties, had managed to establish and equip several hospitals and get the Medical Department in relatively good shape. The regimental surgeons were still left largely to their own devices, although in July Congress allowed them to draw medicines and instruments from the Medical Department. They were still not permitted to requisition special foods, blankets, or any other items necessary for the sick. Before the battles for New York in 1776, Morgan sought to anticipate medical needs, but he found that many regimental surgeons had made no preparation for the expected casualties. The deplorable condition of the sick and wounded following the Battle of Long Island led Washington to recognize the need to upgrade the quality of regimental surgeons and to place them directly under command of the Medical Director. Congress responded by urging the states to be more selective in choosing regimental surgeons and resolving that the Medical Director had full control over all surgeons and surgeons' mates.[12]

These Congressional resolutions did little to allay the dissatisfaction of the regimental surgeons, and they kept steadily undermining Morgan's position with the Continental Congress. During this same summer of 1776, Congress appointed Dr. John Shippen, Jr., as director of the Hospital for the Flying Camp, the name assigned to some 10,000 militia called up from New Jersey, Pennsylvania, and Maryland to protect New Jersey. Shippen's exact status was not made clear, and he soon began encroaching upon Morgan's authority. Meanwhile complaints from regimental surgeons and the inherent weaknesses in the organization of the Medical Department were bringing a great deal of unjustified criticism down on Morgan's head, and Shippen, who had no love for Morgan and was ambitious to boot, was successfully lobbying in Congress to improve his position. During all of this, Morgan was furiously endeavoring to keep his Department supplied, to bring some semblance of order to the various medical units, and to meet the recurrent emergencies arising from the exigencies of war. His efforts availed him nought, and on January 9, 1777, Congress dismissed him from his post.

Morgan, who had worked indefatigably at his job, was taken by surprise by this action and immediately demanded a hearing. His sense of outrage reached new bounds when he learned that his replacement was his old enemy Dr. William Shippen, Jr. The sole benefit which came from this unfortunate situation was Morgan's publication of his work, *A Vindication of His Public Character in the Station of Director-General*, one of the few medical sources to provide an insight into medical conditions during the war.

The events of 1776 made clear the need for an army based upon more than one-year enlistments. In consequence Congress reorganized the military forces and created a new Continental Army for 1777 in which the troops enlisted for three years. By this time both Congress and Washington had become aware of the needless suffering of the sick and wounded and its impact upon the effectiveness of the fighting forces. Consequently Dr. William Shippen took over as Medical Director under far more auspicious circumstances than his two predecessors. In the first place, Morgan had already organized a relatively effective medical staff and a number of hospitals and had demonstrated the role a good medical system could play. In the second, Shippen had a more polished and affable personality and was far more skillful in dealing with people—a particularly useful asset for a Medical Director dependent upon Congress for funding.

At the beginning of his administration Shippen was requested to make plans for strengthening the Medical Department. Shortly thereafter he drew up a proposal similar to one suggested earlier by Morgan, which, like Morgan's, was based largely upon the British system. In submitting the proposal to Congress, Washington made a special effort to urge its acceptance. The proposal involved both a considerable increase in medical personnel and relatively large raises in pay, provisions likely to meet opposition in Congress. Washington stressed Shippen's argument that higher pay was essential to attract able men. Dr. Benjamin Rush, chairman of the Medical Committee for Congress, had already witnessed the American and British army medical services in operation during the fighting around Philadelphia, and he had learned to appreciate the advantages of the British system. Consequently Congress adopted the proposal on April 7, 1777. It established four major geographical sections, each with a deputy director general in charge: a northern division for the Lake Champlain area, an eastern one for the region east of the Hudson River, a middle division for the area between the Hudson and the Potomac, and a southern division. The northern division was headed by Dr. Jonathan Potts, the eastern by Dr. Isaac Foster, and the middle division by Dr. Benjamin Rush. Congress had made Dr. William Rickman of Virginia director of the Southern Department in May 1776 and apparently intended him to remain more or less autonomous. The evidence indicates that Rickman was a poor director, but he had enough political connections to hang on to his job until 1780.[13]

The reorganization also set up a regular chain of command reaching from the regimental surgeons to the director-general. Regional hospitals were established in the districts and a chief medical officer was appointed for each army in the field. In addition to coordinating hospital and medical care, this official theoretically was given supervisory powers over the regimental surgeons. Although the new program, by concentrating more authority in the hands of the director general, was a marked improvement, and Congress, if somewhat belatedly, was finally providing far more generous support, the basic problems still remained. The reorganization plan, like its predecessor, did not clearly define the status of the regimental surgeons nor did it make any provision for supplying them. Eighteenth-century hospitals, and military hospitals in particular, had a horrible reputation, and the sick and wounded were always reluctant to leave their comrades. The British had learned that soldiers recovered much faster and were less likely to catch "hospital fever," the scourge of early hospitals, when they were cared for within their own regiments. By failing to provide for regimental hospitals or regimental surgeons, Congress made a serious mistake, one result of which was to continue the divisive fight between the Medical Department and the regimental surgeons. Moreover, while funds for medical supplies were made available, the Medical Department was not given a commissary general to handle special food and other items needed for the sick.

To make matters worse, as had been the case from the beginning of the war, everyone in the Medical Department with any political influence carried their problems to Congress, and Congress had no hesitancy about intervening in departmental affairs. For example, when serious and apparently justified criticism was made of conditions in the Alexandria hospital under the direct control of Dr. Rickman of the Southern Department, Morgan was prevented by Congress from taking any action. A more serious instance of political interference involved Drs. Rush and Morgan. Lack of discipline was a major problem in the American forces and, as noted, it was an important factor in the high incidence of sickness and disease. Dr. Benjamin Rush, as Surgeon General of the Middle Department, was particularly incensed by his inability to control his patients and by what he considered the general slackness in the army. He was a man of passionate convictions and quick to form opinions. He blamed Washington for the general lack of discipline and as a result became involved with the Conway Cabal. Because Shippen did not or could not remedy certain hospital conditions which Rush brought to his attention, the latter soon engaged in a vendetta with Shippen.

Shippen did not want for enemies; Dr. Morgan was already dedicating himself to this cause and complaints of all types were pouring into General Washington's headquarters and Congress. Rush was serving in Congress at the time he was appointed to his army medical post and was in a position to cause serious trouble. Shippen was not without his own political support, but what probably enabled him to hang onto his job until January 1781 was the vindictiveness of the attacks by Morgan and Rush. Had these two men been less personal in their attacks, they might have driven Shippen from office sooner. As it was, Shippen won the first round, and Rush was compelled to resign from the Medical Department on January 30, 1778.[14] Thus, with sickness and disease rampant in the Continental Army, the Medical Department was crippled by political infighting at the top and in the lower levels by the continuing battle between the Department and the regimental surgeons.

Meanwhile, Director Shippen carefully avoided field campaigns and battles, seldom if ever visited the hospitals, and seems to have had little concern for the men. As if this was not enough, he began profiteering on the sale of hospital supplies to the Army at a time when the sick and wounded were suffering from want of food, clothing, and medicine. When Rush publicly charged him with profiteering, Congress reacted in 1778 by separating the procurement of hospital supplies from Shippen's office. The following year Morgan brought charges of misconduct against Shippen. A long legal battle ensued in which the military court finally acquitted him. Congress reviewed the findings of the court-martial in the summer of 1780 and was not completely convinced of Shippen's innocence. The final resolution which passed Congress merely discharged Shippen from arrest rather than confirming the court's decision to acquit him. Morgan and Rush, still not satisfied, continued their attack, and on January 3, 1781, Shippen, having saved a measure of face, quietly resigned.

The last of the wartime Medical Directors was Dr. John Cochran, a Pennsylvanian who later moved to New Jersey, where he became a founder and a president of the New Jersey Medical Society. On Washington's suggestion, he had been appointed

Physician and Surgeon General of the Middle Department under Shippen. Cochran had collaborated with Shippen in drawing up the reorganization plan in 1777 and was largely responsible for the final overhaul of the Medical Department which Congress enacted in October 1780. Although Shippen was reconfirmed as Director of the Medical Department this same fall, he was already contemplating resigning and it was Cochran who placed the Department on a relatively effective basis. Under the new organization, the semiautonomous geographical divisions were eliminated and full authority was concentrated in the hands of the Director. The place of the regional deputy directors was taken by three chief hospital physicians who could be assigned wherever needed. In March 1781 Congress took a final step and placed the Southern Department under the supervision of the Medical Department.

Dr. Cochran managed to avoid the personality clashes which had troubled the Department since the beginning of the war, and his tenure of office was relatively uneventful. This is not to say that all was well: shortages of all sorts continued to plague the Department; inflation was rampant; and the Continental Congress was scraping the bottom of the barrel for additional sources of funds. From the beginning of his administration Cochran was forced to plead desperately for additional medical and hospital supplies. In March 1781 he reported that one of the hospitals had been compelled to allow ambulatory patients to beg for food, and that conditions were not much better in the other hospitals. On April 2 he mentioned that he had received no pay for twenty-three months. Fortunately in 1781 military action ceased and in the succeeding years the Army steadily dwindled away. Despite many difficulties, Dr. Cochran remained on the job until the peace treaty was signed. By this time the majority of the sick and wounded had been discharged.[15]

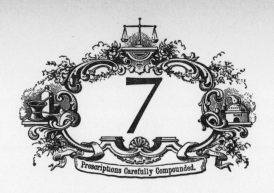

Prescriptions Carefully Compounded.

BENJAMIN RUSH, THE
AMERICAN HIPPOCRATES

THE POSTWAR YEARS

THE rapid expansion in population and wealth which helped the colonies win their independence convinced Americans that theirs was a glorious destiny, as the growing spirit of nationalism emerged in full flower in the early national period. Physicians, along with other American scientists, equated political democracy with the free spirit of scientific inquiry, and they were convinced that American science, untrammeled by political restrictions, would soon lead the world. In part these hopeful utterances, as Brooke Hindle has pointed out, reflected the weakness of the American intellectual position. The new nation had only one scientist with an international reputation and no educational or scientific societies of consequence. All scientific activities had been disrupted by the war, the efforts of the best minds diverted, and the essential contact with Great Britain cut off.

The medical profession in particular had suffered a severe setback. Before the Revolution the better colonial physicians completed their education in the London hospital schools and the universities of Edinburgh and Glasgow. The war severed this connection, and the intense patriotic spirit which followed independence discouraged its renewal. The closing of the two small American medical colleges during the war left medical education largely to the apprentice system. Even worse, the bitter division between the Tories and patriots led many of the best trained physicians to leave the country. Some elected to go with the withdrawing British forces and others were expelled. In the immediate postwar years, a patriotic committee in Charleston, South Carolina, banished thirteen physicians classified as "obnoxious persons" and levied heavy fines on two others. Among those expelled was Dr. Alexander Garden, America's leading naturalist at that time.[1]

To offset these disadvantages, one might assume that the experience gained in dealing with wartime injuries and sickness and the close contact with experienced British and French military surgeons would have provided some compensation, but there is little evidence to this effect. From the standpoint of medicine and surgery no significant advances were made during these years. Drs. Morgan and Shippen, two of the best minds, were preoccupied with their army medical roles, and Benjamin Rush was more concerned with politics than medicine. The latter, a true representative of the eighteenth-century age of enlightenment, at least made a few shrewd observations from his limited military experience. As an avowed exponent of cleanliness and moderation, he argued that the sickness and death which characterized army camps could be avoided by correct hygienic procedures and better food. He warned officers to avoid crowding too many men in a tent and suggested that "unnecessary fatigue" would invite disease. In an age when bathing was commonly assumed to be positively dangerous, he recommended that the soldiers bathe twice a week.[2] He also noticed the psychological effect of victory upon the troops, citing the excellent health enjoyed by officers and men in the British fleet following their decisive defeat of the French in April of 1782. The same held true, he wrote, of the men of the Philadelphia militia who joined Washington's army shortly before the American victory at Trenton. Although they had little experience with an outdoor life, these troops slept in tents and barns—and occasionally without any shelter—during the winter months with scarely any sickness.[3]

Despite the setback caused by the Revolution, the immediate postwar years did see a quickening of scientific and educational activity. Pre-Revolutionary medical societies such as those of New Jersey, Connecticut, New York, and Philadelphia were revived and new ones sprang into existence. Although beset by difficulties, the medical colleges in Philadelphia and New York resumed activity, and Harvard added medicine to its curriculum in 1782. Four years later the Philadelphia Dispensary opened its doors, to be followed in 1791 by the New York Dispensary. Based on the European pattern, these dispensaries were philanthropic agenices designed to give free outpatient care for the poor and at the same time to provide a measure of clinical training for physicians. In 1791 the New York Hospital accepted its first patients, inaugurating an era of hospital building.

Despite the general suspicion of Great Britain, intellectual ties were reestablished, for a common language and culture inevitably led Americans to renew their intellectual allegiance to the mother country. Even that arch-patriot Dr. Rush observed: "What has physic to do with taxation or independence?" The new ties which had been formed with France and the Continent during the Revolution proved too tenuous to threaten the intellectual relationship with Great Britain. Moreover, the Continent was soon to be torn by twenty-five years of revolution and war, and England had temporarily taken leadership in medicine and surgery under the guidance of men such as John and William Hunter.

DR. BENJAMIN RUSH

America had many able physicians at the end of the eighteenth century, but without question one man, Rush, dominated the scene.[4] His importance lies not only in the fact of his rise to preeminence in the American medicine of his day but in his profound influence upon American medical practice, an impact that continued to be felt in the South and West well down to the end of the nineteenth century. While in no sense a typical eighteenth-century American physician, Rush embodied much of the best of his age. His family background, which had embraced a wide variety of Protestant religious concepts ranging from Quakerism to Anglicanism, gave him a strong social conscience and helps to explain his leadership in the humanitarian movement of his day. Although christened in the Anglican faith, his moral ideas were profoundly shaped by the Reverend Samuel Finley, a Presbyterian minister who ran Nottingham Academy, a boarding school where the young Rush spent five years. Subsequently Rush entered the College of New Jersey, or Princeton, and graduated a year and a half later at the age of fifteen. Shortly thereafter he was apprenticed to Dr. John Redman, an outstanding Philadelphia physician and another staunch Presbyterian who would help form Rush's character. In the course of spending five and a half years with Dr. Redman, Rush attended Dr. William Shippen, Jr.'s, lectures on anatomy during 1762 and subsequently enrolled in the lectures given by Shippen and Morgan at the College of Philadelphia.

Medical competition in Philadelphia was keen, and Rush soon realized that he must acquire a European medical degree if he were to succeed. Encouraged by his preceptors and with financial support from his family, in August 1766 he set forth to enroll in the University of Edinburgh. A few weeks after taking his medical degree in June 1768, he headed south to London to continue his studies. Here he spent some five months attending William Hunter's anatomy lectures and making the acquaintance of a wide circle of leading British physicians, one which included Sir John Pringle, the famous army surgeon, and Drs. John Fothergill and John Coakley Lettsom. The latter two are best known for their humanitarian interests and philanthropic endeavors, qualities which appealed to Rush. When Rush learned that Benjamin Franklin was in London, he promptly called upon him. Franklin, always happy to help young Americans, took him under his wing, and in short order Rush was attending receptions and dinners with the outstanding artists and literary figures of the day, men such as Sir Joshua Reynolds, Oliver Goldsmith, and Samuel Johnson.

Armed with letters of introduction from Franklin, early in 1769 he spent several weeks in Paris, where he considered the medicine to be fifty years behind that of England and Scotland, and then set sail for home. With assistance from some of the established physicians, he soon established a successful practice—a practice which received a considerable lift by Rush's appointment immediately on his return from Europe to the position of professor of chemistry at the College of Philadelphia. As the break with Great Britain steadily widened during the tumultuous years of the 1770s, Rush flung himself into politics. His activity in Pennsylvania affairs led to his election to the Second Continental Congress where he signed the Declaration of Independence and developed a taste for political intrigue. During 1777–78 he served briefly in the army, but his fulminations against Dr. Shippen and General Washington soon led to a demand for his resignation. Rush was not solely to blame, but he displayed an unusual rashness and lack of discretion.

In the years following the Revolution, Rush turned his efforts toward moral and humanitarian reforms. He was a strong advocate of both private and public education, and he fought for prison reform, temperance, the abolition of slavery, and the elimination of all forms of tobacco. In the meantime he maintained a substantial practice and continued to play an active role in medical teaching. The combination of his political, philanthropic, and medical activities soon gained Rush a reputation as America's outstanding physician. In lecturing to his students Rush constantly warned against espousing any particular medical doctrine. In 1801, for example, he declared that "undue attachment to great names" had led to the establishment of "a despotism in medicine," and he urged that progress in medicine could only be achieved by free inquiry.

As medicine sought to break away from traditional thinking, physicians such as Thomas Sydenham (1624–89) substituted a nosological approach to medicine, i.e., they began by assuming that disease entities existed and they then sought to classify disorders on the basis of symptoms. Since symptoms and syndromes come in an infinite variety, nosographic texts were soon publishing longer and longer lists of supposed diseases. Instead of clarifying the medical picture the result was to compound the confusion in medical circles. As Rush reflected on medicine over the years, he rejected the nosological approach, or concept of disease entities, and consciously or not, returned to the traditional monistic pathology which explained all diseases in terms of one fundamental cause. At the University of Edinburgh Rush had been greatly impressed by William Cullen, one of the most influential medical professors of his day and a philosopher who believed in systematization. Ironically, two of his students, John Brown and Benjamin Rush, developed medical systems which profoundly, if not disastrously, affected medical practice for two or three generations.

The impetus which led Rush to formulate his medical doctrine was the great yellow fever epidemic in Philadelphia during 1793. Beginning in this year, a series of devastating yellow fever epidemics struck every major American port from Boston southwards. The disease had been absent from America for over thirty years, and the medical profession was at an utter loss to explain or treat the fever. Along with his colleagues in Philadelphia during 1793, Rush was overwhelmed with patients and was desperately seeking some form of effective therapy. At first he tried a cooling regimen supplemented by moderate purging and bleeding, but it seemed of little avail. After fruitlessly consulting the leading authors and trying various forms of therapy, he recalled an old manuscript which Franklin had given him describing a yellow fever outbreak in Virginia in 1741. In it Dr. John Mitchell described how the stomach and intestinal tract in yellow fever was filled with blood and putrefying matter. Until this matter was purged away, he had written, it was impossible to procure a "laudable" sweat. Mitchell further declared that the physician should not be deterred from decisive action by an "ill-timed scrupulousness about the weakness of the body."[5]

Rush was familiar with Dr. Thomas Young's "Ten-and-Ten," a horrendous Revolutionary Army purge of ten grains of calomel and ten grains of jalap, a violent herbal cathartic, but he had qualms about administering it to anyone weakened by yellow fever. Late in August he encountered a yellow fever patient apparently on the point of death who had been deserted by his family and friends. Rush in desperation administered a large dose of mercury and jalap, and to his surprise the man showed signs of recovery. Delighted with the results, he began experimenting with even larger quantities until he was prescribing three doses, each consisting of ten grains of calomel and fifteen of jalap, to be given at six-hour intervals. Along with this, he combined bloodletting and a cooling regimen of cold baths, cold drinks, and cool air. It is likely that the first few individuals on whom Rush tried this therapy did not have yellow fever or else suffered only mild cases. Whatever the case, Rush became convinced that he had solved the problem. He was a warm-hearted, kindly, enthusiastic individual, and once he espoused a cause his enthusiasm was contagious. He immediately proclaimed his new doctrine and, although not without considerable opposition, his views carried the day. Rush's success in promulgating his thesis meant that for many years to come massive purging and bloodletting were to characterize American medical practice.

Rush's purported success in 1793 led him gradually to formulate his concept of the unity of disease. By 1796 he was informing his students that fevers resulted from three factors: a predisposing debility; an external or internal stimulus acting upon the body; and a "convulsive excitement" in the walls of the blood vessels. This "convulsive excitement," he had become convinced, was the essence of fevers and the common feature of all diseases. "Where I formerly said there was only one fever," he declared in a lecture, "I will [now] say there is but one disease in the world." Having concluded that the underlying cause of all illness was vascular tension, Rush assumed that the way to relieve the tension was by bleeding. The centuries-old practice of bleeding had shown clearly that a restless feverish patient when bled sufficiently would within a few minutes lose the flushed skin, delirium, high temperature, and other characteristics of fever. He would, moreover, break out into a copious sweat, long accepted as an indication that the fever was broken.

Since Rush believed that one of the hindrances to the development of medicine had been an "undue reliance upon the powers of nature in curing diseases," a thesis which he blamed upon Hippocrates, he resolved after 1793 to take whatever measures were necessary to save the patient's life.[6] A phrase which one finds repeatedly in early nineteenth-century medical journals epitomizes Rush's approach: "desperate diseases require desperate remedies." He believed that the body held about 25 pounds of blood, over double the actual quantity, and he urged his disciples to continue bleeding until four-fifths of the body's blood was removed. When massive purging caused the bowels to bleed, he felt the purge was doing double duty. The patient's welfare was the prime objective, and if it was necessary to give him violent cathartics and to relieve him of 6 to 8 pints of blood over a two or three day period, Rush did not intend to be faint-hearted.

One of the more surprising aspects of the 1793 epidemic is that Rush's medical views should have gained so many adherents. The evidence is clear that the yellow fever epidemic ran its course in Philadelphia and exacted an enormous death toll. In light of the prevailing medical knowledge, Rush and his colleagues could have done little to reduce the number of deaths, and Rush's heroic therapy undoubtedly compounded the suffering and mortality. Yet Rush emerged as a popular hero from the outbreak. While a number of his colleagues died and several others fled, Rush remained resolutely at his post seeing a hundred or more patients a day. When a slight fever attacked him, he had himself purged and bled, and before he was fully recovered was back seeing patients. The best explanation lies in Rush's personality. He was a warm, humane individual, positive and enthusiastic in his beliefs, and these qualities, plus his reputation as America's leading physician, gave credence to his medical doctrine.

The tragedy is that his personal popularity obscured the views of other more observant and perceptive physicians. Several of Rush's colleagues in Philadelphia—Drs. Adam Kuhn, Edward Stevens, Joseph Goss, and James Hutchinson—were all opposed to purging and bleeding and generally followed a mild supportive policy, the only course which could have been of any help at that time. Dr. James Currie, who was as busy as Rush during the outbreak, wrote a pamphlet describing yellow fever and the best means that he had found to combat it. In contrast to Rush, Currie declared that the disease was a specific contagion spread by contact with the sick or their personal belongings. He decried the burning of gunpowder and tar as a preventive and advised his readers to practice personal hygiene, moderate diet, mild exercise, and to get plenty of fresh air. He, too, rejected bloodletting and purgation and advocated a moderate treatment emphasizing the relief of symptoms and the principle of making the patient as comfortable as possible. Since little could be done for yellow fever patients once the disorder was established, it is unfortunate that these voices of moderation went virtually unheeded.[7]

Rush represents a transition between the eighteenth-century

age of reason and the nineteenth-century age of science. He had a philosophic bent which made him seek fundamental causes, and his medical training encouraged this tendency. Although he was a keen clinical observer, Rush had little interest in pathology and laboratory research. He related to people, and he was happiest when dealing with patients. As indicated, he had broad intellectual interests and dabbled in many fields. His social consciousness may well have been responsible for his political activities. While he had only an imperceptible influence upon political events, his election to various political offices, his status as a signer of the Declaration of Independence, and his brief services as an army medical officer all added to his public exposure and helped enhance his reputation.

By 1800 Rush was considered the greatest American physician of the day. His students were spreading his fame thoughout the United States, and his reputation was adding to the luster of Philadelphia as the leading medical center in the country. When he died in 1813 he was eulogized as the American Hippocrates. As a transitional figure, however, his fame was short-lived. Within ten years of his death his ideas were questioned, and within thirty he was almost universally condemned. In recent times a more balanced picture of him has emerged. By viewing him in light of his age, we can understand the factors which led him into error in his medical reasoning, and we can appreciate his many contributions. While his assumptions may not have been correct, Rush, by emphasizing personal and public hygiene, gave impetus to the public health movement of the nineteenth century. His shrewd clinical observations and ideas with respect to psychiatry were well in advance of his day. For the next century and a half scientists were to withdraw into their laboratories, unlike Rush, who felt that all educated men should participate actively in government. It took the atom bomb to make men of science appreciate the need for Rush's approach.

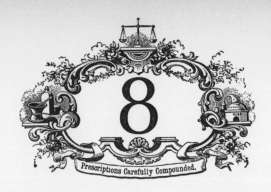

Prescriptions Carefully Compounded.

THE MEDICAL PROFESSION
AND MEDICAL PRACTICE

I N studying the history of medicine one is acutely conscious of two separate streams flowing side by side. One represents the evolution of medical theories, the major figures, the discoveries, and the gradual accumulation of knowledge. Parallel to this, and frequently having little relation to it, was the practice of the average physician. To a cynical observer, it would appear that in each age medical theorists simply sought to justify existing medical practices in terms of the prevailing philosophic or scientific concepts. Until the twentieth century medicine consisted largely of bleeding, blistering, purging, vomiting, and sweating. The agents to procure these results varied and the emphasis frequently shifted from one to another, but the basic therapy remained unchanged. While the theorists argued, the average practitioner, with only a minimum of theoretical knowledge, clung to a vague humoral thesis and sought simultaneously to restore the humoral balance and eliminate the bad or vitiated humors. The only question which troubled him was not whether to resort to bleeding and so on, but to what degree.

By the nineteenth century developments in anatomy, pathology, physiology, and related sciences were preparing the way for
medicine to overcome its lag and catch up with the other aspects of
Western society. To perceptive physicians neither the theories nor
the standard therapeutics seemed of much value, and increasingly
they turned to clinical experience. By this date hospitals were
growing in number and size, and clinicians were able to observe
hundreds of patients. In Paris a group of young physicians using
new techniques and instruments turned diagnosis into a fine art.
Led by Pierre C.A. Louis (1787–1872), they began collecting
clinical statistics on a large scale and tested their diagnoses by
following patients into the postmortem rooms. In terms of medical
practice, their most significant work was the application of statistics
to diagnoses and therapeutics. They soon discovered that the
traditional forms of therapy were not only useless but in many
cases positively harmful.

The impact of the French Clinical School was first felt in
Louisiana where the Creoles still looked to France for intellectual
leadership. Although Louisiana was acquired by the United States
in 1803 and became a state in 1812, its population remained
predominently French for many years. As English-speaking Americans flooded into New Orleans, the two groups inevitably clashed.
American physicians were largely apprentice-trained or else had
taken a relatively easy degree from one of the American medical
colleges. The Creoles carried on the European tradition of university training, which required a physician to spend as much as
fourteen years acquiring his medical degree. With some justification they considered the Americans both crude and virtually
illiterate. To make matters worse, the Anglo-American doctors
generally espoused the doctrines of Benjamin Rush, scorning the
healing power of nature "and firmly believing in direct and drastic
interferences, when confronted" by a sick patient, they gathered
their purges and emetics, couched their lancets, and charged the
enemy, prepared to bleed, purge, and vomit until the disease was
conquered.

The Creole physicians did not completely escape the pernicious influence of the great French bloodletter of this period,
Francois-Joseph-Victor Broussais (1772–1838), but they generally
believed the role of the physician was to assist nature in making the
cure. They were averse to wholesale bloodletting and were reluc-

tant to use calomel and other powerful and dangerous drugs. The wide difference in the medical practices of the two groups in Louisiana can best be seen in their approach to yellow fever. The Société Médicale de la Nouvelle Orléans requested two of its members to report on a yellow fever epidemic which struck the city in 1817. The ensuing report stated that the only methods which had proved of benefit were tepid baths to reduce the fever, "gentle evacuants, acid drinks with cream of tartar, tamerind, orange juice and lemon juice; whey, emollient clysters and purgatives."[1] The regimen recommended in this report was for its day a sensible and moderate one, and it continued to form the basis for the treatment of fevers by the Creole physicians in succeeding years.

As indicated, the Americans had little use for the policy of moderation, and their methods form a sharp contrast to this mild supportive treatment. Dr. M. L. Haynie of St. Francisville, Louisiana, wrote with contempt that the Louisiana French were "extremely adverse to using mercury in any form; and generally, as much opposed to the use of the lancet. . . ." Their "want of correct physiological knowledge," he explained, led them to believe that mercury could never be eliminated from the system and that the quantity of the blood was too small. Confident in his own understanding of physiology, Dr. Haynie stated that bleeding was always required in fevers "to ease the heart and arteries." To relieve the concomitant prostration, mercury was the most effective stimulant: "A few hundred grains (the quantity is not dangerous) introduced into the system" was certain to strengthen the pulse. Dr. Haynie proportioned his dosage to the violence of the disease, usually giving from 100 to 200 grains an hour! He then epitomized what has been called the heroic school of medicine by declaring: "It is but trifling with the life of a man, to give him less of a remedy than his disease calls for."[2]

The existence of two cultures in Louisiana discouraged the mutual exchange of ideas for the first two generations. The Creoles held themselves aloof from the uncultured Americans, maintaining their own societies and French language publications. By the mid-century, however, the better medical men in both groups were recognizing each other's merit, and the Creole practice was exerting a moderating influence upon American practices. Meanwhile, by 1830 the Paris Clinical School was beginning to have a direct impact upon physicians in the East. France had supplanted Great Britain as the mecca for medical students, and American physicians returning from Paris were soon championing the cause of moderation. Some 105 American physicians studied in Paris during the 1820s and another 222 in the 1830s. The list of those studying medicine in Paris in the 1830s is a virtual catalogue of the outstanding names in American medicine—men such as Jacob Bigelow, James Jackson, Jr., Oliver Wendell Holmes, John Collins Warren, Valentine Mott, Alexander H. Stevens, Josiah Clark Nott, and Willard Parker. All told, almost 700 American physicians spent some time in France in the years from 1820 to 1860.[3]

While in Paris these young Americans learned the use of the stethoscope, the art of diagnosis, and took advantage of the unrivaled opportunities for clincial observation and anatomical work. They brought back with them a skeptical approach to traditional therapy which gradually permeated the American medical profession. Jacob Bigelow was one of the first to express this new outlook. In an address before the Massachusetts Medical Society in 1835 he discussed what he called "self-limited" diseases, disorders which once entrenched in the system could not be affected by the art of medicine but which ran their course and eventually disappeared. The existence of these diseases, he said, probably explained why able practitioners employing totally different methods could each claim success for their treatment or why infinitely small homeopathic doses often succeeded.[4] While Bigelow suggested that only a few disorders fell into this category, he made the point that some diseases could be cured by nature alone, a view of medicine directly opposite that which Rush had taught. By the 1850s medical practice among the better physicians had swung away from the policy of active interference to one of caution and moderation. Bloodletting was definitely on the wane and calomel was no longer the mainstay of medication.

It is an oversimplification to ascribe this beneficial change soley to the influence of French and European physicians. Change was in the air, and one can cite any number of physicians who refused to be carried away by a particular system and who relied upon their own powers of observation. Mention has already been made of Drs. Kuhn and Stevens, and the others in the 1790s who opposed Benjamin Rush's debilitating treatment. The medical treatment given George Washington in 1799 has often been cited as an illustration of heroic therapy. Washington, who was suffering from an acute infection of the throat, probably streptococcal, was given the full treatment. He awoke early in the morning of December 14 feeling quite ill and sent for Dr. James Craik. In the meantime he asked his overseer to bleed him. On Dr. Craik's arrival, he blistered Washington's throat with cantharides, ordered an enema, and twice let blood. It was clear that the patient was in a serious condition, and by three in the afternoon two other physicians had been summoned, Drs. Gustavus Richard Brown and Elisha Dick. Although Washington had already been blistered, bled three times, and given several doses of calomel and tartar emetic within the space of a few hours, the two senior physicians, Craik and Brown, over the objections of the young Dr. Dick, decided more bleeding was necessary. On this occasion another 32 ounces was taken, the blood coming thick and slow. Although the physicians continued their efforts, Washington's condition rapidly worsened, and he died at ten o'clock that night.[5] Whether or not Washington at his age and condition could have survived the infection is doubtful, but the debilitating and dehydrating measures could only have hastened the process.

Aside from the picture of orthodox medical treatment provided by these events, a letter from Dr. Brown provides a glimpse into the soul-searching that existed among conscientious physicians. He wrote to Craik subsequently expressing regret over the bleeding and suggesting that Dr. Dick was probably right in opposing it. He described Dick as a sensible man who used common sense rather than books in practicing medicine. Brown's most significant comment indicates that Dr. Dick was literally despairing of medical practice, for Brown concluded: "He is disposed to put up his lancet forever and turn nurse instead of Doctor, for he says one good nurse is more likely to assist nature in making a cure than ten Doctors will by his pills and lancet."[6]

Dr. Jabez Heustis, a military surgeon who served in New Orleans, was horrified at the cavalier way in which mercury was administered to men suffering from yellow fever during an outbreak in 1812. It was not prescribed "by the weight and measurement of grains," he wrote caustically, "that would have been feeble and insignificant, and unworthy the characteristic liberality and boldness of its great advocate and supporter." It was given by the spoonful, and "Few survived to tell the mournful story."[7] Dr. Edward H. Barton of Louisiana in 1832 bitterly criticized all apsects of drastic medicine: "It makes me shudder when I hear of 'heroic practice'; heroism in war is built upon the slaughter of our fellow creatures; it is little less in physic."[8]

The two great epidemic diseases in nineteenth-century America, yellow fever and Asiatic cholera, also played a role in moderating therapy. Yellow fever, which had plagued the colonies for over a century, virtually disappeared from the northeastern states after 1806 but struck with increasing intensity along the South Atlantic and Gulf coasts, reaching its peak in the 1850s. Although a few physicians dissented, bleeding, calomel, and other drastic measures remained the standard treatment for the fever until the midcentury. Since malaria was also a major problem in the South, the introduction of the alkaloid quinine after 1820 proved a boon. Unfortunately, the concept of the unity of fevers was still widely accepted, and it led to the quinine treatment for yellow fever. In the late 1830s it was the vogue to give massive doses of quinine to yellow fever patients, a practice which was at least as bad as the traditional therapy. In 1844 the newly established *New Orleans Medical Journal* commented that there had been a major change in the treatment of fevers by southern practitioners. The use of purgatives and emetics had moderated and been replaced by "the more prompt and bold administration of tonics, above all the sulphate of quinine." "Quinine, instead of calomel," the *Journal* declared, "is now considered in the South, the *Sampson* of the *Materia Medica.*"[9]

A series of major yellow fever outbreaks from 1853 to 1855 finally convinced many southern physicians that active interference in the case of yellow fever merely aggravated the disease. At the end of the great yellow fever epidemic of 1853, the *New Orleans Medical and Surgical Journal* conceded that the quinine treatment, like its predecessors, was of little value.[10] Quinine, bloodletting, and calomel still had their advocates, but there was a rising consensus that a mild supportive treatment combined with good nursing was all that could be done.

The second American scourge was Asiatic cholera, a filth disease which gained a foothold three times in the nineteenth century. Improvements in transportation and the emergence of large, crowded, and dirty cities, which provided an ideal environment for enteric disorders, were responsible for the three major Asiatic cholera epidemics. As with yellow fever, the physicians could neither prevent nor cure the disease. Since dehydration is the worst aspect of cholera, the traditional depletory forms of therapy only intensified the problem. During the first two outbreaks in 1832 and 1849–50, heated debates over medical treatment occurred within the medical profession, but essentially the question was how best to utilize the traditional therapeutics. Opium was standard treatment for enteric or diarrheal complaints, and the arguments raged over the best ways to combine the use of opium with calomel, bloodletting, and emetics. In New York City during 1832 an open clash developed among the various medical groups. The Board of Health's Special Medical Council recommended calomel, opium, brandy, and cayenne pepper. Another group of physicians advised free purging with calomel and aloes or scammony. Still a third group of physicians joined together to publish *The Cholera Bulletin*. On July 23 the editor sarcastically classified his fellow physicians as "the Bleeders, the Calomel Brigade, the Opium Foragers, . . . the Guard of Leechers and Blisters," and so forth. His major criticism, however, was against those who applied one form of therapy either indiscriminately or exclusively, for he concluded that the lancet, opium, calomel, tobacco, and all the other therapeutics were valuable; the problem was—how to use them.[11]

When cholera returned almost twenty years later, the same arguments raged, with each doctor stressing his own variant, but here again, as was the case with yellow fever in the 1850s, one senses a general moderation of practice, a tendency to consider the weakened state of the patient, and to follow a more supportive program. Within a few years this policy was becoming more general, and when Asiatic cholera returned a third time in 1866 the treatment tended to be simpler and more effective. Dr. Warren Stone, a well-known New Orleans physician and surgeon, announced in 1866 that he had found it beneficial to give cholera patients as much ice water as they wished, a great step forward in dealing with a disease which dehydrated its victims.

The almost universal prescription of calomel for cholera patients was based upon long-established beliefs. One was the miasmatic thesis which maintained that a miasma or "noxious substance" arising from filth and putrefying vegetable matter corrupted the natural humors. Calomel, along with jalap and other purgatives, could be counted on to drive out these so-called vitiated humors. Another traditional assumption blamed the liver for a good part of the bodily ills. This belief was strengthened when postmortems revealed that the liver in cholera patients was frequently engorged or congested. The obvious solution was to stimulate the flow of bile by large doses of calomel. So widely held was this belief that calomel continued to be prescribed for cholera patients well into the twentieth century.[12] Other medical theories, too, were cited as justification for the use of calomel. Regardless of the therapeutic value of this drug, it is important to keep in mind that intelligent physicans sought a rational explanation for the use of their therapeutics. And it is precisely this fact that differentiated the medical profession from the empirics or irregulars.

The French Clinical School, the work of skeptical and observant physicians, and the impact of yellow fever and Asiatic cholera all played a role in helping to bring about the transition from excessive and drastic forms of therapy to a policy of moderation and support for the patient. One last factor needs to be mentioned: the role of the public. Medical practice in any society and at any time depends to a considerable degree upon the public wants and demands. While the medical profession today deserves much of the blame for the excessive use of antibiotics, steroids, and tranquilizers, it is equally true that patients expect their physician to do something—and if today's doctor does not give them a shot or a prescription, they are quite likely to look elsewhere. In the nineteenth century most patients were conditioned to calomel and bloodletting, and any physician who failed to resort to them would have been considered remiss. Yet, just as perceptive physicians had their doubts about heroic therapy, so did many laymen. This skepticism increased in direct ratio to the spread of drastic medical measures. In fact the most zealous advocates of bleeding and purging were most instrumental in turning popular opinion against the practice. In America public opinion was one step ahead of medicine in this regard. As much as anything, it was the public's decision to turn from the regular profession to the herbalists, homeopaths, hydropaths, and other medical sects eschewing heroic practices which literally forced orthodox physicians to reconsider their position.

In the care of the insane, American medicine faithfully

reflected European developments. The Enlightenment and the new spirit of humanitarianism which led men such as Philippe Pinel of France and William Tuke in England to offer alternatives to the cruelty and neglect of the insane stimulated a number of sensitive and intelligent Americans to take action. The Pennsylvania Hospital admitted insane patients as early as 1751, and in 1773 the colony of Virginia opened the Eastern State Hospital in Williamsburg to provide for the mentally ill.[13] The first major breakthrough in treatment in America, however, did not come until 1789 when Dr. Rush petitioned the authorities of the Pennsylvania Hospital to provide better facilities for the insane. Rush represented a new school of medical thought, one which considered mental illness a somatic disorder and hence curable. Although we may look askance at the heroic regimen of bloodletting, purging, and so forth to which he subjected his patients, Rush was moving in the right direction.

The late eighteenth and early nineteenth centuries saw the emergence in Europe and America of the so-called moral treatment. An outgrowth of humanitarianism, it assumed that kindness, a cheerful environment, and proper respect for the patient's physical well-being would restore the mentally ill to health. Rush conceded some value to the moral treatment, but he believed the major emphasis should be placed upon medical therapy. The moral treatment was first applied in a few private institutions catering to middle- and upper-class patients, and the results exceeded the hopes of its advocates. Whereas mental patients formerly had been considered incurable and simply chained in dark basements or attics, it now appeared that half or more responded to treatment. At Bloomingdale Asylum in New York, the Pennsylvania Hospital in Philadelphia, the Hartford Retreat, and other institutions, the moral treatment swept the day.[14]

The apparent success of this new form of therapy, which for the first time offered hope for the insane, led to the establishment of a host of state asylums in the period from 1825 to 1860. The individual chiefly responsible for this development was Dorothea Lyndle Dix. In 1841, on becoming aware of the atrocious conditions under which most of the insane poor were kept, she launched a campaign in Massachusetts which led to the expansion and renovation of the Worcester State Hospital. Encouraged by this success, she expanded her activities by going from state to state, systematically exposing the deplorable condition of the insane poor, gaining support from newspapers, prominent citizens, and legislators, and then fighting for the creation of state hospitals. As she swept through the United States, she left a host of insane asylums in her wake.

Ironically, the success achieved by Dix and her supporters almost proved self-defeating. The moral treatment, which seemed to work so well when physicians and asylum superintendents were treating patients of their own class, broke down in the case of immigrants and native-born poor. Mutually acceptable moral values were a fundamental aspect of the moral treatment and required that the healer and the patient belong to the same class; but, when class distinctions were intensified by differences in culture, communication between doctors and patients broke down completely. If this was not enough, the number of insane poor rose in direct ratio to the increasing degree of urbanization. The increase may have been even greater since the problems confronting the newcomers pouring into the cities placed enormous stresses upon them. Consequently, the newly created insane hospitals were overwhelmed with patients from the start, so that even the best-intentioned hospital authorities could do little more than provide custodial care.

Even in the private institutions, by the midcentury it was becoming clear that the moral treatment at best had only limited value. This factor, combined with the almost complete failure in treating the poor, gradually undermined the concept that the insane could be helped. With medicine unable to find a satisfactory explanation for mental illness, the assumption gained strength that it was a genetic or hereditary ailment and hence incurable. The general pessimistic attitude toward the insane in the second half of the nineteenth century meant that, while they were no longer treated with deliberate brutality, neither did they receive active therapy.

Over 100 years elapsed following the decline of the moral treatment before any significant improvements were made in the treatment of mental problems. The work of Freud, Jung, Adler, and their American disciples in the development of psychoanalysis is a complicated and involved subject, and since it is concerned primarily with neuroses rather than psychoses I have chosen not to deal with it. The psychotic are clearly suffering from mental illness, whereas neuroses in some measure seem to characterize all individuals.

Whatever the case, the revolutionary developments in medicine in the late nineteenth century had little impact on the mentally ill, who for the most part continued to receive only custodial care. A few innovations were made in the first half of the twentieth century such as hydrotherapy, electroshock treatments, and various forms of surgery. While some treatments were of limited value, others, such as prefrontal lobotomy, proved disastrous. Not until the development of tranquilizers was any major change made. Beginning in the midcentury these new drugs, by relieving symptoms and enabling patients to function in normal situations, brought a rapid diminution in the number of hospitalized inmates. Advances in biochemistry and physiology are beginning to demonstrate the validity of Rush's view that mental illness is a somatic problem and are beginning to provide more effective means for dealing with it. At the same time, the moral treatment has been revived under new names—halfway houses, milieu therapy, open hospital, and therapeutic community. Much still remains to be done, but the past twenty-five years have seen the first significant steps in the direction of successful therapy for the mentally ill.

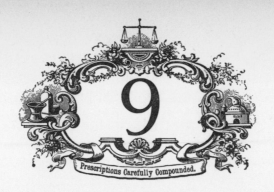

Prescriptions Carefully Compounded.

THE IRREGULARS, FOLK MEDICINE, AND SELF-MEDICATION

THE disastrous results of heroic medical practice and the steady decline in prestige of the orthodox physicians easily explains why the public turned to the irregular medical sects which flourished in the early nineteenth century. There were other factors, however, which help to account for the rise of the irregulars. The colonial period had been one in which any man who could read could be his own physician, lawyer, or theologian. As American society became more complex and specialized and professions began to emerge, a popular reaction developed which took many forms. The egalitarianism of the Age of Jacksonian Democracy was in part an effort to return to those simpler days when every American was self-sufficient—his own lawyer, physician, farmer, carpenter, and so forth. The appearance of organized medical societies with their fee bills symbolized this decline of individual independence. In the good old days medical care had been easily obtainable at little cost by reading medical books or from one's pastor and neighbors.

Despite the inability of most physicians to make a decent living, newspapers and journals in the early nineteenth century constantly inveighed against the high cost of medical care. It was not that medical care was so costly, but simply that home medicine and folk practitioners, a very inexpensive form of medicine, were being driven out by the multiplication in numbers of formal medical practitioners.

THOMSONIANISM

The first individual to capitalize on this growing sentiment was Samuel Thomson (1769–1843). Coming from a poor family in a backwoods section of New Hampshire, Thomson early became interested in botanicals. As a young man he witnessed the death of his mother, an event which he blamed on mercurials and the other harsh drugs of orthodox physicians. When his wife became sick and was subjected to the customary bleeding and drugging, Thomson dismissed the physicians and called in two root and herb doctors whom he credited with saving her life. The medical experiences of his mother and wife turned his attention more firmly to herbals, and he quickly acquired a local reputation as an herb doctor. As the result of his growing reputation, he left farming and in 1805 became an itinerant herbal practitioner, relying largely upon steam baths and botanical remedies.

In the succeeding years he gradually formulated his medical system. Based on a vague misunderstanding of Greek theories, he surmised that there was only one disease, the result of cold, and only one cure, heat. The restoration of heat was accomplished initially by steam baths and then by the use of so-called "hot" botanicals such as cayenne pepper. He likened the digestive system to a stovepipe which occasionally becomes clogged with soot. To clean it out and restore its proper functioning, he resorted to botanic emetics, purgatives, diuretics, and sudorifics.

As Thomson's practice grew, he soon incurred the bitter enmity of the regular physicians. The reaction of the latter was predictable since Thomson constantly denounced them, claiming their medical training was designed to see "how much poison [could] be given without causing death." In addition, he opposed the use of bloodletting and blistering, and the administration of mercurials, arsenicals, and other mineral drugs. Probably the gravest affront to physicians was Thomson's success as a medical practitioner at a time when few doctors could make a decent living. Whatever the case, in 1809 he was thrown into jail after being accused by a regular physician of murdering a patient in Salisbury, Massachusetts. Whatever the merits of the case, the prosecution bungled it by introducing a purported sample of lobelia which turned out to be marsh rosemary, a harmless botanical, and Thompson was acquitted. He first published a brief account of his method in 1812 and gradually expanded this in a series of pamphlets. His culminating work was a book published in 1822 entitled *New Guide to Health; or Botanic Family Physician.* . . .[1]

Thomsonianism had been making slow headway up until this time, but publication of his book gave a great impetus to the movement. And a movement it was—religious, political, and cultural! Thomson, who came from a fundamentalist religious background, acquired a first-rate apostle in the person of Elias Smith. Smith was also a fundamentalist, converted to Thomsonianism in 1816. Suspicious of the legal, medical, and theological professions, Thomson and Smith, the latter now Thomson's general agent, fervently spread the word of Thomsonianism—a cause they equated with that of the common man. The partnership did not long survive, but it did serve to get the movement well underway. Beginning by convincing a few individuals in a given town or area of the value of his method of treatment, Thomson organized them into what became known as Friendly Botanic Societies. With the first publication of his book, he or his agents sold it for $20, bestowing upon the buyer the right to practice medicine in his own family.

As indicated, Thomsonianism was a significant part of Jacksonian Democracy. In advocating seizing medicine from the hands of professionals and returning it to the common man, the proponents of Thomsonianism found a receptive audience. They associated themselves with fighting for the common man. Medical societies advocating licensing laws were accused of trying to achieve a privileged status by means of monopolies. In reaction to these attacks, the physicians did their best to harass Thomsonian practitioners, but public sentiment was against the physicians.

Local judges and juries usually dismissed criminal or civil actions against the irregular practitioners, and state legislatures responded to public pressure by eliminating or negating all licensing requirements. It scarcely needs to be added that Thomsonians spearheaded the fight to repeal medical licensure laws.

As Joseph Kett has pointed out, Thomsonians actively supported a wide range of social movements in the 1830s and 1840s. They supported drives against alcohol, tobacco, coffee, and tea, and espoused the cause of dietary reform. The many-faceted appeal of Thomsonianism enabled the movement to sweep through rural areas in all sections of the country. Thomson published thirteen editions of his book and claimed that he had sold 100,000 family rights to practice medicine by 1839. Whether or not this claim is true—and it well may be—his influence over medical practice was far greater than even these figures would indicate. The movement was so successful it proved self-defeating. As his system was not really new or unique and he was unable to maintain control of his agents, a number of individuals and manufacturing companies quickly seized upon his name and principles for their own benefit. Even more ironically, his subsequent disciples began organizing medical schools and institutionalizing Thomsonian medicine—a development contrary to one of the fundamental principles of Thomsonianism.[2]

HOMEOPATHS

The second major irregular medical sect to make deep inroads into the orthodox practice was homeopathy, a medical theory propounded by a German physician, Samuel Christian Hahnemann (1755–1843). Unlike Thomson, who was largely self-taught, Hahnemann was a well-educated man of considerable scholarship. He studied medicine in Leipzig and Vienna before finally taking a medical degree in 1779 at the University of Erlangen. In between his medical studies, he mastered at least eight languages and worked briefly cataloguing a fine library. For the next twenty-five years or so he wandered around, barely eking out a living from his medical practice, writing, and translating.

Hahnemann was a man of intelligence and erudition, capable of sound judgments, and yet he occasionally wandered out into the wide blue yonder. He showed a great deal of common sense in his judgment of current medical practices, since he deplored the excessive drugging and bloodletting of the day. He was a strong advocate of public and personal hygiene, particularly insofar as it related to communicable diseases, and he recognized the value of moderate exercise, good diet, and fresh air. In addition to criticizing the medical profession for its excessive doses, Hahnemann also deplored the polypharmacy of his day. As mentioned earlier, apparently on the assumption that if one drug was beneficial a combination of them would multiply the benefits, medical prescriptions tended to be long and involved. While this worked to the advantage of the pharmacist or apothecary, its effect on the patient was questionable. Realizing that it was impossible to determine the efficacy of a particular medicine when used in conjunction with several others, Hahnemann decided that tests had to be made on one particular drug. He used the expression "pure," for he discovered a wide variation in the quality of drugs supplied by the apothecaries. As an experiment, Hahnemann swallowed doses of "the bark," as cinchona was called, for several days and experienced what he considered to be the symptoms of fever. It will be recalled that the concept of the unity of fevers was widely held—the belief that there was only one fever (some physicians carried it further and said only one disease). Since cinchona cured fever, Hahnemann reasoned that a drug which could induce a condition resembling a disease in a healthy person would cure that disease in a sick individual.

Over the years he gradually discovered other drugs which appeared to work in the same fashion and was thus led to the first of the two basic principles of homeopathy, *similai similibus curantur*: like cures like. A few years later, while prescribing for some children suffering from scarlet fever, he gave them an infinitely small dose of belladonna and they all recovered. Aside from what he thought was a significant discovery—the use of belladonna for scarlet fever—he believed he had uncovered another medical principle, the value of minute doses. Attempting to account for the success of infinitesimal doses, he assumed that the human organism became extremely sensitive to drugs when sick; hence, what might have little effect upon a well individual would have very positive impact upon one who was sick.

By 1810 Hahnemann had formulated his medical concepts,

and he published them in his *Organon of Rational Healing*, a work which went through five editions and was translated into every major European language. Hahnemann's second principle, the law of infinitesimals, virtually negated the effect of the homeopathic drugs. He was convinced that a dosage of $1/500,000$ or $1/1,000,000$ of a grain was efficacious. Using these highly diluted medicines, he was to all intents and purposes leaving the cure to nature—a course of action which was far better than the rigorous treatment given by most orthodox physicians in his day. Suffice it to say, Hahnemann gradually gained a following and finally became an internationally recognized physician.

Homeopathy arrived fairly late in the United States in the person of Hans Gram, an American of Danish parents, who had studied medicine in Copenhagen and had subsequently been converted to homeopathy. He returned from Denmark in 1825 and settled in New York. Here he gradually began making converts. Meanwhile a number of German physicians were migrating to Pennsylvania, one of whom, Constantine Hering, was both a distinguished physician and scientist. Hering, an enthusiastic homeopath, quickly organized a following and in 1835 established the first homeopathic college in America, the Allentown Academy.

THE ECLECTICS

During these first few years homeopathy grew slowly, although its followers were gradually spreading through the country. It was aided during these years by the development of the Eclectic school of medicine founded by Wooster Beach (1794–1859). Beach received an orthodox medical education but, like Thomson, began emphasizing the value of botanical remedies. He also harbored a general distrust of doctors, lawyers, priests, and political authorities. The Eclectics differed from Thomsonians in their occasional willingness to resort to mineral remedies and, as the name implied, in their willingness to borrow whatever was practical or effective. Eclectic medical colleges began springing up in the 1830s and 1840s, and their existence helped spread the homeopathic doctrine. The receptivity of the Eclectics to new ideas resulted in many of them being converted to homeopathy. Both groups benefited from the spread of Thomsonian doctrines, and by offering more sophisticated versions of botanic medicine the two medical sects gradually replaced Thomsonianism.[3]

THE SPREAD OF HOMEOPATHY

By 1844 the homeopaths were strong enough to organize the American Institute of Homeopathy, the first national medical organization. Yellow fever and Asiatic cholera, two major epidemic diseases which had a great impact upon American medical practice, were also responsible for helping the spread of homeopathy. In the southern states the results achieved by homeopathic physicians in dealing with yellow fever cases were far superior to those of the regular physicians. Since little could be done at that time except to keep the patient comfortable, the homeopathic method which left the cure to nature was far better than the bleeding, purging, and blistering routine of the regulars. Hence it is not surprising that in Louisiana, which was constantly plagued by yellow fever, both French and American physicians began turning to homeopathy. Elsewhere, too, in the southern states homeopathy began gaining ground among orthodox physicians. When the second wave of Asiatic cholera swept through the United States from 1848 to 1853, the homeopathic treatment again demonstrated its advantages over traditional forms of therapy, with the result that hundreds of orthodox physicians began adopting its methods.

The immediate reaction of organized medicine to homeopathy was not unfavorable. Unlike the Thomsonians, the homeopathic physicians were well educated, and they operated from what was apparently a sound rationale. Advocating research, they claimed their findings were based largely upon so-called "provings." These provings consisted of individual physicians testing therapeutics upon themselves to determine what "diseases" or symptoms they caused in a healthy individual. While far removed from the blind and double-blind testing methods of today, in which neither the subject nor the researcher know precisely to which subjects the drug is administered, the "provings" were as valid as much of the research carried on by orthodox physicians in the early nineteenth century. Reviews of Hahnemann's *Organon* in medical journals were not too unkind, and it is evident that the medical profession was reserving judgment. With the profession still in considerable disarray, new forms of therapy or new medical concepts could scarcely be rejected out of hand; even phrenology was accepted as a legitimate aspect of medicine for several years. Indicative of the profession's fairly open-minded approach, in 1832 the Medical Society of the County of New York voted that an honorary membership be awarded to Dr. Hahnemann.

By the late 1830s, however, the attitude of the orthodox physicians began to change, and individual physicians and medical journals began ridiculing homeopathy and castigating its followers. A few of them, more balanced in their judgment, recognized that Hahnemann at least demonstrated that leaving the cure to nature was far better than the rigorous interference of the regular physicians. One of the first to sound a note of alarm against the homeopaths was Dr. Oliver Wendell Holmes. Addressing the Massachusetts Medical Society in 1842 on the subject of "Homeopathy and Its Kindred Delusions," he warned that this doctrine represented a serious threat to organized medicine by denying the validity of existing medical knowledge and rejecting all accepted forms of medical therapy. Oft-quoted as saying, "If all the medicines were thrown into the ocean it would be so much the better for mankind and so much worse for the fishes," Holmes was no blind supporter of contemporary medical practice. He recognized that homeopathy would distract medicine from the pursuit of objective scientific information, and in his address Holmes systematically demolished the doctrines of Hahnemann and the arguments in favor of homeopathy.

Logic was on the side of Holmes, but while he and other regular physicians could see the fallacies in the homeopathic principles, in terms of medical practice they could offer nothing better. Whatever the merits of Hahnemann's theory, it was obvious that homeopathic medicine was more efficacious in practice than the regular or allopathic medicine. This fact was not lost upon observant physicians and laymen, and so homeopathy continued to flourish. Although it was not as great a threat as Thomsonianism in its popular appeal, homeopathy constituted a much more serious menace to the medical profession. To begin with, homeopathy attracted most of its early membership from the ranks of the orthodox physicians; hence the regulars could scarcely ignore the homeopaths as ignorant and unlettered folk practitioners. Further, homeopathy appealed to the middle and upper classes, the main source of income for the regular practitioners—and nothing, it would seem, arouses an individual's moral indignation more than the prospect of an economic loss. Finally, homeopaths could not be dismissed as empirics because they offered a rationale for their practice.

With the formation of the American Medical Association in 1847 the battle lines between the regulars and the homeopaths became more sharply drawn, and the ensuing hostilities lasted well into the twentieth century. The foregoing chapters have shown many reasons why it became necessary to organize a strong national medical association in the 1840s, and certainly the threat from the homeopaths and other irregulars was a major factor in stimulating the initial meetings. In drawing up its code of ethics, the AMA struck the first blow at the homeopaths. The consultation clause stated that no regular physician could consult with any practitioner "whose practice is based upon an exclusive dogma, to the rejection of accumulated experience of the profession." In effect, no physician could consult with a homeopath even at the patient's request. Moreover, a regular physician could not attend any patient, regardless of his condition, unless the homeopath attending the case was first dismissed.[4]

While the intent of the consultation clause was clear, its enforcement was not easy. The AMA itself was a fledgling organization, and the fight against the homeopaths had to be conducted at the state and local level. The problem here was complicated in some cases by the friendly, personal relationships between a number of regulars and homeopaths. Furthermore, refusing help to a desperately ill patient because of a clash between rival medical groups went against one of the most fundamental of all principles of medical ethics. Nonetheless, state and local societies began excluding homeopaths from membership, and in some instances they rigidly insisted upon adherence to the consultation clause. Fortunately for the homeopaths, exclusion from the relatively weak state and local medical societies of that era was no major blow, and their ranks continued to thrive. In New York, for example, where homeopathy was quite strong and where the state society in 1882 rejected the AMA's code of ethics, the homeopaths more than held their ground.

Meanwhile, a second and more successful attack on the homeopaths had been launched with the outbreak of the Civil War. The Army Military Board ruled against the admission of homeopaths into the Army Medical Corps, and, although the homeopaths turned to Congress, they were unable to have the decision reversed. Another area in which the regulars gained some advantages over the homeopaths was in the matter of hospital appointments. The rise of the city brought with it the urban slums, where great masses of overcrowded, underpaid, and poorly fed workers lived in poverty and degradation. Out of necessity, existing municipal hospitals had to be enlarged and new ones built. As the homeopaths began to develop their own colleges and medical societies, they began demanding equal privileges in state and municipal hospitals. As might be expected, the orthodox profession flatly refused to make any concession on this score.

When Chicago prepared to open its municipal hospital in 1857, the homeopaths applied for the right to participate in staffing the institution. Not only was their petition rejected, but they were even denied the use of the hospital facilities. A similar struggle took place in New York City from 1856 to 1858 when the homeopaths applied for the right to staff certain wards in Bellevue Hospital. Strong public support, including that of Horace Greeley, editor of the New York *Tribune*, was mobilized on behalf of the homeopaths, but once more the allopaths (orthodox physicians) won in a closely contested battle. Five or six years later the issue arose in connection with the Boston City Hospital, and here again the refusal of the regulars to serve with homeopaths enabled them to win the day.

During the years from 1850 to 1880, orthodox physicians were generally successful in keeping homeopaths out of the major hospitals. The homeopaths responded by establishing their own institutions, many of which compared favorably with the hospitals operated by orthodox practitioners. In the latter part of the nineteenth century, both groups began raising their educational standards to take advantage of the major advances in medicine. In the process they began drawing together, stimulated in part by a mutual concern over professional standards and a common desire to rid the profession of quacks and unqualified irregulars.

While Thomsonianism and homeopathy were the major irregular sects, they were only part of a general health reform movement in this period which, according to Richard H. Shryock, was "dedicated to the proposition that all men could stay well, if they would but stay away from their doctors." Mention has already been made of the Eclectics, a medical sect which relied extensively upon botanicals but which believed in formal medical education and even established its own colleges. The better Eclectic schools followed the path of homeopathy and eventually either merged into orthodox medicine or simply disappeared. Arising directly out of Thomsonianism were the botanical medical schools founded by Alva Curtis—schools which heralded a movement Alex Berman has referred to as Neo-Thomsonianism. One of Thomson's chief disciples, Curtis broke with him in 1836 and in 1839 chartered his own Botanico-Medical School in Columbus, Ohio. By the Civil War some eight of these schools were established. As Thomsonianism began to fade from the scene, this Neo-Thomsonian medicine took its place, and Curtis' Reformed Medical Association gradually supplanted Thomson's Friendly Botanical Societies. Although this new organization in 1852 sought to define the medical doctrines of Neo-Thomsonianism, it was at best pseudoscientific; and, with the advance of modern medicine, Neo-Thomsonianism soon fell by the wayside. This same fate was also shared by some fourteen or fifteen other botanic medical schools founded in the pre-Civil War years.[5]

One characteristic which all of the irregular sects shared was a healthy distrust of orthodox medicine, and this widespread feeling also played a part in the popular health movement during the years 1830 to 1870. Yet opposition to the medical profession was only a part of the explanation for the widespread interest in health and personal hygiene. These same years witnessed a social and cultural renaissance affecting all aspects of society and bringing into existence a wide range of reform movements—temperance, abolition, women's rights, and so forth. Although leaders in each of these movements tended to ride their own hobby horses, inevitably they and their followers supplied each other with mutual support. A key figure in the popular health reform movement was Sylvester Graham (1794–1851), whose name has since become immortalized by the Graham cracker. Graham, the son and grandson of minister-physicians, entered the ministry and did not concern himself with medicine until he became active in the Pennsylvania Temperance Society in 1830. In the course of preparing a series of temperance lectures he began studying physiology, diet, personal hygiene, and other matters pertaining to daily life. Before long he became the leading exponent of a moderate way of life, which included exercise, fresh air, cold showers, and a diet marked by coarsely ground whole wheat bread, vegetables, and fruits.

Graham appeared on the scene at the right time. Traditionally mankind has lived in an economy of scarcity in which gourmandizing has been a form of conspicious consumption—an indication of relatively high status in society. One has only to read the menus of the seventeenth, eighteenth, and nineteenth centuries to realize what sturdy trenchermen were our well-to-do forebears. Along with excessive eating went a comparable over-imbibing of alcoholic beverages. In early times, the elite quaffed down large quantities of wine and brandy while the poor had to content themselves with beer and ale. The eighteenth century, however, saw the advent of relatively cheap rum, gin, and bourbon; and alcohol, far more than religion, became the opiate of the industrial masses. For those living in abject poverty in city slums, alcohol proved a simple and cheap escape from the drabness of life. As Graham contemplated the ills of his contemporaries, he became convinced that a bad diet, intemperance in eating and drinking, lack of exercise, and poor personal hygiene were largely responsible.

In his call for cleanliness, Graham was again in tune with his times. Bathing has had an interesting history in Western civilization. It was rated highly by the Egyptians, who in turn passed it along to the Hebrews and Greeks. The Romans carried bathing to a high point, by constructing magnificent private and public baths, but the Christians, casting aside all heathen ways, decried cleanliness and made a virtue out of dirt. The anchorites and hermits of early Christianity took an almost sinful pride in having gone unwashed for twenty or thirty years. The Renaissance of the fifteenth and sixteenth centuries saw a revival of bathing, as wealthy Europeans sought to emulate life during the classical civilizations; unfortunately the emergence of public baths coincided with the great wave of virulent syphilis which swept through

Europe in the sixteenth century. Since the baths had turned into a form of indoor recreation involving considerable licentiousness, the public put two and two together and came up with three. Bathing became equated with venereal disease, and the practice rapidly fell into abeyance. By the early nineteenth century people widely believed that it was positively dangerous to get wet all over. As the author can recall from his own childhood in England and America, suspicion of bathing, particularly in wintertime, continued until well into the twentieth century. While it is clear that Graham affected no major revolution in the personal habits of Americans, he was in the forefront of the more liberal elements, and his pleas for washing and bathing found many listeners.

With the evolution of American religious thought, reform movements were literally crusades, and Sylvester Graham preached his gospel of whole wheat grain, moderation, exercise, and hygiene with all the fervor of an evangelist. He believed, however, that personal hygiene must be based on a sound understanding of physiological principles, and he and his disciples were staunch advocates of teaching physiology in schools and public forums. Even in their advocacy of what they called physiological reform, however, the Grahamites believed they were promoting a higher cause. One of them wrote in the Boston *Health Journal* that physiological reform "is peculiarly suited to raise man from a state of sensual degradation and raise him to the rank, which as a rational and immortal being, nature intended he should occupy. . . ."[6]

One last irregular group deserves mention, the hydropaths. Treatment of the sick or ailing by means of internal or external applications of either "pure" or mineral water is an age-old method. After a long period of desuetude, it enjoyed a revival in the eighteenth century and by the mid-nineteenth had achieved a measure of scientific status. The water cure, as a formal medical practice, first reached America around 1840, and within a few years hydropathic practitioners and hydropathic institutes spread throughout the United States.

The reactions of two Mississippi sisters, Kitty and Penelope Hamilton, to the hydropathic treatment explains why the practice spread so rapidly. The two girls were treated by a Dr. Byrenheidt at his institute in Biloxi, Mississippi. Kitty Hamilton commented upon the physician's great "delicacy and consideration for female modesty." Her sister Penelope wrote: "It is a happy change indeed from poisonous drugs to pure cold water. Would to heaven I had come here when I was first taken sick; instead of being butchered by Pill givers. How many hours of pain and anguish I might have been spared. . . ." She added that the doctor used no drugs, but relied exclusively upon cold water taken internally and externally. Both girls mentioned that the doctor recommended dumbbells, skipping ropes, and other forms of exercise. The restricted life of supposedly delicate upper-class females brought on many minor complaints which were often compounded into serious illnesses by harsh bleeding, drugging, and enforced bed rest. For women who had endured this experience, life in a hydropathic institute with its orderly routine, moderate diet, mild exercise, cold baths, and ample quantities of water in the place of drugs must have been a welcome change. In New York City Dr. T. H. Trall broadened the concept of hydropathy to include the ideas of Graham and virtually all other health fads of the day—including the physical culture school and the uses of electricity. By the second half of the century hydropathy had given way to what had become known as the "hygienic system," a form of therapy that embraced most of the ideas of the popular health reformers.[7]

Irregular physicians and popular health reformers often found themselves looked upon askance by conservative laymen, and they encountered strong and bitter opposition from the regular medical profession. Yet in the long run their ideas carried the day. While continuing to denounce health faddists and irregulars, orthodox physicians gradually accepted many of their major principles. The medical profession was forced to concede that excessive drugging, bloodletting, and other forms of drastic therapy were positively harmful; it had to recognize the so-called physiological principles of sound diet and moderate exercise; and it could scarcely deny the value of health maintenance or preventive medicine. The doctors were not the only ones profoundly affected by the popular health movement. Over forty years ago Richard H. Shryock pointed out that the teachings of Graham and the other health faddists had been accepted by a large segment of the American population. He noted the then-prevailing emphasis upon diet and nutrition and commented: "People nowadays are seekers after roughage and the whole grain cereals. They worship fresh air and sun-tan, and the bath room has become the very symbol of American civilization." His words ring even truer today. The thousands of Americans patronizing natural food stores, doggedly performing their daily jogging, or faithfully exercising in YMCA's, schools, or in their homes to televised instructions all bear testimony to the success of the health reformers.[8]

A fact frequently overlooked is that in any day and age a good part of medical practice falls into the categories of folk medicine, self-medication, and quackery. For the vast majority of people, sickness represents a serious economic threat, and their first impulse is to try a folk or proprietary medicine or some practical home technique. Throughout history, and in many rural areas in the world today, individuals with a knowledge of local herbals quickly found their services in demand and their local prestige increased by any minor successes in dealing with human or animal ailments. Men with a degree of tactile sensitivity and manual dexterity often acquire a measure of skill in bonesetting. Older women with a little more experience, and probably even greater confidence, can easily set themselves up as midwives. Since childbirth is a natural process and most illnesses are self-limiting, midwives and purported healers of all types would have little difficulty gaining credibility. As with physicians, those whom they cured remained to praise them, while their failures were often in no condition to complain.

Frequently these individuals passed on their knowledge and skills to a younger person. In Europe most of the midwives, herbalists, and so forth were the product of generations of folk practitioners. Many of these folk doctors crossed the Atlantic, but mobility, social fluidity, and the newness of the American frontier opened the way for anyone interested in medicine to claim a special proficiency in the field. The appeal of the empirics was enhanced by the inability of the regular medical profession to offer a better alternative.

Aside from advertisements by Thomsonians and various other medical sects, the newspapers abound with notices from a wide variety of empirics. In 1837 the *Daily Pittsburgh Gazette* announced that Waterman Sweet, a "Natural Bonesetter," would be in the city shortly to make his services available. A story in another Pittsburgh journal two years later mentioned an E. Warner, described as an

"Old Indian Physician" who had practiced in the city for ten years. Appealing to the growing distrust of calomel and other metallic salts, Mr. Warner explained that he relied solely upon botanical remedies.[9] Much more impressive than E. Warner's modest advertisement were the Indian medicine shows. An old American tradition depicted the Noble Red Man as a simple child of nature living in accordance with its laws, supposedly familiar with medicinal herbs, the natural remedies provided by God. The theme of nature's remedy still survives in advertising today, and Indian medicine shows entertained and bilked patrons of state fairs until well into the twentieth century.

From folk remedies to proprietary medicine was a fairly easy step once newspapers and magazines became common and advertising relatively cheap. In the colonial period Widow Read advertised her well-known ointment for the itch, one that cured quickly, had no offensive smell, and was safe to use on even sucking infants. The Widow Read, who by more than a coincidence advertised in the *Pennyslvania Gazette,* was the mother-in-law of Benjamin Franklin. In Charleston certain "Dutch Ladies" publicized their "Choice Cure for the Flux, Fevers, Worms, and bad Stomach, [and] Pains in the Head."[10] The list of men and women in America who decided to capitalize upon a family remedy is a long one—and so is the number of individuals who merely sought easy wealth by exploiting human suffering. In the nineteenth century the state of medicine permitted nearly every proprietary drug manufacturer to secure the endorsement of well-known physicians and clergymen for his product. In most cases the motives for lending their names were purely economic, but the standard medical prescriptions were often of dubious merit, and it was not hard for a physician to convince himself that a particular nostrum was valuable.

The line between the makers of proprietary drugs and outright quacks is always a fine one. If we define a quack as someone simply trying to get rich, then we legitimize many sincere purveyors of preposterous instruments, techniques and remedies. America's first significant quack was Dr. Elisha Perkins of Connecticut who capitalized on the interest in electricity and magnetism late in the eighteenth century by devising his "Patent Metallic Tractor." The Tractor consisted of two rods, one of brass and one of iron, with which the afflicted part was stroked. Although the device brought considerable wealth to Perkins and to his son, Benjamin Douglas Perkins, it may have led to his death. Convinced of the efficacy of his Tractor, Dr. Perkins took it to New York City during a yellow fever epidemic in 1799 only to die of the fever shortly after his arrival. If sincerity be the test, Elisha Perkins was no quack.[11]

One can only wonder which is most amazing— the greed and callousness of the quacks or the gullibility of their clientele. As with proprietary drugs, quackery flourished in direct ratio to the availability of newspapers and magazines. A large percentage of quack advertising related to venereal or, as they were termed, "secret diseases." The notices usually promised an easy, painless cure and not infrequently assured husbands that they could continue to perform their marital duties without any danger to the wife. Quackery and proprietary drugs played a major role in newspaper advertising. A study of one 1858 New England newspaper showed that almost a quarter of the entire paper and half of the advertising space was filled with quack advertisements.[12] The story of quackery and proprietary drugs in America is both comic and tragic, and it has been well told by Professor James Harvey Young in his two books, *The Toadstool Millionaires* and *The Medical Messiahs.*[13] Suffice it to say that, for good or for evil, proprietary medicines supplied a major part of the self-administered drugs, and quackery was rampant in the nineteenth century.

Another major source of self-medication was the multitude of medical works aimed at the large market provided by the lay public. The first few pamphlets and books of this nature in America were based upon a genuine effort to provide useful medical information. For example, the minister-physician, Thomas Thacher, published his *Brief Rule* for dealing with the "Small Pocks, or Measles" in 1677 with the laudable intent of disseminating vital information. The same can be said of Cotton Mather's pamphlet on measles which he published in 1739, and John Wesley's *Primitive Physick,* the first domestic medical book published in America. This latter book was to go through literally dozens of editions in the late eighteenth and early nineteenth centuries.[14]

Both antedating and occurring alongside of the domestic medical works were the commonplace books in which husbands and wives carefully inscribed recipes for soap-making, preserving, tanning, and curing the ailments of man and beast. Beginning in the eighteenth century almanacs began supplying a good deal of medical information along with meteorological data and a jambalaya of miscellaneous facts. Plantation account books, too, provided a wealth of useful information for their owners, and no subject was of more interest to them than the ever-present sicknesses. Since herbals were the mainstay of medicine and were prescribed by every medical handbook, large plantations usually kept a medicinal garden, and they were quite common even on small farms. Newspapers, too, reflected the general concern with health, and purported cures and prescriptions were frequent items in their columns. Throughout the eighteenth and nineteenth centuries many readers faithfully clipped these stories and pasted them into their commonplace books.

By the nineteenth century the publication of domestic medical books was a profitable business, and these publications were a major source for home treatment. A few were openly intended for the lay public, but many of them were ostensibly designed for the medical profession, although it is clear that their authors had a larger readership in mind. The need for clear and explicit general medical works was great. Medical students whose education was derived solely from attending one or two sessions of lectures at an early medical school were scarcely prepared to deal with patients. Most physicians in this early period merely served an apprenticeship with some local physician until they felt qualified to set out on their own. The better apprenticeships lasted two to five years, but the duration was often much shorter. Hence it was a rare beginning physician who did not rely upon a handful of general medical books until he had acquired a good deal of practical experience.

James Ewell's *The Medical Companion, or Family Physician*, which was widely used in the southern states, is typical of domestic medical works. Published in 1807, it was dedicated to President Thomas Jefferson, a dedication which the President graciously acknowledged. In his preface Ewell appealed first to patriotism, declaring that most comparable books treat diseases "existing in very *foreign climates and constitutions,* which must widely differ from ours." Having disposed of his British competition, he declared that his book had been written by a native American who had practiced successfully for years in the southern states. He thought the work would be "exceedingly useful to all, but especially to those who live in the country, or who go to sea, where regular and timely assistance cannot always be obtained." The medical student, too, "whose theoretical knowledge has only prepared him to commence the arduous duties of his profession," would also benefit from it. An important section, he pointed out, was the "Materia Medica" which describes "those precious simples wherewith God has graciously stored our meadows, fields, and woods, for the healing of our diseases, and rendering us happily independent of foreign medicines. . . ."[15]

The chief medical aid in the West was *Gunn's Domestic Medicine, or Poor Man's Friend,* first published in 1807, and written for the average citizen. On his title page, Dr. Gunn proclaimed that his book discusses "in plain langauge, free from doctor's terms, the diseases of men, women, and children" and "contains descriptions of the medical herbs and roots of the United States." The work covered every aspect of medicine, and Gunn confidently assured his readers they need have no qualms about undertaking medicine or surgery. The section on the amputation of arms and legs best illustrates his direct approach. He asserted that the only difficulty is to know when to amputate—a problem, he assured his readers, which even the most skillful surgeons frequently cannot handle. Once the decision had been reached, the rest was simple: "Now to perform this operation requires nothing but firmness and common dexterity, for any man . . . to perform it well." The few essential instruments consisted of a large sharp carving knife, a penknife, a carpenter's tenon, a shoemaker's crooked awl, a pair of slender pincers, and a dozen or more ligatures made of waxed thread or fine twine. With these, plus "a piece of old linen, large enough to cover the end of the stump, spread with simple ointment or lard," adhesive plaster, bandages, a sponge, and some warm water, Dr. Gunn declared: "You are now prepared fully to perform amputation; which I will so plainly explain that any man, unless he be an idiot or an absolute fool, can perform this operation." The first step consisted of laying the patient on a table covered with a blanket "with as many persons as may be necessary to hold him."[16] The rest of the instructions are equally explicit.

A third medical book worth mentioning is Dr. J. Cam Massie's *Treatise on the Eclectic Southern Practice of Medicine* published in 1854.

Aside from the fact that Dr. Massie represents the Eclectic school of medicine, he illustrates the rise of the southern nationalist, or states' rights, medicine. As sectional conflict intensified in the United States, the South closed ranks and literate southerners sought to justify slavery and to demonstrate that the southern way of life was unique. The medical profession was in the forefront of this movement, and a series of articles in southern medical journals began arguing, first, that blacks were anatomically and physiologically different from whites and hence did not react the same way to diseases, and, second, that the climate and environment in the South modified all diseases. In consequence, physicians trained in the North and medical books written by northerners were not to be trusted in dealing with southern disorders.

As an introduction to his work, Dr. Massie printed a letter from a group of Texas physicians pointing out the need for a book "presenting the various modifications which diseases assume in Texas" and urging him to make one available. In response, he conceded the need for such a work and agreed to undertake the task. He did not propose, he informed his correspondents, to write a work which would "dispense with the necessity of calling for professional aid in all cases of importance." Nonetheless, while the book would be "purely scientific," it would at the same time be "composed in that SIMPLE and POPULAR style which renders subjects, however abstruse, comprehensible and even entertaining to the general reader." Thus it would be "a desirable addition to the library of the practitioner, and moreover a valuable aid to every father of a family. . . ."[17] Dr. Massie was clearly aiming for the best of both worlds, professional recognition and mass sales.

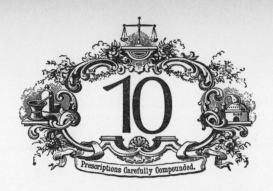

THE BIRTH OF
AMERICAN SURGERY

I N surgery, as in medicine, America made few significant contributions prior to 1860. At the same time it produced a good number of first-rate operators, most of whom practiced in the major medical centers. Surgery in the early nineteenth century was still considered part of the doctor's work, although as the century advanced certain physicians with the talent and inclination began to concentrate upon surgical procedures. In Boston, New York, Philadelphia, and New Orleans, where ample hospital facilities and an abundance of clinical material existed, the level of surgery was equal to, or not far behind, that of the British and Continental centers. American students visiting Paris and London observed the work of such great French surgeons as A.-A.-L.-M. Velpeau and G. Dupuytren, and the English surgeons John Hunter and Astley Cooper, and brought their innovations and techniques back to America. The whole field of medicine was making notable strides these years, and American surgery benefited from both the European developments and its own contributions.

In the opening years of the American nation surgery was still concerned primarily with ulcers and abscesses, gunshot wounds and injuries of all types, the treatment of fractures and hernias, extracting teeth, amputations, and difficult obstetrical cases. The more able operators cut for the stone, removed cancerous breasts and other more obvious cancers, and ligated aneurysms. Pain was inevitable, and operations were performed with little regard for hygienic considerations. If shock and hemorrhage did not kill the patient, his chances of developing septicemia or gangrene were extremely high. Surgery was always a grim and bloody business, and the dread of surgery carried over to the image of the surgeon. Of necessity he had to be a strong, fast, forceful operator, ruthlessly immune to the screams and struggles of the patient. In the early nineteenth century, surgeons took a measure of pride in their stiffened blood- and pus-encrusted coats, proof of their experience in the field. The catlin, scalpel, or other instrument was often wiped on the surgeon's coat sleeve before and after cutting into the patient, and sutures were frequently wrapped around a coat button or occasionally held between the teeth of the operator. Lacking an understanding of germs or infection, surgeons used any convenient method for solving immediate problems. Reporting in the *Boston Medical and Surgical Journal* in 1833, a surgeon described his difficulty in removing a uterine tumor. Having cut away a section of it, "the remaining part could not be separated from the uterus as a distinct substance; still as it was not supplied with nerves, the great part was torn off by the finger nail."[1] Regrettably the patient died.

Operations were invariably public spectacles. Medical students and the public used to fill the surgical amphitheaters when popular surgeons were performing, often crowding around the operating table itself. When surgery was performed at home or in the doctor's office, relatives and friends gathered around to help hold the patient. Considering the many individuals in street clothing jamming into the operating area and the complete lack of hygienic precautions by the surgeons, the wonder is not that so many died in the pre-aseptic era, but that so many survived.

Major surgical procedures were invariably a last resort, and only acute pain, discomfort, and fear could force patients to place themselves in the hands of the surgeon. Some of the prominent surgeons who operated before large crowds required the patient to commit himself to surgery the night before, and then kept him locked in his room until time for the operation. One can only imagine the fears of a candidate for surgery as he listened to the screams coming from the operating room and was hustled from his room into the amphitheater by two husky hospital aids. Here his first glimpse would be the glowing brazier heating up the cauterizing irons and the bloodstained surgeon and his assistants. Small wonder that many were too terrified to move or utter a sound, a few bolted for safety, often with the surgeon and his crew in hot pursuit, and others begged to be allowed to forego the operation. In 1847, Valentine Mott, a famous New York surgeon, commented upon the inevitable relationship between pain and surgery. It was commonplace, he wrote, to see "individuals praying in mercy that we would stop, that we would finish, thus imploring and menacing us, and who would not fail to escape if they were not firmly secured." He concluded that "*to avoid pain* in operation is a chimera that we can no longer pursue in our times."[2] Ironically, even as Dr. Mott was despairing of relieving the agony caused by surgery, the introduction of chemical anesthesia was about to eliminate the grim picture he had drawn.

Before moving to the discovery of anesthesia, it might be well to look briefly at some of the more important American surgeons. Despite what appears to be the relative crudeness of operating conditions and techniques, intelligent and able men were performing innovative and occasionally delicate operations. The results were not always favorable, for few patients would submit to the knife until their diseases were well along. Nonetheless, lives were saved, and the experience gained helped to pave the way for restoring countless other individuals to health in the future. Surgery in America as a specialized area dates back to Dr. Philip Syng Physick (1768–1837), a professor at the University of Pennsylvania who was appointed to the chair of surgery. This position was created in 1805 when the board of trustees voted to abolish the chair of anatomy, midwifery, and surgery and to establish a separate professorship of surgery—the first such position in an American medical school. Physick was no Antyllus or Paré, but he was a first-rate teacher, a fine operator, and the best-known American surgeon of his day. He was famous for his lithotomies (removal of bladder stones), and his success in removing over 1,000 of them from Chief Justice John Marshall firmly established his reputation. He is also known for his introduction of buckskin sutures, and for his improvements in existing surgical instruments. He devised an instrument for tonsillectomies, another for paracentesis or bladder drainage, and a precursor of the stomach pump.[3]

The field of surgery is so broad and includes so many different types of surgical procedures, nearly all of which are in a constant state of modification, that the enthusiastic biographer or regional historian can always claim for his subject or subjects at least one or two so-called "firsts." Hence it is that virtually every prominent American surgeon in the nineteenth century—and many who were not so important—can lay claim to this somewhat dubious distinction. The best surgery in America was done in the areas of bones and joints, the vascular system, and gynecology. A father and son combination, John Warren (1753–1815) and his son, John Collins Warren (1778–1856), are recognized for their work in the excision of bones and joints. The most notable surgeon in the Midwest in this field was Dr. Daniel Brainerd (1812–66), the founder of Rush Medical College in Chicago. He is also credited with the bone drill and with devising new methods for dealing with fractures and deformities.

Insofar as vascular surgery was concerned, aneurysms, caused by syphilis, trauma, or cancer, were the major occasions for surgical intervention, and the operations consisted largely of ligating or tying off major arteries. Here again there are dozens of "firsts," but several of the outstanding surgeons deserve to be mentioned. Dr. Wright Post (1766–1822) of Long Island, New York, was one of the earliest American surgeons to tackle vascular problems. He was probably the first to ligate the femoral artery successfully (1796) and the second American to ligate the external iliac (1814). Valentine Mott (1785–1865) of New York City was a student of the famous English surgeon, Astley Cooper, and, like his mentor, ranks as one of the great pioneers in vascular surgery. In the course of his long career he performed literally dozens of operations involving nearly all of the major arteries. His boldness and daring and the degree of success he obtained are all the more remarkable since most of his operations were performed in the days before anesthesia and antisepsis. A third major figure in vascular surgery was Dr. Warren Stone of New Orleans (1808–72), possibly the top-ranking surgeon in the South. In the 1850s Warren treated two cases of gluteal aneurysms by open incision, a procedure which was both bold and risky at that time. He was also the first to use silver wire for ligating arteries and to insist that the ligature should be tied only tight enough to stop the flow of blood. This latter procedure was designed to avoid the secondary hemorrhage which occurred when the usual ligatures cut their way through the artery. Stone, as with the other surgeons of his day, performed a wide range of surgical operations and was considered an outstanding physician.

A simple listing of names and surgical procedures fails to recreate the milieu in which this work was done, and for this one must turn to contemporary accounts. A newspaper description of an operation performed in New Orleans during the mid-1830s by Dr. Charles A. Luzenberg, a highly skillful surgeon, tells us a good deal about American surgery. Luzenberg had just returned from observing surgery in Europe during 1832 and was putting his newly acquired knowledge to work. The operation consisted of "tying the carotid artery and extirpating a sarcomatous parotid gland, involving the ear and a large portion of the integuments of the cheek and neck" on a sixty-two-year-old male. A number of local physicians witnessed the operation and the patient "sustained the operation, which was unavoidably painful and tedious, with great fortitude."[4] Here we have the classic picture of an American surgeon trained in Europe performing a long and complicated operation without benefit of anesthesia upon a patient for whom surgery was obviously a dire necessity.

A more vivid account was written by a correspondent for *Harper's Weekly* in 1859. At that time New Orleans had two medical schools with a combined enrollment of over 600 students, and the surgical amphitheater in the Charity Hospital was always crowded when a popular professor was operating. The journalist wrote:

One of the most exciting spectacles to be witnessed in the institution [Charity] is seen when fifty or a hundred students crowd the couch of some patient who is about to undergo an important surgical operation. The trembling expectancy of the terrified subject, the nervous pallor of the medical tyros, who are about to see a man's leg or arm whipped off for the first time; the careless nonchalance of the hospital habitues; the giant form of that veteran man of the knife, Dr. Stone, as with cuffs thrown back, eye all ablaze, his lips firmly clenched, he prepares to make the adroit thrust; the quick prefatory whirl of the well-grasped blade; the sudden flash of polished steel; the dull, muffled sound of the yielding flesh, the spirt [sic] of blood, the scrape of the keen edge upon the solid bone, the sharp cry of the patient, followed by the heavy moan of pain—these are the outlines of a picture that thrills and terrifies the uninitiated beholder.[5]

Stone, a powerfully built individual, possessed the physical strength, audacity, and dexterity which were so essential to a surgeon, and he may well stand as a symbol for surgery in the first half of the nineteenth century.

OBSTETRICS AND GYNECOLOGY

The operative field in which America made its greatest contribution was obstetrics and gynecology. Unlike developments in general surgery, which were associated with hospitals and medical centers, the innovations in this field were made by bold, resolute individuals impelled by circumstances to make grave decisions. Nearly all of them practiced in relative isolation—either on the frontier or in rural areas. It is possible that their isolation was an advantage, since they were less likely to have been deterred by traditional beliefs as to what was and was not possible or to have been restrained by the advice of older, more experienced, and more cautious heads. Yet the men who made the greatest contributions were in no sense apprentice-trained empirics with little knowledge of medicine. As will be seen, both Ephraim McDowell and J. Marion Sims received excellent medical training for their day, McDowell in America and Great Britain and Sims in the United States.

Although surgical invasion of the peritoneal cavity was considered a virtual death warrant for the patient, American physicians successfully ventured into this area quite early. Dr. John Bard of

New Jersey reported three cases of laparotomies for extrauterine pregnancy in 1759, and this same operation was performed by Dr. Charles McKnight of New York in 1790. William Baynham of Virginia also operated for extrauterine pregnancy in 1791 and 1799.[6] While these operations speak well for the courage and ability of American surgeons, they were in no sense landmarks—the making of gynecological history was left for Ephraim McDowell.

Ephraim McDowell (1771–1830) was born in Virginia, but moved with his family to Kentucky in 1784 and settled in the small frontier town of Danville. After finishing secondary school, Ephraim elected to study medicine, first under the preceptorship of Dr. Alexander Humphreys, and later by attending lectures at the University of Edinburgh. While at the University during 1793–94, he was influenced by one of the outstanding professors, Dr. John Bell. Returning in 1795 to Danville, McDowell quickly established his reputation as the best surgeon west of Philadelphia, but his opportunity to gain fame did not come until 1809 when he was called as a consultant by two physicians attending a patient whom they thought was slow in delivering twins.

According to McDowell's own account, on examining the patient he discovered immediately that she had a large tumor. He explained the situation, warning her that four of the best surgeons in England and Scotland had asserted that the danger from peritoneal inflammation was so great "that opening the abdomen to extract the tumor was inevitable death." If she was prepared to die and was willing to come to Danville, he would remove the tumor. The patient, Mrs. Jane Todd Crawford, demonstrating even greater courage than her surgeon, unhesitatingly made the sixty-mile journey on horseback in the middle of winter, resting the enormous tumor on the pommel of the saddle. With a minimum of preparation and assisted by his nephew, who had studied medicine in Philadelphia, and a young apprentice, McDowell began the operation. While the patient lay on a table reciting psalms, the abdomen was laid open, the tube ligated, and the diseased ovary, weighing almost twenty pounds, was removed. As soon as the incision was made, the intestines fell out on the table, remaining there for about thirty minutes. It was Christmas Day, McDowell wrote, and "they became so cold that I thought proper to bathe them in tepid water previous to my replacement." He then pushed the intestines back into the abdomen, sutured the incision, and put the patient to bed. Five days later, on looking in on the patient, he found Mrs. Crawford making up her own bed. Twenty-five days after the operation, she drove home, to live for another thirty-one years.

In 1813 and 1816 he again successfully removed ovarian cysts. Following the third operation, he published an account of the three cases, but his article encountered disbelief and was dismissed. In 1819 he described two more successful cases, and this time his work began to achieve some notice. It was not, however, until a letter he had sent to Dr. John Bell in 1817 was finally published in the *Edinburgh Medical and Surgical Journal* in 1824 that McDowell finally achieved the recognition he deserved. By the end of his career, he had performed the ovariotomy twelve or thirteen times with the loss of only one patient—a remarkable record for that date. In 1830 he suffered an attack of what was called inflammatory fever. The onset was characterized by an acute attack of pain and nausea followed by fever. Ironically, it is not unlikely that this pioneer in abdominal surgery died of acute appendicitis.[7]

A fascinating sequel to McDowell's success, and one which may have been far more typical of early nineteenth-century surgery, was the first ovariotomy attempted in Tennessee. In 1818 Dr. James Overton diagnosed a case of ovarian tumor and gained the patient's consent to operate. Delighted at the opportunity to demonstrate his skill, Dr. Overton decided to operate on a pillowed table out in the open in front of the patient's home. In full view of a large crowd, he made his incision, exposing the smooth surface of an unusually large tumor. Before he could make a further incision, some irregular movements in the tumor caused him and his assistant to quickly close the abdomen. A few days later the patient gave birth to a healthy child. Although the case cost Dr. Overton his medical career, he apparently did not lose his sense of humor. He subsequently informed a colleague: "I did not retire from the practice of medicine, I was victorious in defeat. The practice retired from me and left me in triumphant possession of the field."[8]

The second American to achieve international fame in the area of gynecology and obstetrics was another small-town southern practitioner, J. Marion Sims (1813–83). Sims's father was a minor local official in Lancaster County, South Carolina who had visions of his son becoming a lawyer. But Marion had decided to enter medicine and his father, in reluctantly agreeing, made a most revealing comment upon the status of the medical profession: "Well, I suppose I can not control you; but it is a profession for which I have the utmost contempt. There is no science in it. There is no honor to be achieved in it; no reputation to be made. . . ." He then concluded: "and to think that *my* son should be going around from house to house through this country, with a box of pills in one hand and a squirt in the other . . . is a thought I never supposed I should have to contemplate."[9]

The story of Sims's medical education has already been recounted, a brief stint as an apprentice, a session as a student at the Charleston Medical School, and another one at the Jefferson Medical College in Philadelphia. Upon graduation from the latter on March 1, 1835, Sims felt absolutely incompetent to start practice, and consequently enrolled in a month's course of private lectures offered by one of the professors. The lectures turned out to be on the subject of regional and surgical anatomy. Sims later wrote that he knew a great deal about dissection but absolutely nothing about the practice of medicine. After a shaky start, he managed to acquire some reputation in the little town of Mt. Meigs, Alabama. Just as he was becoming well established and his practice was flourishing, a severe attack of malaria forced him to move to Montgomery, the capitol of the state. Here he quickly earned a fine reputation as a physician and an even better one as a surgeon. Discovering he had an unusual aptitude for surgery, he began concentrating in this area, and successfully treated a wide variety of conditions, including clubfoot, strabismus, and harelip.

After about ten years of practice, he was called in consultation to help with a seventeen-year-old slave girl who had been in labor for seventy-two hours. The child's head was impacted in the pelvis, and, although Sims successfully delivered the child with forceps, so much damage was done that the patient, named Anarcha, was left with complete urinary and rectal incontinence. Touched by her tragic condition, he went home and explored the literature, only to find that the condition was considered hopeless. Shortly thereafter he encountered two similar cases of vesicovaginal fistula in slave women, and in both instances told their masters he could do nothing. While he was still pondering about these unfortunate women, he was summoned to attend a large white woman who had fallen from a pony and suffered a retroversion of the uterus. In trying to correct the situation, he placed the patient on her knees and elbows. While trying to push the uterus into place manually, he turned his hand in the vagina, and the uterus suddenly disappeared from his touch. The patient expressed immediate relief, but as she lay down, there was a sudden sound caused by the passage of air. The patient was embarrassed, but Sims quickly realized what had happened. In moving his hand, he had allowed air to enter the vagina, and the normal atmospheric pressure had pushed the uterus back into position.

He realized that if he could place one of his vesicovaginal patients in a knee-elbow position, dilate her vagina with normal air pressure, and use some type of speculum, it would be possible to see the extent of the damage and to devise means for correcting it. One of the patients was still in Sims's small eight-bed clinic waiting to be sent home. Calling on his two medical students to help him, Sims placed her in position and tried the experiment. "Introducing the bent handle of a spoon," he wrote, "I saw everything, as no man had ever seen before. The fistula was as plain as the nose on a man's face."

For the next four years, Sims was to devote most of his energy, effort, and income to a long series of operations on slave women suffering with this condition. The first almost led to the death of the patient, but Sims persisted, gradually gaining more and more experience. Finally, after four years of experimentation, he operated for the thirtieth time on Anarcha, and successfully closed the fistula. Sims then operated on the other two women and quickly restored them to health, demonstrating conclusively that he had devised an effective method for treating this horrible condition. In order to win his victory during the four-year battle, Sims had had to discover the knee-elbow (Sims's) position, devise a special curved speculum (Sims's speculum), make a new catheter to keep the bladder empty while the fistula was healing, and, finally, learn to avoid sepsis by the use of silver sutures. In the process he had to develop new techniques and improve his own skill as a surgeon.[10]

Dr. Sims was a man of perseverance, dedication, and remarkable ingenuity, and he deserves great credit. In his zeal to solve this particular medical problem, he sacrificed a good part of his medical practice, maintained six or seven stricken women slaves at his own cost, and devoted several years to the project. His neglect of private practice caused problems with his family, but he resolutely continued along his chosen course. Note, however, that, had Sims not lived in the South where slaves were available, his "experiments" would not have been possible. These repeated operations were performed for the large part without anesthesia and must have caused considerable suffering. It is highly unlikely that any surgeon, northern or southern, would have experimented on white women in such a way, nor that the patients themselves would have submitted to such a lengthy ordeal— one covering several years.

Sims's major breakthrough in gynecology did not bring him immediate fame. A few weeks after his first successful operation, a severe attack of diarrhea prostrated him, and the disorder continued to flare up. Despairing of a cure and feeling his life was in danger from the climate, he once again broke up his home, and in 1852, moved his family to New York City. About this same time, convinced that he was dying from the disease, he published an account of his operation in the *American Journal of Medical Sciences.* In ill health and with only limited funds, Sims had difficulty establishing his practice in New York City. His career opened up once again when in 1855, with the aid of friends, he established the Women's Hospital of the State of New York. As head physician, he was given ample opportunity to operate and soon earned an outstanding rating as a surgeon and gynecologist.

The rest of Sims's career was a happy and productive one. The honors he received in Europe, where he lived during the Civil War, strengthened his position in America, and henceforth he divided his time between the two continents. While the operative procedure for vesicovaginal fistulas was his major contribution, in later years he devised methods for amputating the cervix uteri, clearly described the symptom complex of vaginitis, was a pioneer in gall bladder surgery, and published a classic work on the problems of abdominal surgery.

THE CESAREAN SECTION

The cesarean section, as its name implies, has a long history, but it was still a relatively rare operation until well into the nineteenth century. During the medieval period it was occasionally used as a postmortem method for saving the child. The idea of operating on the live mother was revived in the seventeenth century, although only the boldest and most skillfull of operators were willing to attempt it. In the late eighteenth century a bitter quarrel developed between Jean Louis Baudelocque, the elder, inventor of the pelvimeter and the father of obstetric pelvimetry, and the supporters of the symphyseotomy, an operation which consisted of enlarging the diameter of the pelvis by dividing the cartilage connecting the pelvic bones. The latter was, and still is, a complicated and dangerous operation. Fortunately a number of successful cesarean sections by French surgeons during this period swung the tide in favor of the cesarean.

While all this seems a little far removed from American medicine, these events had a direct bearing on developments in early nineteenth-century Louisiana, where French-trained surgeons performed a series of cesarean sections. The man who introduced this operation into Louisiana was Francois Marie Prévost (1771–1842), who was born in France and studied medicine in Paris during the Revolution. His student days in Paris coincided with the clash between Baudelocque, who was elected professor and chief surgeon-accoucheur at the Maternité in 1794, and his rivals, and Prévost may have heard the arguments put forward as to the relative merits of the two obstetrical procedures. We know little of Prévost's earliest medical career but by 1800 he was serving as an Officer de Santé in Haiti. The great slave insurrection there caused him to flee to Louisiana, where he settled near Donaldsonville. Although a small town in rural Ascension Parish, Donaldsonville had several French surgeons, all of whom had been trained in France, and at least two had served for many years in Napoleon's armies. Hence Prévost was familiar with contemporary developments in medicine and surgery and had the encouragement of able colleagues.

Reflecting inadequate diet and other conditions, cases of pelvic deformity were not uncommon in the nineteenth century, and the slave population in the South was particularly affected. While midwives handled most normal obstetrical cases, in difficult deliveries physicians and surgeons were usually called in, and Prévost, along with his colleagues, must have seen many young mothers labor in suffering and agony for days before succumbing to pain and exhaustion. Sometime between 1820 and 1825 Prévost was faced with the decision of what to do with one of these slave women who was unable to have a normal delivery. We might well wonder how many of these cases he had already seen and what it was that led him on this occasion to attempt the radical step of performing a cesarean section. Whatever the case, he performed the operation and saved both mother and child. When the mother became pregnant once more, Prévost again delivered the child by a cesarean section. In 1825 he performed a third cesarean section upon another slave, but on this occasion, although he saved the child, the mother died.

It is possible that some other Louisiana surgeon may have preceded Prévost in delivering a child by cesarean section. Early in 1824 a St. Franciscille, Louisiana, newspaper published a medical fee bill signed by fifteen physicians and surgeons, all of whose names indicate a British origin. The lengthy fee bill included some 160 items. Of the several fees relating to parturition, the most expensive one was simply listed as "Cesarean."[11] Presumably at least some of these surgeons were prepared to perform a cesarean section if necessary. Yet physicians and surgeons in those days frequently sought to build their reputations by offering to do far more than they intended, and there is no evidence that the cesarean section was ever performed in the St. Francisville area.

Stimulated by Prévost's success, a number of cesarean sections were performed in Louisiana in the ensuing years. A compilation of all such surgical procedures in the United States between 1822 and 1877 made by Dr. Robert P. Harris showed a total of 79. Of these 15 were performed in Louisiana between 1822 and 1861. Both Dr. Harris, who published his findings in 1878, and Dr. Rudolph Matas, who confirmed them over sixty years later, commented on the relatively high degree of success obtained by Louisiana physicians. The 15 operations resulted in saving 11 mothers and 8 children—a high recovery rate which is all the more surprising since the evidence indicates that none of these early operators practiced uterine suture. As Dr. Matas wrote, they followed the traditional practice and left the healing of the uterine incision to the unaided "efforts of Nature."[12]

It is worth noting that all of the cesarean sections in Louisiana were performed on slave women. The usual practice in cases where the pelvis was deformed or too small was to resort to craniotomy, cutting up the head of the fetus in order to facilitate delivery. The fear of abdominal incisions was so great that it was generally considered much safer to destroy the child than sacrifice the life of the mother. The high risk which was involved in any abdominal surgery makes it more than a coincidence that so many of these early patients were slaves, and clearly indicates that southern surgeons and physicians were far more willing to try new procedures upon slaves than upon other women.

The second American physician to perform a cesarean section was Dr. John Lambert Richmond. Richmond, a typical product of the West, had worked at various jobs before becoming a Baptist minister and then a janitor in the Medical College of Ohio. Taking advantage of the opportunity, he enrolled in the school and was graduated as a physician. With this degree, he was, like the colonial preachers of old, able to minister to both the physical and spiritual wants of his congregation. While preaching in a small town across the river from Cincinnati in April of 1827, he learned that a woman across the river had been in labor for thirty hours and was about to die from repeated convulsions. The night was stormy and windy, but he crossed the river, examined the patient, a large black woman pregnant with her first child, and decided to take the baby by cesarean section. In his report on the operation three years later he stated that he began operating at one o'clock at night with "only a case of common pocket instruments. . . ." The wind was blowing directly through the unchinked walls of the log cabin so that his assistants had to hold up blankets to stop the drafts from blowing out the candles. Despite these handicaps, he was able to save both mother and child.[13]

The circumstances which led Prévost and Richmond to resort to a cesarean section must have recurred many times on the American frontier. One can only wonder how many other American physicians confronted with similar emergency obstetrical situations dealt with the crisis in this fashion. Each of the early operators waited several years before informing his colleagues or publishing a report of his operation or operations. America was primarily rural, and a good part of it was still frontier. Moreover, the isolation and the relatively low educational standards among American doctors were scarcely conducive to their reporting case histories. In any event, by 1830 the American medical profession was beginning to learn that the cesarean section could be performed successfully. Yet while the work of Prévost and Richmond may have inaugurated a new era for the cesarean section, the operation remained a rarity until well past the Civil War. Most physicians, when faced with the decision, preferred the safer course of craniotomy.

WILLIAM BEAUMONT AND
THE PHYSIOLOGY OF DIGESTION

In terms of international recognition as an original contributor to medical science, the American who ranked second to J. Marion Sims in the nineteenth century was an obscure army surgeon who, when a remarkable opportunity was presented to him, had the initiative and intelligence to seize upon it. William Beaumont (1785–1853) was born in Connecticut, acquired a medical education through an apprenticeship, and, after gaining a medical license in Vermont, enlisted as a surgeon in the army in 1812. After serving honorably during the War of 1812, he returned to private practice and business until 1819 when a former comrade persuaded him to reenlist. Beaumont was ordered to Fort Michilimackinac on an island between Lake Huron and Lake Michigan.

In June 1822 Beaumont was summoned to attend a French-Canadian trapper who had been hit in the side by an accidental shotgun blast at close range. The victim, Alexis St. Martin, was horribly mangled, his chest was torn open; the left lower lung, the diaphragm, and the stomach badly lacerated; and the flesh burned to a crisp. Mixed in with blood, bone splinters, lead shot, wadding, and bits of clothing were the contents of the stomach. Serious stomach wounds were invariably considered fatal, and to Beaumont the case was clearly hopeless. Nonetheless, he cleaned and dressed the wound as best he could and tried to make the patient comfortable. Almost miraculously, St. Martin survived, but his recovery was long and slow. After a year in the military hospital the wound was still open and a gastric fistula refused to close. The military authorities felt they had done enough for him and decided to ship him back to Canada, his native country. Beaumont, realizing that the journey would probably be fatal for a man in St. Martin's condition, remonstrated, and when this failed he took the man into his own home. Here for two years he nursed and cared for his patient, who slowly gained strength. Although the wound healed, St. Martin was left with a permanent gastric fistula.

The nature of digestion at that time was still only vaguely understood. The seventeenth century had produced two schools of thought about it. One, the iatrophysical group, argued that digestion was a mechanical process in which the churning action of the stomach broke down the food. Another, the iatrochemical school, maintained that the process was essentially a chemical one. By the eighteenth century it was recognized that the stomach produced some type of fluid which prevented fermentation and which was capable of dissolving food. In the early nineteenth century experimental physiologists were beginning to feed samples to animals and, after a certain time, to kill and dissect them to see what had happened to the food. In other experiments animals were forced or induced to swallow sponges on a string in order to retrieve some of the gastric juice. Beaumont saw that the gastric fistula gave him easy access to St. Martin's stomach, and he realized that here was an opportunity to determine precisely how the stomach functioned.

The fistula opened up just below the left nipple, making it possible for Beaumont to look directly into the stomach. In giving St. Martin the usual purges which were basic to nearly all medical treatment, Beaumont wrote that he gave them "as never medicine was before administered to man since the creation of the world—to wit, by pouring it through the ribs at the puncture of the stomach." He found that he could pour water directly into the stomach with a funnel or spoon in food and then draw the contents of the stomach back out with a syphon. He began experimenting with pieces of meat and other food items which he would tie on a string and suspend in the stomach for varying time periods. He was thus able to ascertain precisely how long it took to digest a particular food item and to ascertain what the gastric juice did to each of them.[14] St. Martin obviously derived little intellectual pleasure from the experiments, and understandably he was a most unenthusiastic human guinea pig. He constantly objected to the experiments and occasionally disappeared. In 1825 he apparently disappeared for good, leaving Beaumont with a great many questions still unanswered.

Almost four years later Beaumont learned that St. Martin had returned to Canada and married. Even though he now had two children, Beaumont persuaded him to return, paying all transportation costs and other expenses. The experiments were renewed in August 1829 and continued to the spring of 1831. By this time St. Martin had two more children, and Beaumont allowed St. Martin and his family to go home on condition that they would return when asked. In the fall of 1832 St. Martin reported back to Beaumont, who signed him to a contract. Early in 1834 family pressure and a strong personal distaste for his role caused St. Martin to return to Canada and nothing could be done to persuade him to return to his role as a human guinea pig. The experiments apparently did him no harm since he lived to the age of eighty-three, outliving Beaumont by well over twenty years.

By the time St. Martin returned to Canada for good, Beaumont had completed his major research, and although he would have liked to continue the experiments, he had acquired enough knowledge to give a fundamental explanation of the digestive process. He had been in contact with Dr. Robley Dunglison of the University of Virginia, who made some valuable suggestions. Dunglison, along with a colleague, also analyzed a sample of gastric juice and identified it as free hydrochloric acid. The two men also suggested the presence of a second digestive factor, which was subsequently identified as pepsin. In 1833 Beaumont published his classic work, *Experiments and Observations on the Gastric Juice and the Physiology of Digestion*, which laid the basis for our present understanding of the gastric process.[15]

Beaumont began by surveying the existing knowledge of digestion and then gave a detailed account of some 238 experiments. He described accurately the appearance of the mucous membrane, both normal and pathologic, noted the movements of the stomach through the digestive process, showed that the gastric juice is secreted only when food is present and that it contained free hydrochloric acid. His remarkable experiments on the effects of gastric juice upon various foods helped lay the basis for future dietetic studies. The work was hailed in scientific circles and received good reviews, although the book was privately printed and the author received no financial benefit. Only 1,000 copies were printed, and Beaumont had difficulty in disposing of them. A subsequent German edition and one published in England showed that European scientists appreciated his findings, but these editions, too, provided no financial assistance to enable Beaumont to continue his research.[16]

Beaumont had been fortunate in an earlier army appointment since Surgeon General Lovell had given him every assistance with his research. This happy state of affairs ended in 1836 when Lovell died and was replaced by Colonel Thomas Lawson. Lawson, a surgeon general with a long and undistinguished career, virtually forced Beaumont out of the army in 1839.

THE DISCOVERY OF ANESTHESIA

The greatest boon America has given medicine was chemical anesthesia, and its discovery clearly fits within the American empirical tradition. From earliest days mankind had sought the means to alleviate pain, and in the process had learned about a great many analgesics. Willow bark, which contains salicin acid, and a great many other herbals were widely used for this purpose, and opium and alcohol were in common use by the early nineteenth century. Traveling quacks and dentists knew the value of distracting the patient's mind from what was happening to him, and on a more scientific basis a few dentists and surgeons were experimenting with hypnotism, a popular fad in this period. Hypnosis—or mesmerism, as it was also called—was still in its infancy, and required amenable patients and time and effort on the part of the physician or surgeon. Had chemical anesthesia not been introduced for a few more years, it is quite possible that the history of hypnotism might have been quite different. As it was, hypnotism was pushed into the background.

Inventions and discoveries usually follow when two conditions exist: one, the proper technology, and two, a significant demand. On this basis anesthesia should have appeared somewhere around the beginning of the century. By 1800 two of the three basic chemical anesthetic agents had been known for many years. Although not given its present name until the eighteenth century, ether was discovered by Paracelsus in the sixteenth century, and, under the name of "sweet vitriol," may go back as far as the thirteenth century. The second agent, nitrous oxide, was discovered by Joseph Priestly in 1772. In the 1790s a series of experiments with these gases showed that both of them had the potential for relieving pain during surgery. The famous chemist Humphrey Davy began experimenting with nitrous oxide as a young surgeon's assistant, and in 1800 he published his classic work, *Researches, Chemical and Philosophical; Chiefly concerning Nitrous Oxide.* . . . In it he described how he had relieved the pain caused by an erupting wisdom tooth through inhaling nitrous oxide. Later on he wrote that, since the gas "appears capable of destroying physical pain, it may probably be used with advantage during surgical operations in which no great effusion of blood takes place." A few years after this, one of Davy's students, Michael Faraday, made a number of experiments with sulfuric ether and suggested that it, too, might be used to ease the pain of surgery.[17]

The third of the anesthetic agents was discovered by an American chemist, physician, and farmer, Samuel Guthrie (1782–1848). Guthrie learned his medicine through an apprenticeship with his father and through two terms of lectures, one at the College of Physicians and Surgeons in New York City in 1810–11 and another one at the University of Pennsylvania in 1815. He settled in New York, spending most of his life in Sacketts Harbor, at that time a frontier section in the northern part of the state. He was one of those rare individuals with an inventive and practical mind. Intrigued by chemistry, he dabbled in many areas, and in the process of his experiments he produced what he called "chloric ether" or chloroform. Shortly thereafter the substance was discovered independently in both Germany and France.

By 1831, then, there were three chemicals available which were suitable for anesthesia; in effect, the technological problem had been solved. At the same time, the demands for some means to relieve pain were steadily increasing. Developments in gross and pathological anatomy and the rise of localism in medicine were encouraging surgeons to operate more frequently and to perform longer and more complicated surgery. As surgeons became more venturesome, they encountered a greater reluctance by patients to face the almost unendurable agony of a long operation. Moreover, a patient struggling and writhing in pain was scarcely a suitable subject for delicate surgical excision or repair. Hence surgeons were casting about in search of means to ease the dreadful agony caused by the knife and the cauterizing iron. At the same time, surgery traditionally had been associated with pain and suffering, and any surgeon who did not quickly adapt himself to it could scarcely expect to remain in the profession. In consequence the older, experienced surgeons, as indicated by an earlier quotation from Valentine Mott, accepted it as inevitable.

While the surgical patients often submitted to the knife under the threat of death— *i.e.*, either die in pain from their disease or take a chance that the surgeon could effect a cure— the dentists were in an entirely different position. Other than babies who were often assumed to have died from "teething," nobody was believed to die from toothache. If one bore the ache long enough, the tooth would eventually rot out, and the problem would be solved. The gums and teeth are extremely sensitive, and as dentists made the transition from itinerant tooth-pullers to a professional class, the need to ease pain was even more important than in surgery. The aching tooth could be borne, whereas the spreading cancer, the growing pulsating aneurysm, and the urinary calculi which blocked the urethra forced their victims to turn to the surgeon. An equally important consideration was that the dentist hoped to see his patient many times, whereas the surgeon rarely expected to see his patient again.

In the eighteenth century France and England held leadership in dentistry, but by the nineteenth American technical skill and mechanical ingenuity enabled the United States to forge ahead. At first training was largely empirical or gained through an apprenticeship, and it was not until 1825 that the first formal lectures in dentistry were offered in the medical school of the University of Baltimore by Professor Horace H. Hayden. In 1840 Hayden joined with several other dentists to organize the first American dental school, the Baltimore College of Dental Surgery. This same year saw the establishment of the American Society of Dental Surgeons, the first attempt to create a national professional organization. By more than a coincidence it was about this time that a number of dentists began experimenting with methods to eliminate or reduce the pain during dental surgery.[18]

Precisely at the time when surgeons and dentists were becoming more concerned over the problem of pain, nitrous oxide and ether were becoming fairly easy to obtain, and one of the fads which swept the country in the second quarter of the century was the so-called "laughing gas" parties. Medical and chemistry students first began inhaling ether or nitrous oxide at social gatherings, and as news of their euphoric effects spread "laughing gas" parties or "ether frolics" became quite popular among middle- and upper-class groups. On many occasions individuals hurt themselves stumbling around under the influence of one of the gases and were not aware of it until the effects wore off. Considering how frequently this fact was reported, it is surprising that it took so long to apply this insight to the relief of surgical patients.

Beginning in the early 1840s a number of dentists and at least one surgeon began experimenting with ether and nitrous oxide. As with many advances, it is impossible to give exclusive credit to any one individual for discovering anesthesia. Possibly the first man to administer ether as an anesthetic was William E. Clarke. In January 1842 he gave ether to a patient while her tooth was being extracted by a dentist, Dr. Elijah Pope.[19] Unfortunately, neither Clarke nor Pope realized the significance of what they had done, and so they receive only brief mention by historians.

Without question the first individual to use ether as a surgical anesthetic was Dr. Crawford W. Long (1815–78) of Jefferson, Georgia. Long was a relatively well-educated physician. He had graduated with honor from Franklin Academy, the forerunner of the University of Georgia, had attended the Medical Department of the Transylvania University in Lexington, Kentucky, and then transferred to the University of Pennsylvania, where he took his medical degree in 1839. Following this he spent some eighteen months "walking the hospitals" in New York City. He returned to Georgia in 1841 and settled in the small town of Jefferson. As a medical student he had participated in the ether and "laughing gas" parties and, stimulated by the appearance of an itinerant showman, introduced ether parties to the city of Jefferson. During these parties, Long observed how individuals became insensitive to pain while under the influence of the gas, and he decided to apply this observation to his surgical practice. On March 30, 1842, he removed a small wen or tumor from the neck of one James Venable while the patient was under the influence of ether. A month or two later he excised a second tumor from Venable's neck under similar circumstances. In July of this same year he amputated the toe of a young black boy using the same painless method. In the next three years he performed three more operations using ether as an anesthetic.

Unfortunately for Dr. Long's fame as an innovator, he did not report any of his operations until 1849, over three years after the first public demonstration of surgical anesthesia by Morton and Warren. As a well-educated physician, Long should have realized the significance of his discovery. On the other hand, he lived in a relatively isolated area, and he may well have felt that reports of minor surgery performed by a rural physician would receive little credence in more sophisticated medical circles. As a physician in a sparsely settled area, his opportunities to perform surgery were limited, and he may have been waiting to compile more evidence before publicizing his work. It seems reasonably clear that he used ether for anesthetic purposes at least six times prior to Morton's demonstration in 1846. With this much experience, why he did not report his work to one of the medical journals is difficult to say, but this failure to do so places him in a category with Clarke and Pope.[20]

The next character in what was to become a tragic quest for the credit of discovering anesthesia was Dr. Horace Wells, a leading dentist in Hartford, Connecticut. Wells may have become interested in the effects of nitrous oxide as early as 1840, but he was stirred to action on witnessing a demonstration in December 1844 by a popular lecturer, Gardner Q. Colton. Wells noted that a member of the audience who volunteered to take the gas injured his leg while jumping around, yet showed no evidence of having felt pain. Wells, who needed one of his own teeth extracted, talked to Colton after the performance and asked about the possibility of using gas in the operation. The upshot was that Colton came to Wells's office and administered nitrous oxide while an associate of Wells's, Dr. John M. Riggs, removed the molar. Wells was delighted that he felt no pain and had Colton show him how to manufacture and administer the gas. After successfully using anesthesia to extract several teeth, early in 1845 Wells went to Boston and through his former partner, Dr. William Thomas

Green Morton, was given an opportunity to demonstrate his method before Dr. John C. Warren's medical class. For one reason or another, the patient yelled when the tooth was extracted, and the medical students booed and hissed, causing Wells to retire in mortification. Wells returned to Hartford where he continued to experiment with gas in his dental practice.

The third major figure in the anesthesia controversy was the aforementioned Dr. William Thomas Green Morton (1819–68), Wells's friend and former partner. As a student at the Harvard Medical School, Wells had had as his preceptor Dr. Charles A. Jackson, a physician, chemist, and geologist. Jackson, an intelligent and controversial figure, had recommended to Morton in 1844 that he might reduce the pain from dental work by applying drops of sulfuric ether to the gums. The method was of some benefit, and Morton then turned to the use of ether as an inhalant. When he administered the gas to two of his dental assistants, they became too excited for him to work on them. He again consulted Jackson, who recommended that he use pure sulfuric ether. After experimenting on himself, Morton was eager to try ether on a dental patient. On September 1846 he painlessly extracted an ulcerated tooth from a patient using sulfuric ether. Wisely, he saw to it that an account was published in the following day's newspaper.

Convinced that he had found the answer to surgery without pain, Morton contacted Dr. John C. Warren, Boston's foremost surgeon, to arrange for a demonstration. Suffice it to say, arrangements were made for Morton to test his anesthetic on a young man, Gilbert Abbot, who was to have a tumor removed from the left side of his neck. On October 16, 1846, Dr. Warren, with Morton serving as the anesthetist, gave the first successful public demonstration of surgical anesthesia. The following day Morton again successfully anesthetized a surgical patient, proving that his initial success was no accident. In the meantime the medical community around Boston was searching for a name for the condition produced by "Letheon," Morton's name for the gas. The answer was supplied by Dr. Oliver Wendell Homes, who wrote to Morton in November suggesting that the name of the condition be called "anaesthesia" and that the adjective be "anaesthetic."

News of Morton's discovery spread rapidly, and, with a few minor exceptions, it was generally hailed as a major advance.

Before the end of 1846 ether had been administered in both Paris and London, and within a year its use had spread throughout the entire United States. In November 1847 a famous British physician, Dr. James Young Simpson, introduced chloroform into his obstetrical practice. Since chloroform was easier to handle, it quickly became the anesthetic agent of choice throughout the United States. While a few objections were raised to surgical anesthesia, it was the use of anesthesia for obstetrics which aroused the greatest complaints in America and England. As might be expected, fundamentalist ministers constantly sniped at this interference with God's design, but the real opposition came from within the ranks of the medical profession. Dr. Charles D. Meigs, a prominent Philadelphia obstetrician, was one of those leading the attack against obstetrical anesthesia. The pains of childbirth, he wrote, were part "of those natural and physiological forces that the Divinity has ordained us to enjoy or suffer." He argued that the nature of labor pains had been exaggerated and cheerfully stated that few women "lose their health or their lives in labor. . . ." He could not help feeling astonished at reading about cases of midwifery that had "been treated during the profound *Drunkenness* of etherization." "To be insensible from whisky, and gin, and brandy, and wine, and beer, and ether, and chloroform," he declared firmly, "is to be what in the world is called Dead-drunk."[21]

Whatever physicians and ministers may have felt about it, parturient women had no doubts, and since patient demand helps shape medical practice anesthesia swept the field. In England Queen Victoria placed the stamp of approval upon it in 1853 by taking chloroform during the birth of her eighth child, but in England and America popular demand was the major factor. The reaction of parturient women to the use of chloroform was the subject of a paper read before the Massachusetts Medical Society in 1856. The author, Dr. John G. Metcalf, stated, "in every case, if I am called to a succeeding labor, the first question has invariably been, 'Have you brought the chloroform?'" Three years later a Philadelphia physician expressed a similar view, declaring that he had never found "a single instance where a patient would consent to its discontinuance after commencing its inhalations." The universal cry, he added, "has been, 'give me more!'"[22]

The immediate and widespread recognition accorded the

introduction of anesthesia should have brought prestige and rewards to those who pioneered in it. Alas, such was not the case. Within a few months a violent quarrel broke out among the various claimants to the honor of having discovered it, one which contributed to the tragic deaths of at least three of them. Up to this point three major figures have been discussed: Crawford W. Long, Horace Wells, and Samuel T. G. Morton. The fourth individual to assert priority in discovering anesthesia was Charles Thomas Jackson (1805–80), the Harvard professor who suggested the use of ether to Morton. Shortly after Morton's demonstration Jackson wrote to the French Academy of Sciences claiming full credit for discovering anesthesia, and early in March 1847 he made a similar statement before the American Academy of Arts and Sciences. Morton indignantly responded, and the clash between the two men widened into a four-way battle when Morton, having gained nothing from his patent, pressured the United States Congress to give him a suitable reward. Bills were introduced into Congress to award $100,000 to the discoverer of anesthesia. This brought Horace Wells into the fray, and in 1854 Senator W. C. Dawson of Georgia introduced the name of Crawford Long. The debates over the claims and counterclaims of these four individuals continued in Congress until 1863 when the unresolved issue was finally dropped.

Wells, the most unfortunate of the four claimants, was barely embroiled in the controversy before he committed suicide. After seeking to prove his pioneering work, he opened an office in New York. However, while experimenting with chloroform, he was arrested in January 1848 while under its influence and placed in prison. Embarrassed, ashamed, and depressed, Wells committed suicide by cutting his thigh with a razor. Morton continued his legal battle, much of it against Jackson, for another twenty years, impoverishing and frustrating himself in the process. According to John F. Fulton, he died of a stroke in 1868 brought on by reading one of Jackson's attempts to undermine his position.[23] Jackson himself was no more fortunate. This erratic genius spent much of his later life embroiled in various controversies. These did not end until his mind gave way in 1873, causing him to spend the last seven years of his life in a mental institution. His overweening desire for fame deprived him of the satisfactions which should have come from some real accomplishments. The life of the fourth claimant, Crawford Long, ends on a much happier note. While he assiduously gathered evidence to justify his priority, he maintained his successful medical practice, lived a normal life, and died suddenly in 1878 while aiding in the delivery of a baby.[24]

In trying to evaluate the four conflicting claims, those of Jackson can be dismissed. Crawford Long undoubtedly was the first to perform surgery on an anesthetized patient, but his failure, for whatever reason, to inform the medical world until three years after the Morton–Warren demonstration—and seven years after his first use of ether—relegates him to a minor role. Horace Wells deserves far more credit, and but for a mischance might well stand alone as the discoverer of anesthesia. In any event, his work paved the way for his former partner, William T. G. Morton, to carry on the experiments and bring the project to fruition. While Morton deserves the major credit, there is no question that the time was ripe, that the technology available—and that even without Wells or Morton chemical anesthesia would have appeared on the scene within less than a decade.

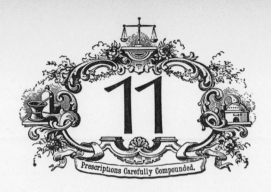

Prescriptions Carefully Compounded.

EARLY NINETEENTH-CENTURY PHYSICIANS AND SURGEONS

O NE can scarcely write about medicine in the years between the Revolution and the Civil War without discussing such outstanding medical figures as Rush, McDowell, Beaumont, and Sims, but a great many more physicians left a permanent imprint upon American medicine, and several of these are worthy of special notice. In Boston the Warren family has been associated with medicine—and Harvard Medical School in particular—since before the Revolution. Joseph Warren (1741–75), a Boston medical practitioner, was killed at Bunker Hill. His brother, John Warren (1753–1815), helped establish the Harvard School of Medicine, where he served as the first professor of anatomy and surgery and was one of the founders of the Massachusetts Medical Society.

His son, John Collins Warren (1778–1856), succeeded to his father's professorship at Harvard and taught surgery for forty years. When Harvard Medical School moved from Cambridge to Boston in 1810, Dr. Warren, along with Dr. James Jackson, took the initiative which led to the founding of the Massachusetts General Hospital. In their appeal to wealthy Bostonians, the two physicians pointed out that the hospital would "afford relief and comfort to thousands of the sick and miserable" and then asked: "On what other objects can the superfluities of the rich be so well bestowed?" Dr. Warren was active in medical journalism and was one of the leaders in establishing the *Boston Medical and Surgical Journal* in 1828, a journal which resulted from a merger of the *New England Journal of Medicine and Surgery* and the *Medical Intelligencer*. Close to the end of his teaching career he performed the classic operation with W. T. G. Morton which introduced anesthesia. Warren's prominence and prestige as a surgeon undoubtedly helped to establish anesthesia as a legitimate surgical technique.[1]

New York was the home of many able physicians, and a fine representative of these was David Hosack (1769–1835). His education was characteristic of that of the best trained physicians—an apprenticeship, courses at two American medical schools, and two years of study in Edinburgh and London. He had just started his medical practice in New York in 1795 when a series of yellow fever outbreaks began. In opposition to Benjamin Rush, Hosack argued that the disease was imported and that bloodletting and drastic purging were fruitless. In 1796 he was appointed professor of materia medica at Columbia and continued to teach throughout his career, subsequently holding positions at the College of Physicians and Surgeons and later on at the short-lived Rutgers Medical School.

While serving as resident physician for the New York Board of Health in 1820, one of many temporary health boards appointed prior to the establishment of the Metropolitan Board of Health in 1866, Hosack lectured to medical students on yellow fever, which was again threatening the city, and upon what was called medical police, a term which encompassed sanitation and public health. His proposals, which included major sanitary reforms and large-scale city planning, were too far ahead of his time, but they reveal him as a humane, perceptive, and intelligent citizen.[2]

His active social life may have been responsible for his selection as Alexander Hamilton's surgeon on the occasion of the tragic Burr–Hamilton duel. In the days of formal dueling, each participant brought his own physician, one of whose duties was to examine any wounds to determine whether or not the participant was too badly injured to continue the fray. In Hamilton's case, Hosack recognized that the wound was fatal. All he could do was to make his patient as comfortable as possible during the "almost intolerable" suffering Hamilton endured for the remaining thirty hours of his life.

The career of Dr. Daniel Drake (1785–1852) presents a sharp contrast to that of the two sophisticated Easterners just described. Drake was essentially a product of the frontier. He was raised under typical frontier conditions in Mays Lick, Kentucky. At the age of fifteen his father took him to Cincinnati and apprenticed him to Dr. William Goforth. On Drake's completion of his four-year apprenticeship, Goforth took him in as a partner. Realizing his medical shortcomings, Drake headed for the Medical College of the University of Pennsylvania in Philadelphia late in 1805, a journey of eighteen days by horseback. Here he attended the lectures of Benjamin Rush, Philip Syng Physick, William Shippen, and Caspar Wistar. When the semester ended early in March 1806, Drake returned to his home and began practicing. Anxious to move onward and upward, he migrated to Cincinnati in 1807.

In 1810, Drake published his book *Notices Concerning Cincinnati*, in which he described the town, its population, and its diseases, the first such work to appear west of the Alleghenies. In it, Drake gave the earliest description of milk sickness, a disease caused by drinking the milk or eating the flesh of cows that had ingested white snakeroot or rayless goldenrod. Later on this disorder became a major problem in the Midwest. In 1815 he returned to Philadelphia, where he took a second course of lectures at the University of Pennsylvania and obtained his medical degree. As his reputation spread, he was invited to become professor of materia medica and botany in the Medical Department of Transylvania University, Lexington, Kentucky.

Realizing the desperate need for trained physicians, and having positive ideas about medical education, in 1819 Drake returned to Cincinnati and secured a charter for the Medical College of Ohio, the forerunner of the Medical School of the University of Cincinnati. Here, as president, he spent a stormy three years embroiled in quarrels with some of his faculty. A contemporary book dealer and author wrote that the early history of the college could be aptly styled "a history of the Thirty Years War." The quarrels among the professors and the town's medical faculty became quite bitter. On one occasion, after a Dr. Oliver B. Baldwin had published a bitter attack on Drake, the latter entered Baldwin's house early in the morning purportedly armed with a club to force the owner to retract his statement. Baldwin claimed that Drake seized him by the throat and threatened to beat him. In the ensuing struggle, Baldwin's shirt was torn and he fled into the street. Drake, while denying Baldwin's version, admitted he entered the house "to remonstrate against the publication," and, when Baldwin became alarmed and left in haste, Drake said: "I ran a few steps after him to get him fairly under way." A local jury, on the testimony of bystanders, convicted Drake of assault and fined him $10.

As if Drake was not having enough troubles, in January 1820 Dr. Coleman Rogers, the college's vice-president and professor of surgery, challenged him to a duel after Drake dismissed him from the college faculty. Drake wisely refused. After further wrangling, the faculty expelled Drake. Although pressure from local towns-people forced his reinstatement, by this time Drake was ready to give up. He resigned in 1823 and accepted a position at his former school, Transylvania University. His stay in Lexington was more or less uneventful, but for some reason he elected to return to Cincinnati in 1827. Here he helped found *The Western Medical and Physical Journal* and was the prime mover in establishing the Cincinnati Eye Infirmary. Always restless, he accepted an appointment in 1830 to the Jefferson Medical College in Philadelphia.

In the meantime he had been mulling over the problems of medical education and publishing his ideas in essay form in his medical journal. In 1823 he collected these articles and published them in book form under the title *Practical Essays on Medical Education and the Medical Profession.* In this work Drake urged the need for a solid background in Greek and Latin, required attendance at lectures, a four-year period of medical training, and stricter examination of candidates for graduation. Few intelligent medical professors questioned Drake's ideas—but, as indicated earlier, the colleges wanted students and the students merely wanted easy degrees. Drake's hopes of being able to put his ideas on medical education into effect led him to leave Jefferson in 1831 to found a new medical college in connection with Miami University. Insurmountable difficulties soon caused its dissolution, and the following year Drake was again on the faculty of the Medical College of Ohio. For the next twenty years he moved back and forth between Louisville, Lexington, and Cincinnati, finally returning once more to the Medical College of Ohio, only to die shortly after the opening of school in 1852.

Notable as this achievement may be, Drake's chief claim to fame lies in his great two-volume work, *A Systematic Treatise, Historical, Etiological and Practical, on the Principal Diseases of the Interior Valley of North America, as they appear in the Caucasian, African, Indian and Esquimaux Varieties of its Population.* This study was the result of a life-long interest in the subject. As early as 1808 he had published *Some Account of the Epidemic Diseases which Prevail at Mays-Lick in Kentucky,* and his two following studies, *Notices Concerning Cincinnati* (1810) and his *Picture of Cincinnati* (1816) show how he was broadening his interest to include the population and environment.

To appreciate Drake's interest in this subject, we must remember that virtually nothing was known about communicable and epidemic diseases. As it became evident in the eighteenth and nineteenth centuries that distinct and separate disease entities did exist, the search for a causal factor or factors turned to meteorological phenomena and the physical environment. The quest was not new, for Hippocrates had suggested such a relationship in his *Airs, Waters, Places* centuries earlier. Two eighteenth-century American books which clearly show the revival of interest in the Hippocratic thesis are Lionel Chalmers's two-volume work, *An Account of the Weather and Diseases in South Carolina* (London, 1776) and William Currie's *An Historical Account of the Climates and Diseases of the United States of America . . .* (Philadelphia, 1792). Public health in the nineteenth century to a large extent was equated with sanitation, and the sanitary movement was profoundly influenced by the various attempts to explain disease in terms of climate and geography. Hence, Drake's study of the people and diseases in the Mississippi Valley was in a well-established tradition.

Throughout his career Drake seized every opportunity to travel in what he termed the great central valley of North America, observing every conceivable phenomena, and in 1844 he began writing his comprehensive study. The first section was a detailed account of the topographical and hydrographical features of the valley. The second dealt with climatic conditions and included tables showing such phenomenena as winds, rainfall, snow, and humidity. The third section described the people—diet, housing, occupations, clothing, and so forth. The final section was a thorough account of the diseases. The first volume appeared in 1850 and the second was published posthumously in 1854. Reviewers were unanimous in their praise, and the book was hailed as a major work in the field of medical topography. Researchers may no longer scan Drake's work searching for clues as to the nature of febrile diseases, but the descriptions of the topography, climate, people, and diseases of the Mississippi Valley make it an invaluable historical source.[3]

It is fitting that the next physician and surgeon discussed be closely associated with Drake in the field of medical education. Dr. Samuel David Gross (1805–84) began his study of medicine as an apprentice but quickly realized the need for a more formal education. He left his preceptor and, after finishing at an academy, entered the newly established Jefferson Medical College in Philadelphia. Upon graduating in 1828 he began private practice in Philadelphia. With only a few patients and a great deal of time on his hands, he busied himself translating various French and German medical books, a project that was educational but not particularly remunerative. Unable to build a decent practice, he returned to his home in Easton where he continued his research and publications. In 1833 he was offered the post as demonstrator in anatomy at the Medical College of Ohio. His success as a teacher and his growing medical reputation led to an invitation two years later to move to the Cincinnati Medical College as professor of pathological anatomy. While there he published his classic study, *Elements of Pathological Anatomy,* the first comprehensive work on this subject in the English language. This book, published in 1839, spread Gross's fame throughout America and Europe. The following year he was appointed professor of surgery at the University of Louisville, where he remained for the next sixteen years save for a brief interlude in New York. In 1856 he was invited to return to his old school, Jefferson Medical College, and spent the rest of his long life in Philadelphia.

Gross was an indefatigable worker, maintaining a large surgical practice, teaching, and pouring out a stream of articles and books. While at the University of Louisville he wrote three major works: one on intestinal lesions, a second on diseases of the bladder, prostate, and urethra, and a third on *Foreign Bodies in the Air-Passages*. In 1859 he brought out his two-volume textbook, *A System of Surgery, Pathological, Diagnostic, Therapeutic and Operative*, a work which remained standard for many years. As with all great surgeons, he was keenly interested in the history of his field and in the work of his predecessors, and in 1861 he edited *The Lives of Eminent Physicians and Surgeons of the Nineteenth Century*. He was a founder of the American Medical Association and was active in establishing several pathological and surgical associations. Most of Gross's career antedated the emergence of the era of abdominal surgery, but he was a pioneer in the field and his work helped lay the basis for subsequent developments.[4]

One of the more able nineteenth-century physicians, Oliver Wendell Holmes (1809–94), is best known as a poet and essayist. Yet Holmes was an outstanding teacher of anatomy and made one of the few significant American contributions to nineteenth-century medicine. Holmes, born in Cambridge, Massachusetts, came from an old New England family. After graduating from Harvard, he briefly studied law and then switched to medicine, beginning his studies at a private medical institution and enrolling in courses at the Harvard Medical School. He then headed for Paris, the mecca for American medical students, where he spent two years observing Pierre Louis, Baron Larrey, Dupuytren, and the other outstanding French clinicians. He returned to Boston, took his medical degree from Harvard, and began practicing. He had already published literary essays in the *New England Magazine* and in 1836 he issued his first volume, *Poems*. As he moved into his medical career, he wrote several prize-winning medical papers. In 1838 he was appointed professor of anatomy at Dartmouth, a position which required only three months a year of his time.

He gave up the Dartmouth professorship in 1840 and devoted himself to literature and his medical practice until his appointment in 1847 as Parkman Professor of Anatomy and Physiology at the Harvard Medical School. It was in this position that his graceful use of English, his wit, and his skepticism endeared him to the students. His reputation as a lecturer was such that he was assigned the last of five morning lectures. Anatomy is a subject which can be deadly to unruly medical students already worn out by a grueling schedule, but Holmes successfully kept their attention for the entire hour from one to two o'clock in the afternoon. Holmes held his chair for thirty-five years, retiring in 1882.

In all likelihood Holmes would have been remembered primarily as a literary figure who was incidentally a great medical teacher had it not been for the publication in 1843 of an article in the *New England Medical and Surgical Journal* entitled "The Contagiousness of Puerperal Fever." In the prebacterial era, puerperal fever was a mysterious disease which periodically swept through maternity wards or struck at parturient women immediately after they had given birth in their homes. The medical profession was at a loss to account for it and was equally at sea as to the means for curing it. Holmes's attention was drawn to this disease when a local physician who had dissected a victim of puerperal fever fell sick and died with symptoms closely resembling those of the fever. After reflecting on this case, Holmes became convinced that the disease was a specific contagious infection which could be passed by direct contact. Since maternity patients had little or no contact with each other, he surmised that physicians were responsible for carrying the disease. Working on this assumption, he urged physicians with patients about to deliver to avoid participating in autopsies of puerperal fever victims or, if they did so, to wash themselves completely, change all clothes, and wait at least twenty-four hours before attending an obstetrical case. If any patient developed the disease, he warned, her physician should take extreme sanitary precautions before visiting another obstetrical case. If two cases of puerperal fever develop under his care, the physician should give up practice for at least a month. Holmes also advised physicians to insist that all nurses and attendants take the same precautions.

Holmes's article was printed as a pamphlet and was reprinted in many medical journals. Although some skepticism was expressed, it was quite influential in encouraging American physicians to practice elementary sanitary precautions in dealing with parturient women. Holmes never doubted the validity of his advice, and when his ideas were attacked early in the 1850s by Drs. H. L. Hodge and C. D. Meigs, two prominent obstetricians,

Holmes republished his article with an introduction reaffirming his position. The significance of Holmes's article is that it preceded the work of Ignaz Philipp Semmelweis by four years. The latter, who is generally credited with discovering the nature of puerperal fever, arrived at his discovery in a manner similar to that of Holmes. Semmelweis, however, met considerable opposition, was hounded from his position in Vienna, and eventually suffered a tragic death in Budapest. The stark tragedy of Semmelweis's life has caused him to loom larger than Holmes in medical history, but Holmes was the first to recognize the role of the physician as the carrier of puerperal fever.

One of the more intriguing of early American physicians is Dr. Benjamin Waterhouse (1754–1846). Although generally credited with introducing vaccination into the United States and being its chief advocate, Waterhouse did not make so favorable an impression upon his contemporaries. It was not until the closing years of the nineteenth century that Waterhouse began to assume a place among the near greats in American medical history. His star shone ever brighter until 1957 when Dr. John Blake reappraised his work and firmly relegated him to a very minor role.[5] Waterhouse became a medical apprentice at the age of sixteen and sailed for Great Britain five years later, where he spent three years living with the well-known Quaker physician, Dr. John Fothergill, while he studied medicine. Edinburgh still drew the majority of American medical students, and Waterhouse spent nine months there in this period. It is a commentary upon the day that Waterhouse, an outspoken American patriot, should have spent the years from 1775 to 1778 in London and Edinburgh. In the latter year he embarked for Holland, where he received a medical degree from Leyden.

Few American physicians had the academic credentials Waterhouse had by the time he returned to America, and in 1783 he was offered the professorship of the theory and practice of physic in the newly organized Harvard Medical School. Waterhouse might well have fallen into historical obscurity had he not received a copy of Edward Jenner's book in 1799 giving an account of his discovery of a new and safer smallpox preventive, "variolae vaccinae" or cowpox. Waterhouse summarized Jenner's work and published it in the *Columbian Centinel*, a Boston newspaper. Along with several other physicians, he managed to get some of the cowpox virus and in July

1800 he vaccinated his son. He then tried it on six other persons
and found that the vaccine did provide immunity from smallpox.

The traditional account states that Waterhouse was besieged
with requests for vaccine from physicians, but that he rejected
them on the grounds that he wanted to be sure the vaccine was
administered correctly. Blake has shown that Waterhouse was far
more concerned with establishing a monopoly over the vaccine than
with establishing safeguards, for he soon began offering it to select
physicians in return for a guarantee of one quarter or more of the
revenue derived from it. Before Waterhouse could set up his
distribution system, a number of other American physicians began
receiving vaccine from English sources.

With a strong demand for the vaccine and a variety of supplies
coming in from England, abuses inevitably crept into the practice
of vaccination. A series of unfortunate accidents caused a reaction
against vaccination. To Waterhouse's credit, he fought to clarify
the situation and he prompted the Boston Board of Health to make
a public experiment of the vaccine. In August 1802 the Board
vaccinated nineteen young volunteers and demonstrated that they
had been successfully immunized against smallpox. Whether Dr.
Waterhouse was apprehensive about spurious vaccination because
he thought it would undercut his profits or whether he was
humanely concerned is difficult to say.

Throughout his life Waterhouse constantly pushed his claim
of having been the first to administer vaccination in the United
States. In doing so he disregarded the many other physicians who
had imported vaccine matter themselves and who had not hesitated
to share it with their colleagues. His attempt to make money out of
the vaccine and his subsequent denials that he had tried to do so did
little to endear him to his colleagues. Within a few years his
relations with the Massachusetts Medical Society became embit-
tered, and he became involved in an equally unsavory quarrel with
his colleagues on the Harvard Medical Faculty, one which led to his
dismissal in 1812. Benjamin Waterhouse did play a role in bringing
vaccine virus to America and he was one of its most ardent
advocates, but he has no place in the pantheon of American medical
leaders.

In sharp contrast to Waterhouse was Dr. John L. Riddell, a
student and friend of Daniel Drake, who served as professor of

chemistry at the Medical College of Louisiana from 1836 to 1861. He dabbled in many areas of science, ranging from his early interest in natural history to physics. In the course of his long career he drew up a proposed bill providing for a geological survey of Louisiana, analyzed the local drinking water, designed a method for filtering and softening it, and then turned his attention to the construction of microscopes. Early in the 1850s he designed the first binocular microscope, publishing a detailed description of it in the *New Orleans Medical and Surgical Journal* in November 1853. The following spring he informed members of the Physico-Medical Society that he was constructing a new kind of objective for the microscope. By making the objective "in two vertical halves," Riddell explained, he anticipated that with "ordinary (not erecting) eye-pieces, the binocular image produced [would] be both erect and orthoscopic." Riddell has generally been overlooked by medical historians, but he was one of the better physician-scientists of the early nineteenth century.[6]

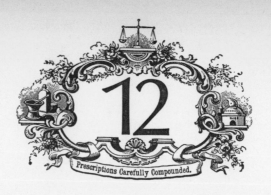

Prescriptions Carefully Compounded.

MEDICAL EDUCATION, LICENSING AND FEES BEFORE THE CIVIL WAR

ALTHOUGH medical schools began flourishing in the nineteenth century, the apprenticeship system still remained an integral part of the doctor's training. Ordinarily the student paid a fee of $100 per year and agreed to remain with his mentor for a period of from two to five years. Daniel Drake's father, for example, apprenticed his son for four years, agreeing to pay Dr. William Goforth the $100 standard annual fee. Apprentices lived with the physician, and their duties ranged widely, varying from currying his horse to compounding medicines. Frequently prominent physicians accepted several young trainees. (Dr. Benjamin Rush took on seven apprentices at one time).[1]

Medical school professors, who lectured and carried on an extensive practice, were more likely to refer to their apprentices as private students. During the year 1807–8 Dr. David Hosack had four private students in addition to those pupils enrolled in his course. The regulations he prescribed for his private students clearly indicate that they were in effect apprentices. The students were expected to be in his office from 9 A.M. to 9 P.M. except when at the hospitals, attending lectures, or eating meals, and they could not leave the city or be absent from the office without permission. Their duties involved taking care of the office, preparing and dispensing medicines, and keeping a register of the weather. Dr. Hosack, recognizing that the devil finds work for idle hands, required all conversations and reading done during office hours to pertain to medicine.[2] Physicians strongly supported the apprentice system, since it provided both an added income and a measure of cheap labor for them. The apprentice system and the medical colleges, as William G. Rothstein has pointed out, worked harmoniously until the college began to offer clinical training, a development which did not occur on any appreciable scale until after the Civil War. One consequence of the continued existence of an apprentice training program was a relatively high percentage of physicians without any formal medical training as late as 1900.

The most remarkable development in the years from the Revolution to 1860 was the phenomenal growth of medical schools. The two pre-Revolution institutions survived the war years—but not without considerable difficulty. The Medical College of Philadelphia managed to reopen, but it was threatened by competition from the newly created University of Pennsylvania. The problem was solved in 1791 when the two schools merged to form the present University of Pennsylvania. Columbia Medical School (King's College) had even greater problems when it was revived in 1792. Part of the trouble was a personality clash between Dr. Samuel Bard and Dr. Nicholas Romayne, the "stormy petrel" of New York medical politics. Romayne resigned from Columbia and established a private school in the late 1780s, making arrangements for his students to receive medical degrees at Queen's College (Rutgers) in New Jersey. In 1807, assisted by Drs. David Hosack, Samuel Latham Mitchell, and several others, Romayne established the College of Physicians and Surgeons under the auspices of the University of the State of New York. In the meantime Columbia was struggling to survive, granting only thirty-four medical degrees between 1792 and 1811. By 1810 both schools were beset with problems, and the following year the Regents of the State University decided to merge Columbia into the College of Physicians and Surgeons.[3]

While the schools in Philadelphia and New York were trying to solve their problems, new medical colleges began appearing on the scene. In 1782 Harvard established a medical department with three professors, and in 1798 Dartmouth formally established a medical school. It should be noted that the latter school consisted of one professor, Dr. Nathan Smith, and an assistant, Lyman Spalding. It was not until 1810 that the Dartmouth trustees appointed a second professor.[4] Transylvania University in Kentucky created a Medical Department in 1799, but it was 1817 before any official courses in medicine were given.[5]

Medical education received a notable setback in 1788 as a result of what was termed the Doctors' Riot. A brash young medical student engaged in dissection in New York City reportedly waved a dissected arm at a group of young boys. One of them peeped into the window and was told it was his mother's arm. Since his mother had died recently, the boy was horrified and ran to tell his father. The father visited the grave and discovered it had been robbed. He gathered a group of fellow laborers and literally tore the dissecting rooms apart, destroying an anatomical museum which Drs. Richard Bayley and Samuel Clossy had been in the process of creating. The mob then started looking for medical students and doctors, some of whom took refuge in the jail. Their anger and frustration intensified by social problems, the mob raged for over two days before being brought under control.[6]

The destruction of the anatomical museum was a bitter loss because of the difficulty of securing subjects for dissection. Out of necessity, physicians and their pupils in the antebellum period were compelled to resort to grave-robbing, a practice which did not endear them to the public. In some cases medical students were responsible for acquiring their own subjects, but most medical schools relied upon professional "resurrectionists," "sack-'em-up men," or "body-snatchers," who charged a standard fee according to the age of the subject and the condition of the body. Since any medical school of consequence had to give its students a chance to dissect, and since it was virtually impossible to secure bodies legally, there was a justifiable public suspicion and resentment against medical schools. Public reaction to grave-robbing varied from area to area, with the consequences ranging from relatively mild fines and prison sentences to violent mob action. Accusations of grave-robbing led an unruly mob in Maryland to burn down the University's first medical building in 1807.[7]

The shortage of subjects made medical students quick to seize any opportunity that came their way. When news of John Brown's Raid was first heard, the entire student body of Winchester Medical College in Virginia boarded the next train for Harper's Ferry, eventually some of the students chanced upon a dead body and shipped it back to the college. There papers on the body revealed it was John Brown's son Owen. Undeterred by this fact, a dried preparation was made of the body, and it was added to the other anatomical specimens used for demonstration purposes. According to Wyndham Blanton, the Union commander learned about this on entering Winchester in 1862, recovered the body, and burned the college buildings to the ground in retaliation.[8]

The first state to pass an anatomy act was Massachusetts, where public outrage over body-snatching in 1830 led the Massachusetts Assembly to legalize the granting of bodies to medical schools. Unfortunately, Massachusetts was an exception to the rule, for it was not until the midcentury that other states began following suit. Some legislatures did not act until near the end of the century. Pennsylvania, for example, did not pass an anatomy act until June 1883.[9]

The one place where the medical profession had no difficulty procuring subjects was New Orleans. The city's Charity Hospital, opened as a private institution in 1736 and taken over by the state in 1811, was designed primarily to provide medical care for the poor. As New Orleans was a major seaport, the vast majority of patients were outsiders. By 1849 the hospital was admitting over 18,000 patients annually at a time when hospitals were largely places of last resort and when a case fatality rate of from 10 to 12 percent was considered quite satisfactory. Precisely because the majority of those who died were poor and homeless, or poor and away from home, their bodies were usually consigned to the potter's field; consequently, there was no one to object when the bodies were assigned to physicians or medical schools for dissection purposes. The notices and advertisements sent forth by the New Orleans medical schools invariably stressed the ample clinical material at Charity Hospital and the unlimited number of subjects for dissection.

As of 1800 the United States had only four small medical colleges to serve a fast-growing population of over five million. Two more were added in 1807 when Romayne established the College of Physicians and Surgeons and Maryland chartered the College of Medicine in Maryland. This latter institution was largely the work of John Beale Davidge, a Baltimore physician who had been giving private lectures in obstetrics and surgery. The state legislature left the operation of the school largely to the professors, except for authorizing a series of lotteries in 1808 to help with the construction of a school building. The new building was not ready until 1813, and in the meantime the professors lectured successively in an old warehouse, a church, and a theater.[10]

While medical schools had been slow in appearing during the first thirty years of the new nation's history, their numbers increased rapidly after 1810. No less than twenty-six were founded between 1810 and 1840, and another forty-seven between 1840 and 1875.[11] Since neither clinical training nor laboratory work was considered necessary for a medical degree, all that was required to start a medical college were several lecturers and a lecture hall. A good many medical schools obtained a charter first and then started looking for quarters. The promoters of these schools usually consisted of a group of from four to seven young physicians. Once a charter was obtained, they would borrow, hire, or rent a lecture hall until they could raise enough money to buy or erect a building. A good part of the building funds were contributed by the founding professors, and for the rest they usually appealed to the state legislature and/or private charity.

Tulane University School of Medicine is a fine example of how the early proprietary medical schools began. The originators were three young men, not one of whom was older than twenty-six years. Two of them, Drs. Warren Stone and Thomas Hunt, arrived in New Orleans in 1833. Warren was the product of a poor Vermont family, while Hunt came from a well-to-do Charleston background. Shortly after their arrival, the two men encountered Dr. John Harrison, a former Marylander who had recently come to New Orleans. All three were interested in establishing a medical school, and Hunt, who had an excellent classical education, was selected to serve as the spokesman for the group and the first dean of the college. They recruited four other prospective professors, and in 1834 secured a charter for the Medical College of Louisiana. An announcement that the school would open in January 1835 led to some sharp denunciations by the French-language papers. The French-speaking physicians, many of whom held French university degrees, argued that a medical school was impossible in New Orleans since the city did not have a university.[12]

Untroubled by these arguments, Dean Hunt gave his inaugural lecture on January 5 in the church of the Reverend Theodore Clapp.[13] The faculty also borrowed a room in the State House, but they were soon able to rent a lecture hall for $25 per month. Appeals for funds were made to the state legislature, but these efforts were not successful, and the school continued to operate in temporary facilities. For example, Dr. John L. Riddell, the professor of chemistry, taught his class during the 1838–39 session in the basement of the Methodist Church. Finally, in 1843 the medical professors offered to provide all medical care in Charity Hospital and to admit one poor student free of tuition from each parish (county) in the state in return for a building site for their school. The legislature acquiesced, and by the end of 1843 the college was housed in a three-story building in the typical classical style of the day—complete with two Corinthian columns dominating the front. The first floor contained a large lecture hall, a chemical laboratory, and a small library; the second was occupied by a surgical amphitheater, a museum, and two small classrooms; and the third was used as a dissecting room.

Two years later in 1845 the legislature chartered a state university and specified that the Medical College of Louisiana would become the Medical Department of the University. Subsequently this same body appropriated funds to erect a new and larger building for the Medical Department. Although the legislature continued to give financial support, the medical school remained under control of the professors and was to all intents and purposes a proprietary institution.[14]

In this respect, and in others, the medical school was typical of its day. Despite a rising enrollment, which exceeded 400 in 1860, the number of professors remained at its original figure of seven. The school term ran from November 1 to the end of March, and students seeking a degree were expected to attend the same lectures for two successive sessions. An additional year's experience in a physician's office was also required, but the certificates attesting to this were often worthless. For conscientious students it was possible to acquire the rudiments of a medical education, but for those simply seeking a medical degree life was much simpler. Dr. Stanford E. Chaillé, an 1853 graduate who subsequently became dean of the school, wrote that "students could enter very late and leave very early, [and] there were instances of cases in which little more was required than one's presence, payment of the entrance fees, and attendance at the final examinations." Even the examinations were nominal, since the students visited the seven professors for an oral quiz within the space of an hour and a half. And it was customary for each professor to spend a few minutes inquiring about the student's plans and his family. Chaillé added that he himself graduated with a unanimous vote of the faculty only seventeen months after he had first entered the study of medicine.[15] Significantly, the University of Louisiana was the leading medical college in the Deep South and ranked as one of the better ones in the country.

The vast majority of medical schools organized during the nineteenth century were proprietary institutions, a term which needs explanation. As of 1800 it was obvious that the number of graduates from the existing medical colleges was hopelessly inadequate for America's burgeoning population. This vacuum in medical education was filled by small groups of ambitious young practitioners who brashly took it upon themselves to establish schools. Under these conditions, the traditional concept of professional medical training as an academic discipline simply had no validity. Entrance requirements were virtually eliminated, and the emphasis was placed upon practical skills and knowledge. Many of the professors were themselves the product of the apprentice system, and they could see little value in laboratories or libraries.

The caliber of these schools varied widely, depending upon the educational background and conscientiousness of the professors, but, as already indicated, even in the best schools it was possible to acquire an easy degree. From a professional and economic standpoint, physicians had much to gain by an attachment to a medical college. Students paid a matriculation fee usually ranging from $5 to $10 and a graduation fee of from $25 to $35. In addition, they purchased a ticket at a cost of about $20 from each professor whose class they wished to attend. A popular professor could also expect to attract the public to some of his lectures; hence a professorship could mean a substantial addition to a physician's income. The matriculation and graduation fees were generally applied to overhead costs, and the professors paid any extra expenses out of their lecture fees. More important than the income from teaching was the prestige attached to it. A physician's standing in the community was enhanced by a professorship, and consultation fees from former students tended to grow during long teaching careers.

In his classic study of American medical education in 1910, Abraham Flexner blamed the University of Maryland for the introduction of proprietary schools—a system, he wrote, which divorced American medical schools from universities and led to a progressive lowering of educational standards. It is clear, however, to anyone who studies conditions in early nineteenth-century America that the universities to which medical schools might have been grafted simply did not exist. When the Maryland legislature established the College of Medicine of Maryland, there was no university within the state. The same was true in 1845 when the Louisiana legislature transformed the Medical College of Louisiana into the Medical Department of the University of Louisiana. The University existed only in name. Moreover, even in the case of schools such as Harvard and the University of Pennsylvania the medical school professors collected their own fees and remained virtually autonomous for much of the school's history.[16]

Yet Flexner was right in attributing the decline in standards to the rise of these schools. The ease with which medical colleges could be established and the fact that many professors were more concerned with collecting fees than with providing a medical education led to a keen competition for students. As this competition sharpened, there was a tendency to lower standards, both for entrance and graduation. Yale presents a fine illustration of this point. When medicine was first offered in 1813, the course was six months. After losing students to institutions offering much shorter courses, Yale gradually reduced the academic year to four months.[17] In later years, when demands for medical reform were growing, the occasional college which sought to raise its requirements quickly found its student body slipping away and was forced to conform to the general mediocre level.

Despite this discouraging picture, the situation was not without its redeeming qualities. In the first place, these schools supplied America with doctors and surgeons whose empirical skills were not too far behind those of their European contemporaries. Conscientious students learned a great deal from their preceptors, broadened their medical knowledge by reading, and, if they could afford it, supplemented their training abroad. In the second place, these proprietary medical colleges established the principle that medicine was a profession which required advanced formal education. While the caliber of these schools remained low during the antebellum period, they laid the base for an effective system of medical education.

If the attempts to reform medical education prior to the Civil War proved fruitless, it was not for want of trying. In 1825 the Vermont State Medical Society circularized a number of state societies and medical colleges urging that the requirements for medical degrees and licenses be raised. The result was a meeting in Northampton, Massachusetts, which included representatives from medical societies and four medical schools in five New England states. Apparently only Yale sought to conform to the recommendations stemming from the meeting, and it was forced to back down when its enrollment began to decrease. In the succeeding years a number of other abortive attempts were made by medical societies in Ohio, New Hampshire, and New York. The most persistent efforts were those of the New York State Medical Society, and although the Society did not achieve its aim, its efforts toward reform did lead to the formation of the American Medical Association in 1847.[18]

At the first National Medical Convention in 1846 (the forerunner of the AMA), a committee was appointed to study medical education and to recommend any needed changes. After having made contact with about half of the existing schools, the committee recommended lengthening the academic year to six months, requiring students to attend lectures for two six-month terms, and insisting that the students must present clear evidence of having served an apprenticeship with a qualified physician. College faculties were to have seven professors, each of whom was to be capable of providing instruction in one of the seven branches of medical science. In essence these branches were medicine, surgery, anatomy, physiology and pathology, materia medica and pharmacy, midwifery and gynecology, and chemistry and medical jurisprudence. The committee further recommended that the students must spend three months dissecting and that the college provide clinical instruction and hospital practice.[19]

Carried away by the enthusiasm displayed at the Philadelphia meeting in 1847 two schools lengthened their courses to six months, the University of Pennsylvania and the College of Physicians and Surgeons in New York. The net effect in Philadelphia was to increase the enrollment of the Jefferson Medical College at the expense of the University of Pennsylvania. The latter school continued the experiment for several years, but was eventually forced back to the four-month term.[20] The experiences of these two schools illustrate that, while most medical colleges favored reform in principle, they had no intention of raising standards at the cost of student enrollment—and fees! During the 1850s the rise of sectarian or irregular colleges may have even aggravated the situation. Dr. Richard Arnold of Savannah in 1857 denounced "the growing abuse" of "taking a winter student, hurrying him through a Summer Course and turning him out a Doctor in less than a year. . . ."[21] Whether or not the level of medical education declined during the 1850s, it is clear that the movement to reform medical schools came to nought. It might be noted that the Medical Department of the University of Louisiana (the present-day Tulane) met all of the recommendations of the AMA educational committee except for the six-month course of instruction. Yet, as Dr. Chaillé had observed, it was still possible to slide through with a minimum of medical knowledge.

MEDICAL LICENSURE

Influenced in part by the relative shortage of physicians, American colonial officials made few efforts to require the licensing of physicians. The first licensure law in the colonies was enacted in 1760 for New York City. The early and unsuccessful efforts in this direction by New York City and the colony of New Jersey have already been discussed.[22] The New York licensing law was reenacted in 1792 and five years later made applicable to the entire state. Incidentally, the preamble to the 1792 law justified the need for licensing on the grounds that quackery was rife and "many ignorant and unskilful persons presumed to administer physic and surgery . . . to the detriment and hazard of lives of the Citizens themselves.[23]

As state and local medical societies blossomed in the early national period, state legislatures tended to turn licensing over to them. New Jersey adopted this policy in 1790 and was followed by New York and most other states. Louisiana, where the French and Spanish regimes had consistently maintained strict controls over physicians and surgeons, reenacted and eventually broadened a licensure law shortly after it came under American control. Shortly after Louisiana gained statehood, the legislature in 1816 established a state board consisting of four physicians and one apothecary. The following year the act was amended to establish two separate boards, an Eastern and Western board. The Eastern Board, which served the New Orleans area, continued to grant medical and pharmaceutical licenses until 1854. The Louisiana licensing boards survived much longer than their counterparts in the other states, but even so the acquisition of a license was more a matter of prestige than a legal requirement, for there is little evidence to show the prosecution of unlicensed practitioners.[24]

The emergence of state medical societies as licensing agencies led to an immediate clash with the medical-degree-granting institutions, which assumed that a degree automatically gave its possessor the right to practice. The matter first came to a head in connection with Harvard University. In a public examination of candidates for licenses, the Harvard medical graduates were so much better prepared than the other candidates that the Massachusetts Medical Society, which had insisted on examining all candidates, was forced to back down. The issue was finally settled in 1803 when the society agreed to accept a Harvard medical degree in lieu of an examination. The policy of the Massachusetts Medical Society of establishing a dual system—a medical degree or an examination— was soon followed by most state societies and licensing boards. While virtually all of the older states passed licensure laws of one type or another, few of these measures prescribed penalties for noncompliance. In most cases an unlicensed practitioner was simply denied the legal right to collect fees—a dubious punitive measure, since the licensed physicians themselves were constantly protesting their inability to collect fees. Even in those states where licensing boards existed, it was still relatively easy to obtain a license. Licensing agencies only collected a fee if they granted a license, a situation likely to discourage them from rejecting candidates; all the more so, since an individual rejected by one board could often apply to another. License fees proved a substantial source of income for some medical societies. For example, they constituted 27 percent of the Maryland State Medical Society's income during the year 1827—a fact of life which undoubtedly encouraged its licensing board to be lenient.[25]

By 1820 the public was becoming increasingly skeptical of the medical profession and equally suspicious of what it referred to as "monopolies." In part it was a reflection of the Jacksonian spirit of egalitarianism, one aspect of which was a distrust of intellectuals and learning. This democratic spirit also implied the right of any American to choose his own doctor or lawyer—and the right, too, if he wished, to practice medicine or law. In the newly created states west of the Appalachians the legislatures rejected all attempts at professional licensing, and, in the older states where licensure laws had existed, most of them were repealed. As of 1845 ten states had repealed their licensure laws and another eight states in the West had never enacted any. In the early 1850s only Louisiana, New Jersey, and the District of Columbia were making any effort to regulate the practice of medicine, but these areas, too, were not immune to the laissez-faire movement. In 1852 the Louisiana Legislature repealed all existing license laws and by 1864 New Jersey took away the authority of the state medical society to license physicians. In so doing she joined the rest of the states in opening the practice of medicine to anyone. Thus by the outbreak of the Civil War not a single state had an effective medical licensing law.[26]

THE PHYSICIANS' EARNINGS

While a few prominent physicians could make relatively large incomes from teaching and medical practice, the vast majority of doctors either eked out a bare living from medicine or else used it as a supplement to farming or business. Dr. Goforth of Cincinnati, to whom Daniel Drake was apprenticed, was considered an excellent physician, but he could scarcely have accumulated any substantial capital. According to Drake, he charged 25 cents for bleeding, 25 to 50 cents per visit, and a dollar for sitting up all night with the patient. For country patients an added charge of 25 cents per mile was added to the bill. A fee bill drawn up by seven Nashville physicians in 1821 showed the following charges: visit in town, $1; obstetrical case, $20; prescription at shop, $1; amputation of thigh, leg, or arm, $50; vaccination, $2; and blister, $1. Fee bills issued by Louisiana doctors showed that the rates were roughly comparable to those throughout the other southern and western states.[27] Charges by physicians in the small towns and rural areas in the East were not too different from those in the West and South.

As might be expected, the highest charges were made by physicians in the major eastern cities, most notably Boston and New York. An 1817 Boston fee bill listed a first home visit from $2 to $5 and each succeeding visit at $1.50. Vaccination cost $5. Charges for major surgery were slightly lower than those given in the Cincinnati fee bill, however. A New York fee list about this same time showed a home visit at $5 plus extra charges for any distance traveled. Bleeding by cupping glasses or the jugular vein was listed at $5, although bleeding at the arm, probably the most common, was only $2. A great many major operations were included for which the charges generally ranged from $50 to $150. Lithotomy, for example, cost $150, while surgery for aneurysms, depending upon the type and location, could run as high as $200.[28] Keen competition in the medical field meant that in most cases the fee bills represented what the physicians hoped to get rather than what they actually charged. Few medical associations were able to maintain the published fees. In many cases adverse public reaction forced the doctors to rescind the fee bill, and in others enough physicians refused to subscribe to make the fee bill inoperative.

The failure of most of the efforts to establish standard charges was only one of the financial problems besetting the physician. Particularly in small towns and rural areas, cash was always in short supply, and doctors had to accept produce and personal service. What was much worse was the even greater difficulty of collecting bills in any form. Since farm income depended upon the annual sale of crops, in rural areas the doctor's bill was often paid on an annual basis. In the South and some of the other areas, too, it was not unusual to let a medical bill run for years, often until the death of the patient.

In part because of the difficulty of collecting fees, the contract system of medical practice spread widely. It gained its greatest foothold in the South, where it was aided by the plantation system. Unless a young physician could be accepted as a partner by an established practitioner, he found it difficult to make a start. By contracting with one or more plantations he was assured of a minimum income and a chance to gain needed experience. In urban areas these same inducements led young practitioners into providing a flat annual rate for members of labor unions, social organizations, and other groups. Since the contract system, at least in theory, emphasized keeping patients well, it should have appealed to medicine, a profession which claims to want to do so. The fee system, however, is based upon the profit motive, and physicians have traditionally made more money from treating the sick than from maintaining health. Hence every medical society in the last 200 years has consistently fought against the contract system, and this attitude is still reflected in the violent opposition by organized medicine to health maintenance organizations today.

During the pre-Civil War era, medical professors and practitioners alike agreed that there was little money to be made in medicine. They also agreed that the root of the problem lay in the excessive number of doctors. *The Western Journal of the Medical and Physical Sciences* asserted in the late 1820s that wherever one went he would find twice as many lawyers or doctors as were needed. A survey of New York State in 1831 showed that it had 2,549 physicians, 1,742 lawyers, 1,300 clergymen. Cincinnati in 1839 with a population of 50,000 had 100 physicians—or one for every 500 residents.[29] As long as the profession remained overcrowded and disorganized, medical degrees easy to obtain, and entrance to medical practice open to anyone, little could be done to improve the average physician's income. While major efforts were made to solve all of these problems in the second half of the nineteenth century, it was not until the twentieth century was at hand before any significant improvement was made.

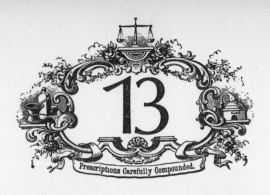

Prescriptions Carefully Compounded.

THE DOCTOR
AND SOCIETY

S INCE social status is determined by many variables and
physicians can be found at all levels of society, any generalization
about the medical profession can scarcely apply to individual
doctors. Two of the most important determinants of social position
are education and money. In the nineteenth century those who
could afford to go to college and medical school, and then on to
Europe to complete their medical training, were usually the ones
who held the best positions as medical professors and enjoyed the
most lucrative practices. Between their fees from medical students,
consultation fees from former students, and their own practice,
these individuals could make well in excess of $10,000 a year, a
substantial sum in that period.

Below this top group were a fairly large number of physicians
holding reputable medical degrees who were able to make a
comfortable living. Their role as a physician guaranteed them
a certain respect in the community, and, once they had achieved a

successful practice, this respect was reinforced by their educational background and economic position. Still further down the social and economic scale was the large number of physicians whose training was derived from an apprenticeship or from one of the many second- and third-rate medical schools. While able individuals could rise from this group and reach a top position, they were exceptions. Many of them were barely literate, a situation which did little to enhance the reputation of the profession. Only a few could make a living from medicine, and they supplemented their incomes by farming or business—one might almost say they supplemented their business income by practicing medicine.

The majority of those who depended upon medical practice exclusively lived in towns and cities. Although the University of Pennsylvania ranked among the top medical schools, Benjamin Rush advised students planning to practice in a rural area to purchase a farm to keep them busy during slack periods. Even students from reputable schools often had great difficulty establishing a practice, since the ratio of doctors to the population was quite high and competition was always keen.[1] In 1847 a survey of the physicians practicing in Virginia showed that about one quarter had neither medical degree nor license. In the new states west of the Appalachians where life was even more freewheeling, it was estimated that half of the practitioners had no formal qualifications.[2] Illustrative of this, in 1850 a cursory survey of 201 practicing physicians in East Tennessee showed that only 35 had medical degrees, 42 had attended one course of lectures at a school but had not graduated, 95 claimed to be orthodox physicians but had never received any formal training, and another 29 professed to be Thomsonians or homeopaths.[3]

The rise of the irregular medical sects added still more to the numbers of illiterate or semiliterate practitioners and further lowered the popular image of the medical profession. Far too many physicians fitted the description given by Daniel Drake of one of his colleagues in a frontier town:

. . . his medicines unlabelled, and thrown into a chaos . . . bundles untied and bottles left uncorked, or stopped with plugs of paper; dead flies in the ointment within his jars, while others are wading through that which has lain so long spread over his counter, that their feet are blistered by its rancidity; his spatulas, foul and rusty; . . . his surgical instruments oxidating and rusting away, like his mind; his study-table, covered with loose papers and medical journals . . . his walls overspread with a tapestry of cobwebs; his windows opaque from dust as the painted glass on an ancient cathedral; his foul candlestick standing all day on his lexicon, and his floor spotted over with the blood of his surgical patients, and his own tobacco juice.[4]

Small wonder that J. Marion Sims's father was almost in despair when he discovered his son wanted to enter the medical profession.

To make matters worse, it was axiomatic that medical students, even in the best schools, were a coarse, crude, uncouth lot. President Charles W. Eliot of Harvard wrote in one of his annual reports that "until the reformation of the School in 1870–71, the medical students were noticeably inferior in bearing, manners, and discipline to the students of other departments. . . ."[5]

As if the handicap of having a large mass of semiliterates practicing medicine was not enough, the profession faced a great many other difficulties, some of which it created for itself. The major handicap for the profession arose from the sheer lack of medical knowledge. Despite great strides in anatomy and other areas, physicians still had little comprehension of the cause of most diseases, and out of necessity they continued to rely on traditional methods. When these proved inadequate to deal with the great fever epidemics, in desperation they applied their therapeutics even more rigorously. Heroic medical practices have already been described and little further need be said about them, other than the wholesale bloodletting and dosing finally reached a point in the 1830s and 1840s where it not only gave pause to sensible physicians but brought a strong public reaction. Medical journals, newspapers, and private diaries and correspondence are replete with horror stories of repeated bloodletting and the disastrous results of excessive and prolonged administration of mercurials, arsenicals, and other dangerous drugs. Thomsonians, hydropaths, and the other irregulars all seized upon this issue and based their appeal to the public on the grounds that they did not resort to drastic therapeutics. One could say that the rise of the irregular medical sects bore a direct ratio to the increasing administration of drugs by the orthodox physicians.

A second major disadvantage suffered by the medical profession was the constant quarreling and bickering among all levels of physicians. This, too, resulted in part from the lack of a rational basis on which to treat patients. While the nineteenth century saw a rising skepticism with respect to all medical theories, intelligent physicians recognized the need for some basic principles. Unfortunately discovering them was not all that simple. As the theory of the unity of diseases set forth by Rush was gradually discarded and the realization dawned that the answers to all medical questions were not to be solved by the discovery of some grand principle, medical men fell to disputing over the cause and treatment of particular disorders.

Men of strong convictions soon gained disciples and the profession found itself divided into warring groups, each one passionately affirming a particular medical viewpoint or course of treatment. Aside from the element of ego involvement in these clashes, the work of the physician was no abstract intellectual endeavor. He was dealing with suffering and dying human beings and was desperately seeking some way to provide relief and save lives. Understandably those doctors who thought—as did Benjamin Rush, for example—they had found a way to save lives enthusiastically promoted their particular form of therapy. State and local medical societies, which generally included only the more educated physicians, were constantly rent by bitter arguments or by personal quarrels. In addition to denouncing each other's medical views, the arguments frequently degenerated into violent personal quarrels. Opponents wrote letters to the newspapers, printed pamphlets, and on occasions resorted to fisticuffs, knives, and duels.

It will be recalled that, when Dr. Benjamin Waterhouse quarreled with the Massachusetts Medical Society in 1806, he began by attacking his colleagues in a letter to one of the local newspapers. An even more flagrant example of these public quarrels involved Dr. Charles A. Luzenberg of New Orleans. In 1838 he was accused of professional misconduct by the Physico-Medical Society of Louisiana for permitting a rather embellished account of one of his operations to be published. After an exchange of correspondence, the Society expelled Luzenberg, published a pamphlet defending its position and scathingly denounced him as "abrupt in speech, uncouth in manners, irritable and petulant in temper, and arrogant and overbearing in his demeanor."[6]

Not content with this denunciation, the Society printed a signed statement by a Dr. John J. Ker that prior to fighting a duel with a Dr. J. S. McFarlane, Luzenberg was "in the habit of suspending bodies of persons who had died under his care whilst House Surgeon of the Charity Hospital, and shooting at them as marks with pistols, in order to improve his skill as a marksman in his expected contest with Dr. McFarlane." Astonishingly, although an exchange of correspondence in the New Orleans newspapers continued for some time, alternating testimonials published by the Society with retaliations by Luzenberg, Luzenberg did not deny the charge. The New Orleans medical faculty split wide open over the Luzenberg case, with prominent physicians to be found on both sides. In the midst of it all, Luzenberg issued challenges to two members of the Medical Society, both of whom declined to accept. Luzenberg's seconds promptly placed a paid notice in one of the newspapers proclaiming one of the men refused the challenge to be "a most consummate coward, and a dastardly poltroon." He replied the following day: "The infamy which has been stamped upon Dr. Luzenberg's character cannot and shall not be wasted away in my blood." The upshot of this long and bitter controversy was the dissolution of the Physico-Medical Society, and a general lowering of public esteem for the medical profession.[7]

The clashes which disrupted medical societies were only one part of the violent public quarrels between members of the medical profession. With competition among physicians keen, accusations of stealing patients were frequently leveled. In the South, where dueling persisted right up to the outbreak of the Civil War, a number of duels were fought over this issue. Louisiana was notorious for dueling, and its physicians fought at least their share. One occurred in 1856 between two leading surgeons, Dr. Samuel Choppin and Dr. John Foster. One of Choppin's medical students was injured in a student brawl and taken to Charity Hospital. He asked for Dr. Choppin, who came and dressed his wound. When Foster, the house surgeon, heard of this, he indignantly ordered the nurse to throw out Choppin's prescription and to redress the injury. The result was a shotgun duel between the two physicians. Fortunately both principals missed, and the affair seemed settled. Three years later they quarreled over a patient suffering from an aneurysm in the right external clavicle who was admitted to Foster's ward. Choppin wanted to operate, but Foster refused to release the patient. After some troubled relations, the two men met at the gates of Charity, both well armed. Following an exchange of angry words, they drew their weapons. Foster got off the first shot, the bullet entering Choppin's neck cutting the exterior jugular vein in two and causing Choppin's first shot to go wild. Foster fired again, this time hitting Choppin in the iliac region. Bleeding badly from two serious wounds and with his guns empty, Choppin drew his bowie knife and staggered toward Foster; fortunately by this time the medical students separated the two men. Since dueling was illegal within the New Orleans city limits, Foster was arrested. Choppin, who recovered from his wounds, refused to press charges and Foster was released after a night in jail.[8]

One of the most amusing duels, which has a comic opera touch, occurred between a celebrated French heart specialist, Dr. Joseph Rouanet, who had come to New Orleans, and a Creole physician, Dr. Charles C. Delery. Rouanet, who was given to expounding with great authority, was presented with the heart of a goose which had died of cardiac disease and asked to give his opinion of it. Without hesitation, Rouanet pronounced it to be the heart of a young baby and spoke of its pathology at some length before learning the truth of the matter. Upon hearing of this, Dr. Delery composed a satirical poem in French verse entitled "The Doctor and the Goose." The Creoles, always irritated by the condescension of the French physicians, gleefully circulated Delery's poem. When Rouanet heard of it, he challenged Delery to a duel. Happily both shots barely grazed the two opponents, and their seconds declared that honor had been satisified.[9]

The intense rivalry between medical schools for students, and the public fights between professors within the same schools has already been alluded to. In addition, there was a clash during much of the nineteenth century between the medical schools and the medical societies. The first source of irritation was the matter of licensure, a power which many states had given to the state medical societies. The colleges assumed that their degrees were an automatic license to practice, and this assumption that eventually carried the day. Another cause of friction was the threat which the colleges posed to the apprenticeship system. As mentioned earlier, apprentices were both a source of income and a form of cheap labor for the physician. Originally medical school courses were designed to supplement apprentice training, but this situation changed when college professors began offering private clinical instruction and eventually incorporated these private courses into the medical school curriculum. The effect was to cause the traditional apprentice system to wither away.

Since the best general education was offered in eastern schools such as Harvard, Yale, Princeton, and Columbia, the percentage of well-educated physicians was much higher in the East than was true for the West and South. Understandably, educated easterners tended to be condescending to their counterparts in the West, and even more understandably westerners resented this patronizing attitude. As medical centers developed in Cincinnati, Lexington, and Chicago, the medical faculties were critical of the alleged superiority of the eastern schools. Many western physicians reacted by becoming highly nationalistic and accusing easterners of being subservient to foreign science.[10]

The recurrent epidemics and the public disputations between physicians as to the causes and means for preventing these outbreaks brought further discredit on the profession. Without going into the details, the major issue in nineteenth-century public health was whether diseases were specific entities brought into a locality or whether they were spontaneously generated whenever the correct combination of filth, crowding, and meteorological conditions existed. (There were, of course, many additional variants of these two theses.) Physicians could be found on both sides of the question, although the majority, conditioned by their experience with malaria and yellow fever, were inclined to support the anticontagionist or sanitationist viewpoint, which considered quarantines to be useless. The long series of yellow fever and Asiatic cholera epidemics which ravaged large segments of the population in this century aroused a tremendous furor and helped to focus public attention upon the inability of physicians to agree. A New York physician in 1822 advocated the appointment of a city board of health, but the majority of members, he said, should be laymen since if the board was "exclusively made up of medical gentlemen there is too much reason to fear that their different opinions might lead, as too often happens, to interminable disputes, and to most disastrous consequences." In New Orleans a law creating a board of health in 1848 specified that practicing physicians could not constitute a majority of the members, and, when a sanitary commission was organized the same year, the law excluded practicing physicians and engineers from membership. A commission studying the New Orleans yellow fever epidemic of 1853 during which 11,000 people died reported that the medical faculty had not cooperated. The loss was not too great, the committee added, for the few who "deemed the subject worthy of their consideration . . . [did] not agree together."[11] The creation of the New York Metropolitan Board of Health in 1866 is a landmark in municipal health; its membership, too, was deliberately balanced in favor of lay personnel.

The medical profession had no illusions about the wrangling and discord which characterized its membership. Dr. J. Augustine Smith in 1828 warned the readers of the *New-York Medical and Physical Journal* to beware speculation and theories. Since speculation was easier than collecting and systematically organizing factual knowledge, he wrote, there had been no change or improvement in medicine for centuries. Frustrated by this lack of progress, the profession had grown querulous. "Let half a dozen medical men be required to give their professional opinions to the public," Dr. Smith asserted, "and they certainly disagree about their facts, and almost as certain fall to calling each other hard names." Dr. H. H. Childs in giving an introductory lecture to the medical class at Willoughby University in 1844 declared: "Need we be surprised that intelligent men extend to the profession a hesitating and doubtful confidence, when educated physicians differ so widely among themselves, avowing the most opposite views, both in theory and practice. . . . That 'Doctors disagree,' has passed into a proverb."[12] A few years later the *Cincinnati Medical Observer* commented: "It has become fashionable to speak of the Medical Profession as a body of jealous, quarrelsome men, whose chief delight is in the annoyance and ridicule of each other."

Newspapers and magazines happily joined in the attack upon medicine. Sarcastic or satirical editorials and stories of malpractice and excessive bleeding and drugging were common. When New

Orleans was threatened by yellow fever in 1839 the *Courier* advised unacclimated residents to leave town or arrange for good nursing. "We mention nurses more particularly," the editor added, "inasmuch as we are convinced that the recovery of the sick depends more on their attention and discrimination than on the skill of the physician." Another Louisiana newspaper deploring the disunity among physicians asserted: "There is just as much uncertainty and confusion among medical men as among Theologians and Politicians." The Philadelphia *Item* in 1858 accused the profession of "poisoning and surgical butchery," and one can cite dozens of similar quotations showing clearly that the public viewed the profession with a mixture of derision and amused contempt.[13]

The prestige of the medical profession was scarcely high at the end of the eighteenth century, and if any change occurred in the first half of the nineteenth century it was probably for the worse. Fortunately, many forces were at work to remedy this situation. The observations of perceptive physicians, the impact of the French Clinical School, the pressure from irregular sects, and developments on the broad front of advancing science were all helping to modify medical practices and pave the way for major strides in medicine. In America a rising demand among physicians for improvements in medical education and for a measure of professional unity led to the formation in 1847 of the American Medical Association. While the AMA remained comparatively ineffective during the nineteenth century, it was one of many factors that enabled medicine to achieve true professional status by the beginning of the twentieth century.

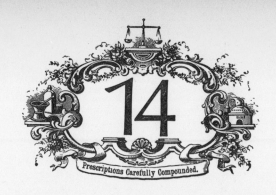

Prescriptions Carefully Compounded.

THE EMERGENCE
OF ORGANIZED
PUBLIC HEALTH

FROM earliest times communities have sought to promote the health and welfare of their members. Whether this involved observing taboos, performing rituals, sacrificing to the gods, or, as in the early twentieth-century fight against tuberculosis, rigidly enforcing the antispitting ordinances, the object was always to increase the general health and prosperity. And it is well to note that health and prosperity have always been associated. Although Western civilization had become infinitely more complex and had entered what has been termed the age of rationalism, the general attitude toward disease in the seventeenth and eighteenth centuries was not too far removed from that of men in primitive societies. Pestilences and other catastrophes were widely held to be punishments sent by God; and, without exception, every major epidemic resulted in the proclamation of days of fasting, humiliation, and prayer.

Yet the advent of variolation in the 1720s and the beginnings of sanitary reform in the late eighteenth century foreshadowed a new approach to human ills. The older concept of a wrathful God striking out at man for minor infringements of his laws gradually gave way to the belief that sickness resulted from man unwittingly breaking moral laws established by God or nature. Possibly influenced by the ideas of Lord Herbert and the Deists, who envisioned a mechanistic universe into which God had placed man after giving him the divine spark of intelligence or soul, the new approach held that man, through his intelligence, could learn the rules of nature and so move toward a more perfect society. In accordance with the nineteenth-century emphasis upon moral order, it was reasoned that sickness, disease, and poverty resulted from immorality; conversely health, wealth, and happiness were proof of one's adherence to the moral laws. It was this assumption which enabled a prominent New Yorker during the 1832 cholera outbreak to thank God that the disease remained almost "exclusively confined to the lower classes of intemperate, dissolute, or filthy people huddled together like swine in their polluted habitations." At the same time, a minister proclaimed that the epidemic was promoting "the cause of righteousness by sweeping away the obdurate and the incorrigible. . . ." A Special Medical Council appointed by the Board of Health during the outbreak lent its authority to this belief by asserting that the disease was confined "to the imprudent, the intemperate, and to those who injure themselves by taking improper medicines. . . ."[1]

Although many individuals adhered to the traditional concept of disease as a punishment from God, increasingly the blame for disease was attributed to the failure of the lower classes to observe the moral laws—personal cleanliness, temperance, hard work, thrift, and an orderly life. The proof was clear to every observer, for the chief victims of disease were invariably found among the dirty and intemperate poor crowded together in the filthy slums. The relative freedom of the middle and upper classes from cholera, typhoid, and other disorders served further to confirm the value of middle-class morality. It was this bland assumption of moral superiority which enabled the well-to-do to wash their hands of the lower classes in the early nineteenth century.

One other factor contributed to what now appears to have been a rather callous attitude on the part of social and political leaders. As noted in the first chapter, the American continent was hailed as pure, undefiled, and healthy, with its air, water, and native inhabitants free from the impurities and diseases of the Old World. Once the initial settlements had become firmly established, the average colonist began to enjoy better health and a higher economic status than his contemporaries in Europe. The endemic pestilences of Europe such as smallpox appeared only occasionally in the colonies; the food supply was both more plentiful and variegated; society was more fluid; and for the thrifty and hard working, economic opportunities were far greater. Americans have traditionally gloried in the seemingly boundless resources of their country and assumed that its rapid growth was based in part on the healthfulness of the environment. As public health historian Barbara Rosenkrantz has pointed out, even today health is regarded as indigenous to our soil and sickness and disease as alien.[2]

The events of the nineteenth century seemed to confirm this thesis. As immigrants began pouring into the major seaports and rural workers were drawn into urban areas, out of necessity they were forced to crowd into the older areas, for the rapidity of urban expansion meant that the construction of housing never kept pace with the influx of newcomers. In the crowded conditions which ensued, sanitary conditions rapidly deteriorated. Most newcomers to the cities, foreign or native, came from rural backgrounds where the sparsity of population enabled nature to take care of human wastes and garbage. They brought with them their rural customs of defecating and urinating wherever they happened to be, and in short order the slums became incredibly filthy. City administrations, too, were incapable of dealing with this massive influx of population and made virtually no provisions for adequate water supplies, decent food, or the removal of human wastes. Under these conditions, mortality rates began rising in American towns and cities during the first half of the nineteenth century and reached a peak around the Civil War years.

As indicated, few immigrants had any substantial resources and out of necessity they were forced into the worst housing. If they had not already been exposed to infectious disorders, they soon encountered smallpox, typhus, and a host of other contagions on their journey to the New World. Those who did not bring diseases with them could scarcely avoid infection in their new homes. Handicapped by language difficulties and often lacking any special training, immigrants were pushed into the lowest-paying jobs, adding economic woes to their many difficulties. Small wonder that their infant mortality rate was enormous, that endemic sicknesses abounded, and that every epidemic disease which swept through the cities wrought its greatest havoc among the crowded immigrant poor.

To comfortable middle-class Americans, the sight of these disease-ridden immigrants huddled together in almost indescribable conditions of dirt and degradation was proof that disease was largely an imported phenomena, one foreign to America. They overlooked the fact that cleanliness and personal hygiene were impossible for a family jammed into one room, who often shared a single well or water hydrant and one or two filthy privies with fifteen or twenty other families. They failed to realize, too, that alcohol offered almost the only escape from the bleakness of the slums, and that the intemperance of the lower classes was an inevitable result of the brutal degradation of their life. Since it was assumed disease and sickness resulted largely from the failure of the poor to obey the natural laws, the major health reform efforts were designed to raise moral standards. This also held true throughout the nineteenth century for the various philanthropic agencies seeking to help the economically depressed. Their solution to poverty was to attempt to teach the moral principles of temperance, hard work, and thrift. As with sickness and disease, poverty, too, was considered the fault of its victims—and this assumption had a long European tradition.

As the nineteenth century advanced and the sanitary movement gained strength, the reformers came to realize the role of environment in the poverty cycle. Pioneer health workers were the first to become aware of the association between sickness, debility, and poverty, and in promoting public health measures they appealed to the public on economic grounds. A healthy population was a productive one, and hence any public funds spent for health measures would repay the community many times. They were no longer content to attempt to reform the poor and sick as individuals but looked to social and sanitary engineers to devise laws and techniques to correct the social imbalance and to create a milieu favorable to health and its corollary, prosperity. By the end of the nineteenth century, the advent of bacteriology and major developments in sanitary engineering convinced many health leaders that the way was now open to abolish communicable diseases, poverty, and other social evils. The problems, as later generations were to discover, were not all that simple.

Whatever the prevailing attitude toward sickness and disease, the American people made a remarkably rapid recovery from the destruction and death of the Revolutionary War years. Despite some difficulties, the major cities experienced a large measure of prosperity and an equally great expansion. New York City, for example, which had suffered two major fires and several years of wartime attrition, expanded so rapidly in the postwar period that its reorganized city government was almost overwhelmed. Following the British evacuation of the city late in 1783, the population was reduced to about 12,000, yet by 1786 it had jumped to 23,614. Within another four years it was over 33,000. Even under normal circumstances it would have been difficult for civic leaders to have provided the necessary water, sewerage, and other facilities for such an influx, but neither New York political leaders nor any other civic officials at this time were conditioned to accept these responsibilities. The result was that New York City turned from a relatively quiet and clean colonial town into a large and dirty city by the end of the century.[3]

Typical of its day, New York in the 1790s had no sewerage or water system. The liquid matter from privies either drained into cesspools or else simply seeped into the ground. Solid waste was theoretically removed by scavengers, but on the occasions when privies were cleaned, the waste matter was usually dumped onto the closest river bank or into the nearest slip in the dock areas. Surface drainage was handled by open drains or kennels which flowed down the middle of the main streets. Street cleaning and garbage removal was left largely to individual householders, with the results which might be expected. The water was obtained from shallow wells located at street corners or else from venders who got it from a spring outside of the city known as the Tea Water Pump. The latter was located near a large body of water called Fresh Water Pond. Unfortunately by the 1790s the expanding city population was already encroaching on the Fresh Water Pond, and its water was becoming polluted. A newspaper correspondent complained in

1784 about nearby residents throwing "all their sudds and filth" into the pond along with "dead dogs, cats, &c. thrown in daily, and no doubt, many buckets [of human wastes] from that quarter of the town."[4]

It was this situation which led the city to attempt to provide a water system on the eve of the Revolution. A British engineer, Christopher Coles, obtained support from the City Council in 1774 to dig a deep well and pump water into the city through hollow logs. Before all the engineering problems could be solved, war broke out, and another quarter of a century elapsed before a water system was put into operation. Even then, chicanery on the part of Aaron Burr and his associates deprived New Yorkers of a good water supply for another forty-odd years.[5]

While conditions in New York were probably worse than in Boston, Philadelphia, and the other major towns, the general picture was much the same. Boston—which grew from about 16,000 residents before the Revolution to nearly 25,000 by 1800— was able to adjust to the expansion more easily, in part because housing construction nearly kept pace with the population influx. In addition, the city officials appear to have been more conscious of the need to keep the city in a sanitary condition. Local citizens were still responsible for sweeping the streets and cleaning the gutters in front of their homes, but the city appointed scavengers to enforce this regulation. The municipality also provided for the removal of garbage, either by impressing carters or else by hiring them, and by the early nineteenth century regular contracts were made for the removal of garbage. Although many complaints were made, visitors to Boston generally were impressed with the town's sanitary condition. One declared in 1818 that the streets "exhibit a degree of order and cleanliness which will in vain be looked for in New York." The state of the other large towns and cities tended to fall somewhere in between New York and Boston in the immediate postwar years. Philadelphia, the largest city and the first one to be ravaged by the wave of yellow fever outbreaks which began in the 1790s, promptly overhauled its sanitary regulations and followed the example of Boston rather than New York.[6]

Up until the twentieth century, the major preoccupation of medicine was how to treat what we would now term communicable diseases, and the exclusive concern of public health was how to deal

with the major epidemics. Familiar dangers hold little terror—
today for example, we accept an annual toll of 50,000 or 60,000
deaths and several hundred thousand casualties from automobile
accidents as a matter of course. So it was that in earlier days the loss
of 30 to 50 percent of children below the age of five from summer
fluxes, teething, convulsions, and related disorders and the many
fatalities among adults from fevers, fluxes, "pleurisies," "pneu-
monies," and cancers were viewed as the inevitable work of a
mysterious Providence. What could not be accepted so casually was
the disastrous and destructive impact of the great killer diseases—
yellow fever, smallpox, diphtheria, Asiatic cholera, and so forth.
These pestilences appeared in some unexplainable fashion, struck
indiscriminately, left permanent scars on some of their victims, and
brought death in a horrible fashion to many others. The degree of
fear they aroused was almost proportional to the infrequency of the
epidemics. Smallpox, which appeared only at long intervals for
much of the colonial period, and yellow fever, only an occasional
visitor, were the two disorders which struck the most terror in the
hearts of early Americans, although they rank well down the list as
causes of morbidity and mortality. Yet they illustrate perfectly the
qualities necessary to arouse public concern—they were mysterious, unfamiliar, caused intense suffering among their victims, and
proved highly fatal. Precisely as a result of these characteristics,
these two plagues were responsible for the earliest quarantine
measures and for the first comprehensive sanitary programs.

While temporary health boards, usually consisting of city
council members or selectmen, had been appointed during some of
the early colonial epidemics, the first impetus to the development of
more permanent city health agencies was given by the yellow fever
epidemics which ravaged American ports from Boston to New
Orleans in the years from 1793 to 1822. The disease had been
absent from North America since 1762 and was reintroduced in
1793 by a large influx of refugees fleeing from a revolution in Santo
Domingo. The disorder first gained a foothold in Philadelphia,
where the appearance of this strange and violent fever completely
mystified the local physicians. In August, however, Dr. Benjamin
Rush recollected an outbreak which had occurred when he was a
medical apprentice and diagnosed the disease as bilious yellow
fever. This news, along with the rapidly mounting toll of sickness

and death, spread consternation throughout the city. Many who could afford it immediately took flight; in the process, some of them carried the disease into neighboring areas. As news of Philadelphia's plight spread, barriers and quarantines were hastily erected by adjacent communities and towns. By the time cool fall weather brought an end to the outbreak, some 5,000 of the city's 55,000 inhabitants had died.[7]

While the Philadelphia outbreak was the worst one suffered by any American city during this period, several epidemics occurred in every major port and in many smaller ones. In almost every case the city government was disrupted and volunteer citizens' committees began assuming responsibility for public health and welfare. The first reaction of civic leaders to the threat or imminence of yellow fever was to institute rigid quarantine measures. The next one was to begin a massive sanitary campaign: gutters were cleaned; stagnant pools drained; garbage and offal removed from the streets; and slaughterers and other nuisance trades were pressured to keep their premises as clean as possible. Since major epidemics always brought normal economic activities to a halt, civic officials and voluntary groups were forced to make provision not only for the sick poor and their families but also for the vast numbers of workers temporarily unemployed.

Because public health is in effect the application on the community level of existing medical knowledge, the yellow fever outbreaks in these years were important also for their impact upon medical thought. Since neither the role of pathogenic organisms nor of insect vectors was understood, yellow fever was a completely strange and inexplicable disease. During the debates over its nature and cause, physicians and laymen divided into two major schools, one which believed the disease to be a separate and distinct entity imported from abroad, and a second which argued that yellow fever was simply a normal summer fever transformed by certain meteorological and environmental conditions into a pestilential disorder. These two opposing viewpoints were not new, but under the impact of the epidemics they hardened into schools of thought. As might be expected, the contagionists argued for strict quarantine measures to keep the disease out of the city, while the anticontagionists or sanitationists advocated elimination of the dirt, filth, and crowding which characterized the older waterfront areas.

The majority of physicians in this period tended to support the sanitationist argument. In the first place, the fever generally began in the crowded and dirty housing around the docks and slips. In the second place, the quarantine regulations did not appear effective, for, despite their most rigid enforcement, the disease seemingly overrode all barriers. For businessmen influenced by economic considerations, there was little choice between quarantine and sanitation. Quarantine measures bore heavily upon trade and commerce, and merchants and shippers could always be counted on to bitterly oppose them. On the other hand, a sanitary program required large expenditures of public funds, and the regulations placed some economic burden upon slaughterers, butchers, tanners, and all the other so-called nuisance trades. While the medical and economic arguments raged, the public never doubted the infectious nature of epidemic diseases, and the mass exodus from towns and cities precipitated by even rumors of a pestilential outbreak bore testimony to this fact. In light of what we know today, those citizens who fled from yellow fever in the 1790s were using admirable judgment.

With the question of the nature of yellow fever unsettled and the medical profession divided, the temporary health committees and health boards which sprang into existence at this time wisely elected to operate on both assumptions; hence they espoused both quarantine and sanitary measures. In glancing over the period from the Revolution to the Civil War, the story in most instances is one of belated precautions. Strong objections from commercial and shipping interests usually delayed the application of effective quarantine measures until too late, and the reluctance of city councilmen to vote funds for sanitary programs meant that little was done until the fever was already raging. Part of the problem lay in the temporary nature of existing health agencies. Local health boards or committees ordinarily were appointed in response to a specific epidemic or series of epidemics. These boards were expected to function only during the yellow fever season, and even in cities where permanent boards had been created by state laws, the members had to be reappointed every spring. If two or three years passed without a major epidemic, the tendency was to let the boards lapse into desuetude. This same situation also held true when Asiatic cholera began striking the United States in 1832.

Once the immediate danger was over, the health laws and agencies created in response to the outbreaks soon disappeared.

As has been shown, in nearly every city the initial action against yellow fever was taken by volunteer citizens groups. These groups were soon given official status or else were incorporated into an official health committee, and from these beginnings came the appointment of more permanent health officials. New York City is a fine case in point. When yellow fever struck Philadelphia in 1793, a citizens committee, fearing that the New York City Council was not taking firm enough protective measures, took upon itself the authority to hire two physicians to assist the local health officer in examining incoming vessels suspected of harboring disease. In addition, the committee stationed inspectors at all wharves and ferries to prevent the entrance of anyone coming from Philadelphia. When committee members conferred with the mayor and council, the latter legitimized the committee's activities and appointed an official seven-man committee to cooperate with the volunteer group. The following year the governor of the state formally appointed an official health committee consisting of the same volunteers and councilmen who had served the previous year.

While the chief function of the New York Health Committee was to strenghten the quarantine regulations, when an epidemic developed in 1795 the committee, in addition, assumed responsibility for the sick and the poor, took over Bellevue Hospital, and initiated a sanitary campaign. On the advice of this committee, in 1796 the Legislature created a permanent health office, consisting of a practicing physician as health officer and several health commissioners. The health office was primarily a quarantine agency, but the law creating it authorized the city to enact certain types of sanitary regulations. To provide for cooperation with the health office, the city council established a health committee of its own. Two years later the authority of the health office to make sanitary regulations was broadened.[8]

This same year, 1798, saw New York's worst yellow fever epidemic, one which killed some 2,000 people. As a result, a new state law in 1799 turned over all authority for handling sanitary matters to the city council and restricted the health office to quarantine activities. The city council promptly appointed from its own membership a health committee, and for a few years this body functioned exceedingly well. Aside from keeping a close watch over sanitary conditions, it provided medical care for the sick during epidemics and performed a wide range of welfare activities.

Recurrent yellow fever outbreaks during these years led to one further step in 1804, the establishment of the office of city inspector. The purpose of this office was to gather information about public nuisances and prepare tentative ordinances for removing or correcting these conditions. Subsequently the council instructed the city inspector to keep mortality records for the city and to establish a register of births and marriages. Under the direction of John Pintard, an able individual who set the pattern, this office made an excellent start, and, although limited in authority, power, and funds, for over half a century it proved quite effective in drawing attention to the steadily worsening health and social conditions.

The following year, 1805, the city decided that it needed a formal board of health and submitted to the state legislature a proposed law to this effect. The latter responded by enacting a measure in 1805 which created a city health board and gave to it all sanitary powers which had formally been invested in the health office. This new board consisted of the mayor, aldermen, and the commissioners of the health office (now strictly a quarantine agency). The board of health performed notably during the yellow fever outbreak of 1805, and it remained quite active for a year or two following. As the threat from the fever receded in the succeeding years, however, the board's efforts, along with its budget, gradually dwindled away. For example, in 1805 the city appropriated $8,500 for the health board, but by 1818 this figure was reduced to $900. A minor yellow fever epidemic in 1819 and another in 1822 temporarily revived the health board. Shortly after 1822 it again lapsed into inactivity until the advent of Asiatic cholera in 1832.

In surveying public health administration for New York City during the first sixty-five years of the nineteenth century one can see that three agencies were involved. The first and oldest was the health office, essentially a quarantine establishment under control of the state. The second was the City Inspector's Office, an agency designed to gather statistics—but one which later assumed considerable supervision over sanitary matters. The third was the board of health, established in 1805 and consisting primarily of the mayor and city council acting in a health capacity. It was intended to function only in the event of a major epidemic or other health emergency, and under normal conditions its duties were nominal. Since the health office was supported by fees collected from incoming vessels and provided its officers with a rather handsome income, the quarantine system was relatively effective for its day. The City Inspector's Office had little power for most of the period, but in the hands of capable men it often proved an effective gadfly. In the midcentury, however, it was given charge of street cleaning. Unfortunately, instead of reforming the sanitation department, the City Inspector's Office itself became corrupted. In summary the brave start made in health administration during the yellow fever epidemics soon came to nought. The only agency which might have attempted to deal with the ever-worsening slum conditions and the rising morbidity and mortality rates, the board of health, remained a minor and insignificant body. By the midcentury conditions had grown so bad that they led to a new sanitary reform movement, but it took another fifteen years or more of agitation before the city obtained an effective health department.

Possibly as a result of Boston's more homogenous population and a slower rate of increase, that city's officials reacted with a relatively high sense of civic responsibility during the yellow fever epidemics. When the initial outbreak occurred in Philadelphia, the Boston selectmen began enforcing fairly rigid quarantine restrictions and taking measures to improve sanitary conditions. In this they had the backing of the governor and the General Court or state legislature. In 1797 the General Court authorized towns to appoint health officers or health boards whose duty it was to attend to sanitary matters. Boston contented itself with simply designating its selectmen as a health board, until a serious yellow fever outbreak in 1798 led a citizens committee to urge the establishment of an elected health board. The General Court passed the necessary legislation, and in March 1799 a twelve-member board, one man from each ward, was elected. Significantly, not one physican was chosen to serve on the board.

The board of health, whose members were unpaid, was given broad powers over quarantine and sanitation; and it was not averse to using them in emergency situations. It enforced a rigid quarantine against both yellow fever and smallpox, and gradually extended its jurisdiction into many areas of concern to the sanitationists. The board also kept careful watch on the markets, the nuisance trades (slaughtering and so forth), the condition of the streets, and the removal of human wastes. As early as 1807 it recognized the need for sewers and cautiously moved into the construction of a sewerage system. Believing that the city's graveyards were a source of contamination, the board obtained full authority over them in 1810, and then used this power to insist that the sextons make weekly reports on burials. In consequence the board was able to start publishing bills of mortality.[9]

As the century advanced, Boston began to face the problems arising from mass immigration and too rapid growth and consequently was not able to maintain its excellent health record. In 1841 Lemuel Shattuck, an outstanding health pioneer, showed that during the previous twenty years the mortality rate in Boston had increased. The situation did not improve in the succeeding years, for the great wave of impoverished Irish which deluged every American city after 1845 drastically changed social conditions for the worse. The classic work commissioned by a Massachusetts State legislative committee and published under the title, *Report of the Sanitary Commission of Massachusetts, 1850,* was largely the work of Shattuck. In it he pointed out that from 1845 to 1849 some 125,000 newcomers were added to the Boston population, making enforcement of health regulations virtually impossible.[10]

In summary, one can say that nearly every major city or town in the United States, under the threat of or presence of epidemic disease, appointed one or more temporary health boards in the years between the Revolution and the Civil War. These boards, with an occasional exception, were considered emergency bodies. Even the more permanent ones only served during the summer months when the threat from pestilential fevers was greatest. Their major concern was quarantine, and, omitting the Boston Board of Health and the City Inspector's Office in New York, the only permanent officials appointed during these years were the quarantine officers. All of the boards urged sanitary precautions, but, although under the immediate threat of an epidemic they often succeeded in temporarily eliminating the worst sanitary abuses, they were unable to affect any major changes. The boards were largely advisory, and without the backing of the city council, which they seldom received, they could accomplish little in the way of sanitary reform. As cities grew larger, social problems multiplied, and municipal governments became more inefficient, the health reformers increasingly found themselves to be voices crying in the wilderness.

As already noted, the grave health and social problems of the cities were compounded in the midcentury by the Irish potato famine and the large-scale migration from the German states. The impoverished Irish migrants, suffering from malnutrition and diseases, were unloaded by the thousands into every American port city from Boston to New Orleans. The resident poor were already jammed into dilapidated older buildings, and the influx of thousands of destitute immigrants created tenement conditions almost defying description. Shattuck noted in Boston that, whereas the average single dwelling held eleven persons in 1845, by 1850 there were parts of town in which the average had jumped to thirty-seven. Only two or three cities had any kind of decent water system, and even in these the best that the lower-income groups could hope for was one hydrant for every fifteen families. No city had a sewerage system worthy of the name, and the reek of overflowing privies in the impoverished sections must have been beyond imagination. Adding to the foul atmosphere were the dairies, stables, manure piles, and heaps of garbage scattered through the towns. Butchers and slaughterers frequently let blood flow into the gutters and simply piled offal and hides on vacant ground next to their places of business. Tanners and fat- and bone-boilers gathered offal and hides in open wagons, thus adding further to the already pungent city aromas. Rivers, creeks, streams, and brooks flowing through the cities had all become open sewers by midcentury. Shallow wells, which still supplied most city-dwellers with water, were polluted beyond redemption. The wonder is not that mortality rates were soaring but that so many of the poor survived.[11]

The decade of the 1850s was a prosperous one for America, although the shadow of the approaching sectional conflict was lengthening. It was also a period that witnessed the second great wave of Asiatic cholera and a series of major yellow fever outbreaks. New Orleans alone lost between 15,000 and 20,000 residents to yellow fever in this decade, and the disorder ravaged every port city in the South and swept far up the Mississippi Valley and the other navigable southern rivers. Public-spirited citizens and civic leaders were already becoming aware of the need for sanitary measures, and the two epidemic diseases forced every city to establish at least temporary health boards. While yellow fever was primarily a disease of the South, Boston, New York, Philadelphia, and other northern ports remembered only too well the earlier devastating outbreaks, and the growing intensity of the yellow fever attacks on the South created general fear and alarm. Without doubt, it was the ever-present danger from epidemic disease which led to the first attempt to establish a national public health organization.

With health reformers increasing their ranks and the AMA's Committee on Public Hygiene having demonstrated that the basic causes of the rising mortality and morbidity rates were common to all urban areas, it was only a matter of time before someone took the initiative to organize a national meeting. The advocates of quarantine were particularly distressed by the wide diversity of quarantine regulations, and they hoped to standardize procedures. The proponents of sanitation saw in a national meeting a chance to promote their own theory of disease causation and an opportunity to exchange ideas and information. In addition, the failure of the AMA to take leadership in promoting public health showed the need for a separate public health organization. A general feeling developed that—since sanitation was largely a matter of engineering—the way to improved public health lay in the joint work of social-minded laymen and physicians.

The first to take action in this respect was Dr. Wilson Jewell of Philadelphia, a city which had maintained a fairly respectable record on the score of public health. Jewell persuaded the Philadelphia board of health in 1856 to sponsor a national convention the following year to discuss quarantine problems; some seventy-three delegates from nine states, the majority of whom were physicians, attended the meeting held in Philadelphia in May 1857.[12]

True to its purpose, the meeting first concerned itself with deciding whether or not disorders could be imported. The delegates agreed that smallpox clearly fell into this category, but they were not so sure about typhus, cholera, and yellow fever. After considerable debate, a consensus was reached that under certain conditions they could be introduced by incoming vessels. Foreshadowing the direction the future sanitary conventions would take, the delegates declared that these latter disorders could not become epidemic "unless there exist in the community the circumstances which are calculated to produce such disease independent of the importation." Nonetheless, the contagionist faction at this first meeting was clearly in the majority, and resolutions by the anticontagionists to the effect that quarantine measures were not enough to protect a community were sidetracked.

The second meeting was held in Baltimore in 1858 for the purpose of drafting a uniform code of quarantine laws. While the emphasis was still placed upon quarantine, its proponents were obviously on the defensive, the minutes showing a rising concern with what was termed "internal hygiene" and a lessening of interest in "external hygiene" or quarantine. Furthermore, the quarantine advocates were at a disadvantage, since the major epidemic disease under consideration was yellow fever. Although unable to account for its transmission, most southern physicians did recognize that it was not communicated directly from person to person.

By the third meeting, held in New York, the sanitationists were gaining the upper hand, and they succeeded in drafting a general sanitary code for cities. The final meeting assembled in Boston in 1860 with the sanitationists firmly in control. As might be expected, they proceeded to lay out a broad program of their own. The Convention also called for scientific studies on the subjects of sewage, ventilation, and disinfectants; and it urged the formation of local sanitary associations—volunteer groups of physicians and laymen working together to remedy the worst sanitary abuses. The prime example for the delegates was the Sanitary Association of New York City, a group established in the mid-1850s. Its original purpose was to fight for cleaner streets and to eliminate corruption in the City Inspector's Office, the municipal agency in charge of sanitation. By the late 1850s a successor to this organization had joined with the New York Academy of Medicine and other associations in support of a comprehensive public health program, one which involved improving the milk supply, housing conditions, drainage and sewerage, and establishing a separate department of health.[13]

Filled with enthusiasm for their cause, the delegates decided to establish a permanent organization and appointed a committee to draw up a plan for submission at the next meeting to be held in Cincinnati the following year. Seemingly oblivious to the bitter division within the country, when the presiding officer at the last session, Mayor Richard Arnold of Savannah, thanked the Boston representatives for their hospitality, the New England delegates responded with three cheers for Georgia![14] Yet the evidence of dissension was all too clear; Louisiana, which had played an active role in the first two conventions, did not send a single delegate to the last two. Before the proposed Cincinnati meeting could assemble, the outbreak of civil war ended any hope for a national public health organization. While health leaders were able to accomplish little during the immediate prewar years, the sanitary movement was gathering the momentum which would sweep away many of the worst sanitary abuses in the postwar years and prepare the way for permanent state and local health agencies.

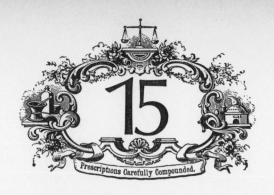

Prescriptions Carefully Compounded.

MILITARY MEDICINE:
THE CIVIL WAR

I N the 200 years of its history the bloodiest loss inflicted on America resulted from the Civil War. This fratricidal struggle caused more casualties than any other military clash between the Napoleonic period and World War I and killed more Americans than any war to date. Over 600,000 American soldiers died from battle wounds, disease, or accidents during the four years of fighting. In the course of the war, the Union Army enlisted about 2,900,000 men and its peak strength stood at 2,100,000. The Confederate enlistments are estimated at between 1,300,000 and 1,400,000. Because of short-term enlistments and thousands of deserters, the strength of the armies varied considerably throughout the war. The records of the Confederacy were destroyed in the burning of Richmond, and any statistics on troops and casualties are at best educated guesses. Dr. Joseph Jones, an indefatigable Confederate Medical Inspector who kept voluminous records, estimated that more than 600,000 men fought on the Confederate side, and that of these some 200,000 were either killed or died of battle wounds and disease. He believed that the ratio of battle deaths to those from disease was roughly one to three: *i.e.*, 50,000 deaths from battle injuries to 150,000 from sickness and disease. The ratio for the Union forces, which were better fed, clothed, and housed, was approximately one to two: 110,000 deaths from battle and 225,000 from disease.

The bitterness of the fighting can readily be seen from the casualty figures. One North Carolina regiment lost 708 men or 85 percent of its strength at the Battle of Gettysburg, and some 63 Union regiments suffered casualties of more than 50 percent of their strength in single engagements. Neither the celebrated Charge of the Light Brigade nor any single battle in World War I caused relative losses comparable to those of the Civil War engagements. Grim as the battle statistics are, the troops faced an even greater threat from sickness. Dr. Jones estimated that each of the Confederate soldiers fell sick about six times during the course of the war. The Union records show over 6,000,000 cases of disease, well over two per soldier. These figures probably underestimate the true number of illnesses, since the widespread distrust of doctors and the incompetence of many army surgeons made soldiers reluctant to report to the medical officer. The common fear of hospitals, and army hospitals in particular, also inclined the men to take care of their own sick. Moreover, on both sides it was not uncommon for the sick to simply go home, a practice which scarcely contributed to the accuracy of the morbidity and mortality reports.

Despite the rising tension, the Federal government and the Confederate States were unprepared for war when the final break came—and both sides were handicapped by the confident thought that victory was merely a few months away. The United States began the war with a handful of military surgeons. As of January 1861 the Army had a total strength of 16,000 men, and a medical staff consisting of a Surgeon General, 30 surgeons, and 83 assistant surgeons. Of these, 8 surgeons and 29 assistant surgeons either resigned to join the Confederate Army or else elected to remain in the South. At the outbreak of hostilities, the entire United States Army Medical Department consisted of slightly less than 100 men. The Confederacy had to start its Medical Department from scratch with a handful of former army surgeons as a base. As it turned out, this proved advantageous since its Medical Department was not handicapped by the red tape and inertia engendered in a peacetime army. Neither side had any experience with mobilizing large bodies of men, and the early army camps were characterized by chaos and confusion. Regiments mobilized by various towns and cities were sent to army camps and military centers only to find no provision had been made for housing or food; some regiments arrived with a surgeon but no medical supplies; and others arrived with neither. To make matters worse, the vast majority of those recruited were young men from rural areas (almost half of the Union troops listed farming as their occupation) where they had experienced little contact with the so-called childhood diseases—measles, mumps, chickenpox, whooping cough, scarlet fever, and diphtheria. The result was that these disorders—measles in particular—spread like wildfire through the army camps in both North and South. In addition, many of the recruits had not been vaccinated, leading to repeated outbreaks of smallpox. The crude vaccination techniques resorted to under army conditions aggravated the situation by transmitting serious bacterial and other infections along with the vaccine matter. Added to these woes were the disorders incident to exposure, poor food, and the incredibly bad sanitary conditions in the camps.

Enough has been said about the level of medical education and the state of medicine in the preceding chapters. One can only add that the army surgeons represented a cross-section of American medicine, ranging from very able individuals to virtual quacks. Most of them had served an apprenticeship and spent some months in a medical school, and sick soldiers received at least as good medical attention as they would have had in civilian life. The major lack was experience with gunshot wounds and trauma. Few of the physicians recruited by the army were qualified as surgeons, and many of them gained their first surgical experience under battle conditions. The Union Medical Department was handicapped during the early war years by a penny-pinching attitude on the part of Congress. The atrocious conditions experienced by the wounded in the first bloody battles were fully reported, and it is difficult to say why Congress took this attitude, but in the early years it consistently reduced requests for appropriations to enlarge the medical staff, provide supplies, and establish an ambulance corps. Undoubtedly the universal distrust of the medical profession played some role in this, although it does not seem to have affected the Confederate government. The attitude of the Federal legislators is all the more surprising in view of the willingness of the Confederate government to comply with requests from its Surgeon General. Unfortunately, while the Confederacy was more generous, it simply did not have the vast resources open to the Federal government.

Reference has already been made to the conservatism and petty-mindedness which characterized the Army Medical Department at the outbreak of the fighting. The Surgeon General was Colonel Thomas Lawson, a veteran of the War of 1812 already in his eighties, whose major interest for many years had been to reduce his departmental budget. It was typical of his thinking that he considered medical books an extravagance. His parsimony was matched by Congress, which, with tension obviously close to the breaking point, voted only $115,000 for the Medical Department in March 1861. Lawson died a few weeks after the opening of hostilities only to be replaced by another aged veteran of the seniority system, Clement A. Finlay, whose army career dated back to 1818. He, too, had spent a lifetime making do with as little as possible, and he could not bring himself to ask for the budget and staff necessary to fight a major war. Like his predecessor, he was imbued with the army's traditional emphasis upon seniority and the rituals of peacetime life, and he simply could not cope with an emergency situation. More important, as a military professional he was sensitive to civilian interference and consistently opposed the activities of the United States Sanitary Commission, a civilian group concerned with the health and welfare of the troops. This opposition led to his downfall, although he helped it along by some rather foolish actions. By December 1861 the disorganization and inadequacies of the Army Medical Department were all too obvious. The Sanitary Commission, capitalizing on the growing dissatisfaction, pressured Congress into a reorganization, and in April 1862 Finlay was removed from office.[1]

The United States Sanitary Commission originated with two prominent New York reformers, Dr. Elisha Harris, a significant public health figure, and the Reverend Henry W. Bellows, a well-known Unitarian minister, but the real impulse came from the thousands of women who were anxious to emulate the work of Florence Nightingale and her cohorts in the Crimean War. In countless towns and cities Ladies' Aid Societies and similar groups were springing into existence, and Harris and Bellows sought to coordinate their efforts. The first meeting was held in the Cooper Union in New York, following which the group formally asked the Surgeon General how it could help. The association's request was dismissed with a statement that everything was fine and no help was needed. A delegation was then sent to Washington where it found the army in a virtual state of chaos. Remembering the almost unbelievable lack of proper sanitary conditions which had characterized the Crimean War, the delegation requested the government to establish an official Sanitary Commission. Despite considerable skepticism on the part of every official all the way to President Lincoln, the United States Sanitary Commission came into official existence on June 13, 1861. It consisted of twelve members: nine civilians and three army men. Fortunately, the military members were so preoccupied with their own duties that they left the operation of the Commission to the civilian members, all of whom were outstanding individuals. The Commission's original purpose was to investigate and to recommend, but under the leadership of its able secretary, Frederick Law Olmsted, it took a far more active role.[2]

The first task of the Sanitary Commission was to fight for sanitary reform. The undisciplined recruits flooding into the Washington area proceeded to befoul their camps in an incredible fashion, and the poorly organized and understaffed hospitals were often in a similar state. One of the Commission's first actions was to print and distribute pamphlets to officers and enlisted men stressing the need for sanitary measures. In general the Army cooperated in the sanitary program, although the degree of cooperation depended largely upon the individual commanders; nonetheless, it took a long educational process before the troops could (a) be required to build latrines, and (b) be forced to use them. In the meantime diarrheas and dysenteries continued to rage among them. Recognizing the inadequacy of Army rations, the Commission collected tons of fresh meat, fruits, and vegetables. It provided thousands of blankets and other supplies, and was a major agency in improving living conditions for the troops and providing care for the sick and injured.

In addition to the Sanitary Commission which operated out of Washington, virtually every town or city had its own committee whose major concern was the welfare of troops from the local area. For example, in June 1862 the Pittsburgh Sanitary Committee sent a delegation of nurses and surgeons to Washington to check on medical care and hospital facilities. The delegates reported that the sick and wounded were receiving good medical attention and that the letters, tobacco, and other items sent to Pittsburgh soldiers had been distributed. Following the Battle of Gettysburg the same Committee posted notices calling on surgeons in Pittsburgh and vicinity "to volunteer their services to visit the fields of the late battles in Pennsylvania, to attend to the wounded." According to the local paper, thirty-four physicians and surgeons promptly reported for duty. The Committee also appealed to authorities to allow wounded Pennsylvania soldiers to be returned to Pittsburgh for treatment. Throughout the war years the national Sanitary Commission continued to receive strong public support and the backing of newspapers. In January 1864 the New York *Times* declared: "No individual— man, woman or child— in all classes of society that have a single luxury, should suffer this winter to pass without contributing something to the great agency for supplying the wants of the army— the Sanitary Commission."[3]

Probably the Sanitary Commission's greatest contribution was the steady pressure for reform it exerted upon the Army Medical Department, the Quartermaster Corps, and other Army departments. It had direct contact with the Secretary of War, and its members could bring political influence to bear upon Congress. It shares a good deal of the credit for the various Congressional measures reorganizing the Medical Department, and the Commission was largely responsible for the appointment of Dr. William A. Hammond to replace Surgeon General Finlay on April 25, 1862. Hammond had served as an Army surgeon for eleven years and had compiled an outstanding record before resigning his commission to accept a professorship at the University of Maryland. Upon the outbreak of war, he reenlisted and, in accordance with the seniority system, found himself at the bottom of the list of assistant surgeons. Fortunately, he came to the attention of the Commission at a time when they were looking for a younger man to head the Army Medical Department.

Hammond promptly appointed a number of able medical directors and instructed them to get the job done, disregarding traditional procedures when necessary. He pressed Congress to enlarge the Medical Department, to create a special hospital and ambulance corps, to raise the rank and pay of surgeons, to establish a medical school, and to place ambulances, medical supplies, and hospital construction under control of the Surgeon General's Office. Congress was in no mood to spend the taxpayer's money on the Medical Department and contented itself with adding about 300 surgeons and assistant surgeons. The proposals for a medical school, a hospital, and an ambulance corps were undercut by opposition from within the Army and from Secretary of War Stanton. Over and above the drastic changes he wrought in the Medical Department, Hammond deserves credit for introducing "ridge ventilation" into the army hospitals, a design guaranteeing a constant flow of fresh air into hospital wards. Hammond also introduced the pavilion hospital. Each structure involved a central unit with wings extending in various directions, thus permitting the segregation of patients according to their medical problems.

While Hammond was fighting for major changes, the medical directors he had appointed were busily straightening out affairs in their respective areas. Jonathan Letterman, one of the most able, reorganized his entire department and created an effective ambulance service for the Army of the Potomac. Hammond's energetic and drastic overhauling of the Army Medical Department outraged too many old hands, and in fighting for needed reforms he soon came into conflict with Secretary of War Stanton. Moreover, Hammond was no diplomat, and his manner irritated many of his subordinates, as well as his superiors. Among his reforms, Hammond had revised the army supply table, but he took one further step—which brought down upon him the wrath of most of his surgeons. In May 1863 Hammond sent out a circular removing calomel and tartar emetic from the supply table. Calomel (mercurous chloride), one of the most widely used drugs, was relied upon both to clean out the bowels and as a general stimulant. Its excessive administration was responsible for a vast amount of acute and chronic mercurial poisoning, and Hammond's action was correct from a medical standpoint. The same holds true with respect to tartar emetic, another dangerous medicine frequently relied upon to remove the so-called poisons from the stomach. Whatever the merit of his circular, it flew into the face of medical tradition and immeasurably added to his unpopularity. The cumulative effect of his actions resulted in his removal from office in November 1863 and his subsequent court-martial for ungentlemanly conduct. By this date his major reforms had taken effect and the able men he had appointed carried the Medical Department through the war. He was replaced by Dr. Joseph K. Barnes. While the latter made no major innovations, he continued the work started by Hammond and performed creditably for the rest of the war years. The example of what had happened to Hammond did not encourage intelligent and aggressive young surgeons to remain in the service, with the result that at the end of the fighting the Medical Department lapsed into its former state of apathy.

The physicians and surgeons who served in the Medical Department fell into four main categories: regular army surgeons and assistant surgeons who were used primarily for staff work; volunteer surgeons and assistant surgeons who were given temporary commissions in the regular army and performed staff duty; regimental surgeons and assistant surgeons commissioned by state governors; and acting assistant surgeons or "contract surgeons," civilians employed by the army largely for general hospital work. With the regular army officers engaged in staff work, medical and surgical care was provided primarily by the regimental surgeons in the field and contract surgeons in the general hospitals. When the first call for volunteers was issued, each regiment was expected to bring one assistant surgeon. The realities of war eventually raised the ratio to a surgeon and two assistant surgeons for each regiment. Theoretically medical commissions were issued by state governors, but in practice most medical officers were chosen by the senior regimental officer. With politics and personal favoritism playing a major role in the selection of regimental surgeons, their quality varied widely. Some states, such as Ohio, Vermont, and Massachusetts, immediately provided examining boards and culled out the most incompetent, but these states were scarcely typical. As the war progressed, however, Army medical examining boards assisted in winnowing the worst of the political appointees and the caliber of surgeons improved. Unfortunately, increasing casualties and unusual demands for medical care created a serious shortage of doctors, forcing a relaxation of the more stringent examining board standards.

For troops wounded in early battles the lack of coordination between the regimental and regular army surgeons, the want of an ambulance system, and the inadequate field hospitals was sheer disaster. At the Battle of Bull Run, or Manassas, in July 1861 the regular army surgeons found themselves unable to exercise authority over the regimental surgeons. To make matters worse, many of the latter assumed that their sole responsibility was to care for men of their own regiments. The civilians hired as ambulance drivers led the retreat and most of the wounded were left lying on the battlefield, some of whom received no medical attention for three days. The situation slowly improved—but not before Second Manassas, when it took a week to clear the field of dead and wounded. The horror and suffering stemming from this bloody battle led Hammond to urge the formation of an ambulance corps, but his appeal was turned down by Commander-in-Chief Henry W. Halleck and the Secretary of War. Fortunately, General George B. McClellan of the Army of the Potomac allowed his Medical Director, Jonathan Letterman, to organize an effective ambulance service which eventually set the pattern for the entire United States Army. Letterman's effective field hospital reorganization and ambulance service functioned fairly well at Antietam (September 1862), and proved its worth at the Battle of Gettysburg (July 1863), where the wounded were removed from the field at the end of each day's fighting. It had taken two years of blundering, bloodshed, and needless suffering, but the Union Army had evolved an effective medical service by this date.[4]

The Confederate Medical Department had two initial advantages. As mentioned earlier, it was a new organization relatively unhindered by custom, tradition, and deadwood. Moreover, almost from the outset it was directed by an intelligent and capable Surgeon General, Dr. Samuel Preston Moore. A second advantage came from the southern victories in the early years of the fighting. By remaining in control of the battlefield, the lack of ambulances was not so acute a problem as was true of the Union Army. On the other hand, the South was always short of transport, both vehicles and animals, and the situation steadily darkened as the war drew on. Once the South had established a system of field, divisional, and general hospitals, its interior lines of communication made possible a greater use of railways for transporting the wounded. The southern railroad system, however, was inadequate for the strains imposed by war, and, as the war progressed, the loss of equipment and the breakdowns caused by excessive use nullified this advantage. Moreover, as the northern armies closed in on the South during the last two years, the medical service was forced repeatedly to relocate its hospitals, straining transport almost to the breaking point.

Surgeon General Moore began building his medical organization immediately upon taking charge. Whereas the Union Army relied largely upon state-appointed regimental surgeons, the Confederate government directly commissioned its approximately 5,800 medical officers.[5] Medical examining boards interviewed all candidates from the beginning, thus keeping the number of incompetents to a minimum. With the exception of a few schools in Virginia, South Carolina, and Louisiana, the South did not have many high-caliber medical colleges, and the average southern practitioner was not as well educated as his counterpart in the North. The situation was aggravated when, in the first wave of enthusiasm for the southern cause, medical colleges were literally depopulated as students and faculty members enlisted in the Confederate forces. Only one school, the Medical College of Virginia, managed to keep its doors open after March of 1862.

As with the Union forces, the first year or so witnessed a great deal of confusion and mismanagement, but the South was quicker to organize a system of field, divisional, and general hospitals. Reflecting the state rights viewpoint, the Confederate Congress in September of 1862 provided that general hospitals be designated according to states, and that when possible the sick and wounded should be sent to those institutions representing their own state. The following year the Confederacy established a number of "way hospitals." These institutions were located along the routes of major railroads and were designed to furnish quarters and rations for troops on their way home who had been either furloughed or discharged because of sickness or wounds.

Surgeon General Moore shared with his northern counterpart,

Hammond, the ability to pick able subordinates. His best appointment was to make Dr. Samuel H. Stout the superintendent of hospitals in the Department of Tennessee. Stout demonstrated the same initiative and executive ability in the Army of Tennessee that Letterman did for the Army of the Potomac. Under Stout's administration, hospital sites were carefully selected and the operations closely observed. In addition, he improved the design of pavilion-type hospitals, made effective use of temporary facilities, and anticipated the possibility that his hospitals would have to be moved. In the face of manpower shortages and a crippled transportation system, Stout managed to withdraw the sick and wounded in an orderly fashion and to arrange facilities to receive them during the long retreat.

The South experienced many of the difficulties which beset the Union Army during the first stages of the war, but, as with the North, it learned by experience. Southern troops were plagued by measles and the other crowd diseases; they were at least as reluctant as northern soldiers to observe sanitary regulations; and they were probably even less amenable to discipline than those from the North. Yet they were fighting for the most part on their own soil, and southern civilians rallied to their support. Local residents often flocked to the temporary hospitals to assist in caring for the sick and wounded, and the Medical Department performed wonders with makeshift facilities. There were justifiable complaints against particular surgeons and certain hospitals, but, once the medical service was organized, it provided as good a care as might be expected.

As indicated, both sides suffered heavily from diseases, and the first year or so saw widespread outbreaks of disorders normally associated with childhood. In 1863 Dr. Joseph J. Woodward of the Union Army referred to measles as one "of the most characteristic diseases of the present war. . . ." He wrote that the official returns greatly underestimated the number of cases and fatalities, since many occurred while the regiments were mobilizing in the states, and that, even after the regiments became part of the regular army, some months elapsed before the regimental surgeons began submitting reports on the sick and wounded. Nonetheless, 21,676 measles cases and 551 deaths were reported in the Union forces during the first year of war. This figure of 551 deaths, however, does not include the many deaths resulting indirectly from measles which were attributed to other causes.[6]

Once the ill-disciplined troops were collected in camps, major sanitary problems emerged—and with them came diarrhea, dysentery, typhoid fever, and a host of gastroenteric complaints. Diarrhea and dysentery were the most common disorders. With a mean strength of 281,000 men, the Union Army recorded 215,214 cases during 1861–62. In citing these figures, Dr. Woodward warned that, while only 1,194 deaths were listed, the actual number was considerably more, since in addition to those dying of subsequent diseases, many extremely sick individuals whose cases probably terminated fatally were given medical discharges. Typhoid, which had been relatively rare in the peacetime army, rose to major proportions in the crowded and unsanitary camps. Approximately 8 percent of all Federal troops suffered an attack during 1861–62, and this figure does not include the thousands of unreported cases nor the large number that was listed under the heading of "typho-malarial fever."

As the war progressed and the troops pushed further into the South, the incidence of malaria rose sharply, disabling and debilitating thousands of men and combining with other diseases to hasten the deaths of many more. Without laboratories to make positive diagnoses, it was difficult for physicians to differentiate between the various fevers. Even for a patient suffering from only one disease, it was not easy to identify the cause purely on the basis of symptoms. In most cases, however, the problem was complicated by a multiplicity of complaints. With bacillary and amoebic dysentery, typhoid, and malaria widespread, multiple infections were common. To complicate the picture further, scurvy in a mild form affected a high percentage of the sick. This latter disorder was of little consequence according to the official records, but a Union surgeon expressed the views of many of his colleagues when he asserted that "both as a distinct affection in its early stages, and as a complicating influence, affecting the other camp diseases of the army, scurvy has hitherto played a large part in the phenomena of disease. . . ." Under these circumstances, it is easy to see why a syndrome broadly classified as typho-malarial fever was considered the major disease throughout the war. The fever was described as one in which "the great majority of cases [show] the well-marked enteric symptoms . . . complicated by malarial and scorbutic phenomena. . . ." These patients obviously suffered from all three or any combination of two of the diseases mentioned— and they may well have had other complications.[7]

It was inevitable that recruits housed in poorly built army camps or tents and constantly subject to exposure would experience a high percentage of respiratory ailments. Almost half of the Union Army was affected during the first year, and respiratory disorders continued to plague the armies throughout the war. Pneumonia was *a* or *the* chief killer, with a case fatality rate of about 20 percent. In addition to respiratory complaints, a vast number of acute and chronic rheumatism and lumbago cases were also recorded. While seldom fatal, these illnesses were responsible for thousands of medical discharges. An analysis by a Union surgeon showed that the majority of patients in this category suffered from either malaria or scurvy complicated by lower back pains. The nominal physical examinations administered to recruits probably allowed many individuals with lower back problems and older men suffering from arthritic or rheumatic conditions to enter the army, and the exposure during military campaigns undoubtedly contributed to their incidence among all age groups.

The diseases which attacked the Union Army bore even more heavily upon the Confederate forces. Many more of the Union troops came from urban areas where they had already encountered measles, mumps, and so forth, whereas the South recruited its forces largely from relatively isolated rural areas. The better-educated recruits from northern cities were also more inclined to recognize the necessity for sanitary regulations and to practice both personal and public hygiene. Furthermore, the Union forces had the advantage of better clothing, housing, and food— factors which guaranteed a higher resistance to infections. The greater susceptibility of southern troops to communicable diseases was evident from the beginning. Measles, one of the first epidemics to plague the northern armies, had a devastating effect upon newly organized southern regiments. One surgeon reported that during a five-month tour of duty in a basic training center he saw 4,000 cases of measles among the 5,000 men. Another southern observer claimed that measles and its sequelae caused more deaths and sickness than any other single cause.[8]

In the warmer climate of the South, enteric infections tended to be both more common and more virulent, and diarrhea and dysentery affected the soldiers from the first mobilization and continued to sicken and debilitate them throughout the entire war. Typhoid had not been too serious a problem in the South prior to the war, although it was becoming more common, but the crowded and unsanitary conditions in the army camps provided it with a perfect environment. Diarrhea is symptomatic of so many ailments, including scurvy, that it is virtually impossible to differentiate between the various enteric disorders attacking the southern troops. Certainly bacillary and amoebic dysentery and typhoid were major medical problems, but it is also true that dietetic disorders and poorly cooked food contributed to much of the diarrhea. For example, an epidemic of dysentery was stopped in one instance when the troops helped themselves to some green corn, and several shrewd observers blamed much of the gastroenteritic problems of the southern soldiers upon their exclusive reliance on the frying pan.

Malaria was endemic throughout much of the South and was the most common of the so-called fevers to plague the soldiers. Although the value of quinine in remittent and intermittent fevers was recognized, for lack of a detailed knowledge of the malarial parasite the drug was used to alleviate the symptoms rather than to eliminate the disease. Moreover, the abundance of mosquitoes insured constant reinfection. Along with enteric disorders and malaria, respiratory infections bore heavily upon the southern troops. Under normal conditions, the South did not experience as much morbidity or mortality from respiratory disorders as was true of the northern states. During the war, however, the poorly clad and ill-fed southern troops apparently suffered more than was the case with Union soldiers.

The Civil War was fought shortly before major breakthroughs in bacteriology explained the cause and nature of infectious diseases, and, although physicians recognized the value of public and personal hygiene in preventing disease, the treatment they accorded patients was only slightly improved over that of the American Revolution. Insofar as surgery was concerned, major strides had been taken in the pre-Civil War years, and a gigantic advance had been made with the discovery of chemical anesthesia.

By making possible longer and more complicated operations, anesthesia was responsible for a vast increase in gangrene and other hospital infections. First-rate surgeons found themselves torn between the wish to intervene surgically and the fear of postoperative infection. These qualms were set aside by the war, since bullet-torn bodies left no alternative but to do surgical repair.

Aside from dealing with occasional cases of trauma, lancing boils, and pulling teeth, the average doctor prior to the Civil War had little opportunity to perform surgery. As a student at a medical college he may have watched a few operations, but it was unlikely that he gained any significant clinical experience. Many young doctors enlisted in the Medical Corps as a means of obtaining surgical experience, and the same held true for quite a few established practitioners. Regardless of their motives for enlisting, army surgeons—often without any prior experience—were called upon to treat serious gunshot wounds and to perform major amputations.

The vast majority of wounds, 94 percent, were caused by bullets. Unlike the present-day steel-jacketed bullets, the widely used Minie bullet was made of soft lead in a conoid shape. Low velocity and a tendency for the bullet to flatten on contact meant instead of neatly zipping through the body as modern bullets do, it often lodged in the tissue, made a larger wound, and usually caused infection by carrying in with it bits of skin and clothing. On impact, the Minie bullet not infrequently shattered a large part of any bone it encountered. Over 70 percent of injuries were to the arms, legs, hands, or feet, one result of which was an inordinately high percentage of amputations, particularly during the first two years. Relatively few surgeons had the knowledge and skill to deal with serious injuries, and amputation was much simpler than complicated repair work. Even after surgeons had acquired more skill and a better technique, overworked surgeons confronted by hundreds of casualties in field hospitals often had no choice but to deal with wounded soldiers as quickly as possible. The almost certainty of infection was another argument for amputation, since hospital statistics showed that cases of primary amputation had a higher survival rate than when the operation was delayed. A primary amputation was ordinarily defined as one which took place within twenty-four hours after the patient had been wounded and before inflammation set in.

The vivid word pictures of surgeons at work following major engagements are almost too painful to recount. Often using makeshift operating tables—the tailgate of a wagon or a door placed upon two barrels—surgeons, with their sleeves rolled up and their arms and clothing covered with blood, cut and slashed and sewed. When the pressure was great, amputated legs and arms were simply tossed on a pile close to the operating tables. Surrounding the surgeons were dozens and sometimes hundreds of seriously wounded men, lying upon makeshift stretchers or on straw placed on the ground, some still quiet in a state of shock, others moaning with pain.[9]

With so many cases awaiting treatment, a patient would be placed on the table, and the surgeon would quickly decide whether or not to amputate. Very likely the man may have been given an opium pill or a drink of whiskey shortly after he was picked up, but in any case ether or chloroform would be administered promptly. Because of its ease of handling and administration, chloroform was the most widely used anesthetic at this time. A folded towel, cloth, or handkerchief was placed over the patient's nose and mouth and chloroform was dropped on until the patient lost consciousness. Considering the crudity of the technique and the weakened condition of so many patients, the deaths attributed to ether and chloroform are surprisingly low. Fortunately, field operations were generally performed in open tents or under a simple canvas cover, thus guaranteeing an ample supply of fresh air. Moreover, with considerable justice, deaths on the operating table were usually attributed to the severity of the injury or injuries.

Antiseptic surgery was still in the future, and the crude techniques of the surgeons have already been alluded to. Penetrating wounds were usually probed with a finger in search of the offending bullet, and it was a common practice for surgeons to wipe their hands on blood- and pus-stained aprons. Dressers customarily used the same basin of water to wash the wounds of several patients and those surgeons who did not wipe their instruments on aprons or coat sleeves simply rinsed them off in a common basin. Bandages and dressings were never sterilized, and the practice of washing and reusing them must have been a major factor in the ever-present hospital infections. Under battlefield conditions surgeons often worked continuously for several days, and reports of swollen feet and blistered hands among them were not uncommon. On both sides civilian doctors rallied to the battlefields to assist the over-worked army surgeons. While these civilians occasionally were accused of incompetence or of coming merely to get surgical experience, they undoubtedly helped to allay some of the suffering.

Despite a vast amount of clinical material, the Civil War brought no major advances in surgery. It did, however, teach several thousand physicians to deal with serious injuries and raised the level of their technical skill. These experiences undoubtedly stimulated an interest in surgery, and thereby contributed to major advances in the later nineteenth century. Whereas before the war only a few of the most skillful and daring surgeons had attempted repair work on major blood vessels, dealing with battle wounds taught thousands of surgeons to ligate great arteries and to treat head and face injuries. Among the few surgical innovations arising from the war was the Hodgen splint, invented in 1863, which, among other advantages, kept the limb in traction while permitting the wound to be dressed, and Dr. J. B. Bean's interdental splint for cases involving a fracture of maxillary bones. Useful as these developments were, probably the most important lesson learned from the war was the need for cleanliness and sanitation in hospitals.

The major hindrance to surgery was the traditional concept of "laudable pus." For centuries the formation of pus was assumed to be part of the healing process, and unless the wound became too inflamed, gangrenous, or showed symptoms of blood poisoning, the infection was allowed to run its course. Disinfectants were employed in treating inflamed wounds, including carbolic acid, bromine, bichloride of mercury, and alcohol, but these were seldom applied until suppuration was far advanced. These same disinfectants were used to disinfect hospital wards and the clothing of the sick. Without a knowledge of the germ theory, however, the application of disinfectants was haphazard and their value was limited. The ever-present flies hovering around the wounds led to the appearance of maggots in the diseased flesh, a situation which was viewed with horror. Whenever possible the maggots were killed with chloroform or some type of disinfectant. Several Confederate surgeons attending southern prisoners in Chattanooga in 1863 for lack of dressings and disinfectants were compelled to leave the wounds alone. They discovered that the maggots ate the diseased flesh, leaving the tissue clean and healthy. This lesson, which had been learned in earlier wars, was soon forgotten, only to be relearned in the bitter experiences of World War I.

The value of female nurses was recognized by both sides early in the fighting, and the Civil War saw them used on a relatively large scale for the first time. As indicated in connection with the Sanitary Commission, thousands of women whose husbands, sons, and brothers had volunteered for the army sought an active role for themselves. Shortly after the outbreak of fighting Dorothea Dix, whose activities on behalf of the insane had made her a national figure, offered her services and was appointed Superintendent of Female Nurses. Subsequently Congress authorized the employment of female nurses in general hospitals. A public controversy immediately broke out over whether or not delicate females should be exposed to the horrors, brutality, and moral dangers of war. Acutely aware of these threats to American womanhood, Dix instituted the same rigorous standards for her nurses that had been applied by Florence Nightingale. Nurse candidates had to be over thirty years of age, plain in appearance and dress, and be willing to subscribe to a host of regulations dictating almost every waking moment of their lives. Dix had won her reputation as a reformer, but she turned out to have little administrative skill. In addition, her exacting personal standards greatly hindered the recruiting of nurses. Since her national prestige and other factors made it impolitic to remove her from office, the Medical Department solved the problem by bypassing her in appointing and directing its nurses.

Army surgeons were generally opposed to the introduction of women into hospital wards as a matter of principle, and they often found justification for their prejudices. The women volunteers came from diverse backgrounds, and few had any experience as nurses; consequently they were frequently more troublesome than helpful. At the same time, most of them were intelligent, emotionally balanced, and capable individuals who quickly made their presence felt. They provided tender care, cleaned up the wards, improved the preparation of food, and contributed notably to improving the morale of the wounded. The Union Army officially enlisted well over 3,000 nurses, but this figure does not include the many women who volunteered their services following individual battles nor those who helped in the general hospitals.

The role of nurses in the South is difficult to assess. Southern women were reluctant to serve as army nurses, yet, since the fighting took place largely in the South, they probably did far more volunteer work. Confederate hospitals faced all the usual problems with male nurses; officers usually assigned the least reliable men to nursing duty, and much of nursing care fell on the shoulders of convalescent soldiers. While northern women eagerly volunteered for hospital duty, southern traditions did not encourage "ladies" to venture into what was considered a man's world. Nonetheless, quite a few southern women on their own initiative traveled to the scenes of fighting during the early months and demonstrated that female nurses could fill a useful role. One of the first of these was the indomitable Miss Sally L. Tompkins. Ten days after the first Battle of Manassas, at her own expense she organized and began operating the Robertson Hospital in Richmond, one of many institutions in the South run independent of the military. Later, when the Confederacy sought to bring these hospitals under military control and ordered that a commissioned officer must be in charge of all hospitals for the troops, Tompkins, whose institution had an enviable record, carried her appeal all the way to President Jefferson Davis, who commissioned her a captain—the only southern woman to hold a commission in the Confederate Army.[10]

Another determined woman was Kate Cumming of Mobile, Alabama. Despite the objections of her family, she and some other women from the Mobile area headed for the Shiloh battlefield in April 1862. On finding a desperate need for help, she elected to serve with the troops throughout the war. The work of Sally Tompkins, Kate Cumming, Ella K. Newsom, and other southern women led the Confederate Congress in September of 1862 to authorize the hiring of females—as matrons, nurses, and cooks—in army hospitals. In Virginia, where so much of the fighting took place, civilian volunteers, men and women, played an important part in caring for the sick and wounded; and throughout the rest of the South, as the wounded were brought into small towns, local people provided food, clothing, shelter, and medical care.

The Civil War did not give as much impetus to women's rights as World War I, but it did help to break down the prejudice against women in the medical area. This prejudice, which applied equally to women as nurses, physicians, and technicians, was firmly rooted, and it took over a hundred years of constant struggle before appreciable gains were made.

One other aspect of Civil War medicine deserves mention—that of medical supplies. Both sides started with virtually nothing, but, whereas the North was producing vast quantities by the end of the war, the South was beginning to face real shortages. As indicated, under Lawson and Finlay, the northern Medical Department never faced up to the realities of the war situation and the need for large-scale supplies, but affairs changed abruptly under Surgeon General Hammond. Upon assuming command in the spring of 1862, he immediately revised the Army Supply Table, making it, as one medical journal asserted, the most liberal for any army in the world. At the same time he saw the necessity for stockpiling medical supplies at major depots. On July 31, he ordered the Medical Purveyor in Philadelphia to acquire and keep on hand enough medicines and supplies to service 100,000 men for a period of six months. The Army demand for huge quantities of drugs created immediate problems. For one thing, prices began rising sharply in response to the growing demand, and, more important, many manufacturers either could not or would not maintain standards of purity. To deal with this situation, in the fall of 1862 Hammond decided that the Army needed its own laboratories for testing and manufacturing drugs. By establishing its own facilities, the Army could assure the purity of drugs bought from private manufacturers, maintain a check on profiteering, and guarantee a constant supply.

The following January (1863) Hammond gave instructions for establishing two laboratories, one in Philadelphia and the other in New York. In addition to producing a large quantity of supplies, the Army under Hammond and his successor, Barnes, bought even larger amounts from private manufacturers. Between those bought from private manufacturers and those produced in its own laboratories, the Union Medical Department was amply supplied during the last two years of the war. With considerable justice, William Proctor, Jr., a man who has been called the "father of American pharmacy," concluded after reviewing the medical supplies made available for the Union Army that never before had military pharmaceutical operations reached such tremendous proportions.[11]

The Confederate government recognized from the start that procuring medical supplies was an immediate and pressing need. In the instructions to its commercial agents the purchase of medical supplies ranked third behind arms and clothing, and almost every blockade runner carried some drugs and hospital supplies. During the first few months the South acquired some supplies by taking over Federal Army depots and through battlefield capture. It was evident that these were only temporary sources, and well before the Union blockade became effective the Confederacy made plans to utilize its native resources.

The leading spirit in this was Dr. Francis P. Porcher, an outstanding Charleston physician, who at the beginning of the war urged in *DeBow's Review* that the South should make use of its native flora and develop its own manufacturing capabilities. Surgeon General Moore followed up Porcher's appeal by circularizing his medical officers in April 1862 calling on them to search the fields and forests for "indigenous medicinal substances of the vegetable kingdom. . . ." He also enclosed a pamphlet entitled *General Directions and List of Plants.* When this proved too limited in scope, Moore requested Dr. Porcher to provide a more complete manual. The result was Porcher's classic work, *Resources of Southern Fields and Forest* published in 1863. It included descriptions of some 35,000 plants and a great deal of useful miscellaneous information—a recipe for making soap, for example. Porcher specified the medicinal value of many plants and suggested the possibilities inherent in others. He also recommended that the southern people raise the more common medicinal plants on their farms and gardens.[12]

Faced with a growing demand for medicinal supplies, the Confederate government sought to guarantee adequate quantities for the army by prohibiting the sale of items such as calomel, opium, quinine, castor oil, and alum except to government purchasing officers. In a day when alcohol was basic to nearly all medical treatment, and it was considered imperative to keep the patient's bowels open, alcohol and castor oil were in great demand. Rising prices led the Confederacy to establish plants and pharmaceutical laboratories for the production of these and other medicines, and a fairly wide range of pharmaceuticals were produced during the course of the war. Individual states also assisted in the production of needed medical items. In 1864 two state laboratories in Louisiana, one in Mt. Lebanon and the other in Clinton, were established. Dr. Bartholomew Egan, in charge of the Mt. Lebanon laboratory, successfully produced substantial quantities of castor oil, turpentine, and a variety of other medicines.

Insofar as the Confederate armed forces were concerned, medical and hospital supplies were never a serious problem until the last few months of the war. In the confusion of beginning hostilities occasional shortages appeared, and medical supplies were scarce now and then in local areas, but from an overall standpoint the situation was satisfactory. Only two items were in short supply throughout the war: surgical instruments and medical books. Surgeon General Moore ordered the publication of *A Manual of Military Surgery* in 1863 and encouraged the publication of several other works. Unfortunately the South was not equipped to produce surgical instruments or printed materials on the scale necessary for a major war, but enough surgical instruments were on hand or were smuggled in to enable the army surgeons to get by. By the end of 1864 increasing complaints about shortages of all types appear in the records. Generally supplies were on hand, but the breakdown of the southern transportation system was making it impossible to distribute them. The war was rapidly winding down, however, and hostilities came to an end before the medical supply situation became too critical.

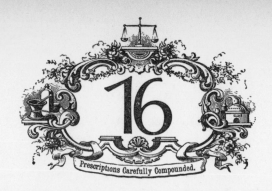

MEDICINE IN THE PAST
ONE HUNDRED YEARS

THE Civil War stimulated both industry and agriculture in the North and provided a major impetus toward making the United States a major industrial nation. One might have expected that the American penchant for mechanics and technology would have carried over into science, but Americans were too preoccupied with economic growth and making money to concern themselves with an abstraction such as basic research. Unless an immediate benefit could be seen, neither business nor government was interested. In consequence, while major advances were being made in chemistry, physiology, and the related medical sciences in Europe, with a few exceptions American physicians were content to concentrate upon their medical practice and, when new viewpoints were set forth, to defend traditional ideas. As will be seen later, the caliber of medical schools was no better in the postwar years than in the early nineteenth century, and it may have been even worse. This fact, combined with the inability of physicians to deal with the major diseases, guaranteed that the medical profession would continue to be held in low esteem.

For various reasons American colleges and universities were not research-minded. Of the three major professions— law, theology, and medicine— the last ranked well below the other two and was least likely to attract funds for either education or research. In 1891 the total endowment for theological schools amounted to $18,000,000 as against only $500,000 for medical education.[1] American medical schools contributed virtually nothing to medical research in the second half of the nineteenth century, and American medical graduates who wished to keep up with the latest in medicine were forced to study abroad. As their predecessors had gone to Great Britain prior to 1820 and to France from 1820 to 1860, American physicians in the post-Civil War period headed for Germany and Austria.

It was not until William H. Welch and others returned from Germany filled with enthusiasm for the possibilities inherent in laboratory research that America began to participate in the worldwide explosion of medical knowledge. In the 1890s Welch shaped the newly established Johns Hopkins Medical School into a research center, setting a new pattern for American medical education. He also encouraged General George M. Sternberg to establish the Army Medical School in 1893 and to promote scientific work by Army medical officers. By 1900 dozens of research laboratories had been established in schools and universities and under the auspices of state and municipal governments, and American medical researchers were confirming the results of European scientists and beginning to make contributions of their own.

The one major American contribution during these years came in the field of medical literature, an area which generally reflected the backwardness of American medicine. In 1876 Dr. John Shaw Billings dismissed the majority of medical theses as hopeless and deplored the fact that medical editing was merely an avocation for busy practitioners and teachers. In writing his student medical thesis Billings had become aware of the need for a first-rate medical library. After service in the Civil War, he was placed in charge of the Surgeon General's Library and was able to use some $80,000 which had been returned with the closing of army hospitals to build up the library's collection. In the 1870s he began work on the *Index Catalogue* of the library, and, with the help of a Congressional appropriation for printing, the first volume appeared in 1880. This work, which eventually ran to three series, is still a major bibliographic tool. In 1879, Billings and his collaborator, Dr. Robert Fletcher, also began the *Index Medicus*, the monthly guide to current medical literature, a work still indispensable to present medical researchers.[2]

The second half of the nineteenth century witnessed a transformation in medicine and surgery. Of the changes taking place, the bacteriological revolution which made possible the conquest or control of the major contagious diseases was the most significant. Although this revolution occurred fairly rapidly, it did not spring fullblown from Pasteur and Koch. Beginning in the 1830s investigations were made of parasites and infusoria, and by the 1850s the causative agents of trichinosis, hookworm, and tapeworm had been identified. Pasteur's work with fermentation in the late 1850s and his demonstrations which settled the question of spontaneous generation had, by 1862, paved the way for the identification of microscopic pathogenic organisms in the latter part of the century.

American medicine remained relatively untouched by these developments. Although a few physicians trained on the Continent brought back the new concept of disease, not until Welch introduced the principle in the 1890s that laboratory training and research were fundamental to medical education did American medicine begin to move into the mainstream of Western medicine. Welch was not alone in this, for he was ably assisted by Dr. T. Mitchell Prudden, who joined with Welch in bringing experimental pathology and bacteriology to America; by Dr. George M. Sternberg, appointed surgeon general in 1893; by Theobald Smith, first director of the Department of Agriculture's pathological laboratory and organizer of the bacteriological departments at George Washington and Cornell universities; and by a number of other intelligent and open-minded individuals.

The most important American discovery in the field of bacteriology during these years was made by Dr. Theobald Smith in connection with Texas Cattle Fever. Beginning work in the late 1880s, by 1889 Smith had identified the pathological agent responsible for the disease. In 1893, along with his collaborator, Dr. F. L.

Kilborne, he had demonstrated conclusively that the cattle tick was responsible for spreading the disease. By confirming the role of insect vectors, Smith helped open a new vista for preventive medicine.[3] The year 1893 was a significant one for American medicine; in addition to the publication of Smith's study on Texas Cattle Fever, Johns Hopkins Medical School opened its doors, George M. Sternberg, a pioneer in bacteriology, was made U.S. Surgeon General, and the New York City Health Department was using its bacteriological laboratory for diagnostic purposes. University, Federal, state, and municipal laboratories were springing into existence, and American physicians and scientists were not only beginning to reproduce the experiments and discoveries of their European counterparts but were preparing to make contributions of their own.

While medical discoveries were being piled one on top of another at an ever-accelerating rate, the average American physician continued the even tenure of his ways, little concerned with what was happening in the laboratories. Many medical journals either disregarded the findings of research men or else expressed considerable skepticism about them. More often than not, the findings of European medical researchers appeared in the newly established scientific journals such as *Scientific American* and *Popular Science Monthly* rather than in medical journals. Long after Pasteur and Koch had been acclaimed for their work, American physicians remained unconvinced. For example, when William Osler worked at the University Hospital in Philadelphia during the 1880s and 1890s, his personal microscope was the only one in use at the hospital. Twenty-five years after Pasteur had laid to rest the theory of spontaneous generation, a graduation thesis at Tulane University in 1887 dealt with a series of diphtheria and typhoid cases that apparently had developed in isolation. The student declared, presumably with the approval of his professors: "From the facts before me, I have been led to the conclusion that both typhoid fever and diphtheria may be spontaneously originated; or, in other words, that there are conditions in which these diseases may arise *de novo* without the transmission of the specific poison from pre-existing cases."[4]

Medical practice in the second half of the nineteenth century did not differ too greatly from that of earlier days, although excessive bloodletting and drugging were no longer the rule. The art of diagnosis was limited to the better physicians, and most practitioners relied largely upon quizzing and observing the patient before prescribing. In fact, the ability to prescribe was considered the real art of medicine. The thermometer and other diagnostic instruments were slowly making their way into the better medical practice, but physical diagnosis remained handicapped by the reluctance of patients, particularly females, to bare their skin to the probing, palpation, or percussion of the physician.[5] In 1862 Dr. Austin Flint wrote of the change that had taken place in medicine during the previous twenty-five years. "Formerly," he wrote, "boldness was a distinction coveted by the medical as well as the surgical practitioner. 'Heroic practice' was a favorite expression, consisting in the employment of powerful remedies or in pushing them to an enormous extent." "Now," he continued, "conservatism has become a leading principle in medicine. . . ." While Flint spoke for the well-trained, intelligent physicians, thousands of other doctors, particularly in the West and South, continued their vigorous assault upon the ills besetting mankind. The treatment given to a parturient black patient by a southern physician in 1887 clearly showed that heroic medicine was far from dead. According to Dr. D. R. Fox's report to the local medical society, within the space of twenty-four hours he cupped and bled the patient of 80 ounces of blood, dosed her with castor oil, gave a purgative enema, and vomited her with tartar emetic every two hours. As a result of his treatment, she was completely "restored to health in about four weeks."[6]

The average physician had only a hazy notion of etiology, and he prescribed largely for such symptoms as fevers, coughs, diarrheas, consumptions, and sore throats. The treatment itself was often hit or miss. While dosage was moderating, quinine, aconite, opium, alcohol, mercury, strychnine, arsenic, and other potentially dangerous drugs still formed the basis of materia medica. Opium, long used for bowel complaints, began to rival calomel as a cureall. It was sold wholesale as raw gum opium, laudanum, paregoric, and morphine and in Dover's Powder and dozens of prescription and patent medicines. In one form or another it was administered for inflammations, sprains, coughs, colds, sore throats, colic, diarrhea, female complaints, and neuralgia. Its administration for chronic and acute pain and insomnia was almost automatic, and medical professors and medical textbook authors seldom warned medical students about the danger of addiction. Attesting to its growing popularity, the annual importation of opium increased from 24,000 pounds in 1840 to 416,864 pounds in 1872. By the 1890s Americans were using half a million pounds of crude opium per year. While a few physicians blamed the growing number of opium addicts upon quacks and irregulars, far more of them conceded that the medical profession by its indiscriminate prescribing was largely to blame.[7]

The old standby, alcohol, was used as a tonic, stimulant, preventive, and cure. Usually prescribed in the form of whiskey or brandy, it was cheap, easily available, and readily accepted by the patient. A popular textbook stated: "alcohol in some form should be used in *every* case of typhoid *from the beginning*. . . ." It was considered equally valuable for chronic and acute diseases, and it was freely prescribed for all ages. A usual dose for infants and children was 1/2 to 2 teaspoonsful every three hours.[8]

Bloodletting, particularly venesection (opening a vein), as noted earlier had begun to fall out of favor in the 1850s, and its use steadily declined as the century advanced. Many older physicians, however, were reluctant to see phlebotomy (bleeding) fall into disuse, and their plaintive appeals on its behalf can be found in medical journals down to the end of the century. Dr. Moritz Schuppert insisted in the *New Orleans Medical & Surgical Journal* in 1882 that in many cases a bold and vigorous use of the lancet was still essential.[9] Even Dr. Flint, an early voice of moderation, asserted in 1886 that within fifty years bloodletting would once again take its place among the physicians' weapons.[10] In 1893, one of America's best-known physicians, Dr. William Osler, declared: "Pneumonia is one of the diseases in which timely venesection saves life," and as late as 1913 Fielding H. Garrison wrote there is scarcely a physician "who may not suddenly encounter some circumstances in his experience in which venesection would turn out to be his sheet and anchor and his patient's salvation."[11]

Although the public image of the physician was rallying from the low point it had reached in the 1840s and 1850s, the average physician enjoyed neither money nor social position. The aim of nearly all young physicians was to establish themselves in a comfortable family practice, preferably among the well-to-do, but the number of physicians far exceeded the demand, and the majority eked out a bare living, supplementing their income by operating a pharmacy or some other business or else by farming. The middle and upper classes expected to be treated in their homes, and the physician who treated the family members and their servants was guaranteed a good income and social acceptability. Young doctors without family connections were forced to rely upon an office practice or else serve as a dispensary physician or visiting physician attending the poor. An office practice itself carried some stigma, since it was the resort of the poorer class who could not afford to have the doctor visit them in their homes. Moreover, the physician with an office practice faced keen competition, not only from his colleagues, but from druggists, who were not averse to prescribing, and from a host of quacks, folk practitioners, and irregulars.

As had been true in the past, a wide gap separated the top physicians from those conducting an ordinary practice. In contrast to the relative poverty and limited status of the usual physician, the leading ones enjoyed both social position and wealth. In most cases these affluent physicians came from well-to-do families and had completed their medical education by studying abroad. They generally held professorships in the medical schools and had the additional advantage of an entré into a middle- or upper-class practice. As the nineteenth century advanced, they also tended to become the specialists in the profession. In this period, however, even specialists maintained a regular family practice.

While the more able physicians were preoccupied with their teaching and medical practices, the demands upon most doctors were not too great, and they had ample time to engage in political and social affairs. In smaller communities they were often among the best-educated citizens, and they frequently gravitated toward political office. In communities without a medical school, physicians on occasion supplemented their income by lecturing. A Pittsburgh newspaper announced on February 19, 1868 that A. O'Leary, M.D., would give a course of physiological lectures on the subject, "Laws of Life, Health, Strength, and Beauty," the lectures to be illustrated by French manikins, models, pathological specimens, and skeletons.[12] Judging by Dr. O'Leary's title, his lectures were clearly designed to appeal to the general public.

The role of family doctor in Protestant America carried with it certain aspects of a father confessor or a moral arbitrator. A good many physicians happily accepted their moral obligations and used the authority of medicine to support the accepted middle-class moral values. They cited anatomical and physiological reasons to explain why females were delicate, sensitive, and dominated by their emotions, and most of them agreed that normal decent females derived no satisfaction from sex other than giving pleasure to their husbands and bearing children. Paradoxically, while holding this latter view, they were uncommonly concerned with both male and female masturbation, considering it a specific disease entity. There is scarcely a symptom, syndrome, disease, or pathological condition that was not ascribed to masturbation— dyspepsia, urethral constriction, epilepsy, blindness, loss of hearing, vertigo, headache, loss of memory, irregular action of the heart, and so forth. Chronic masturbation usually led to moist, clammy hands and feet, stooped shoulders, pale sallow skin, dark circles under the eyes, acne, and a hangdog look. An individual who was nervous, tired, and rundown was automatically suspect.[13] On the basis of these symptoms, it was a simple matter for a physician to closely interrogate—or browbeat—any patient suspected of masturbation and, since few could deny having masturbated, confirm the diagnosis.

As the subject of race became a popular study in the late nineteenth century, the old arguments of southern physicians about the innate anatomical and physiological differences between whites and blacks were revived, and many American doctors in all areas raised their voices in support of Anglo-Saxon superiority.[14] The demand for women's rights was met by scientific medical proof of female inferiority and dire warnings of the disastrous impact of education upon the delicate and sensitive female mind and body. Members of the Medical and Chirurgical Faculty of Maryland in 1881 were alerted by their annual orator to the dangers from the decay of home life and the rise of divorce and abortion. To stop these abuses, they were exhorted to "redeem woman from the bondage of her education and restore her to wifehood and motherhood; to uplift the sexual conscience of the community; . . . and to fill our homes with prattling children—these be the great missions of the physician, missions which he must cheerfully and manfully accept as his Duty of the Hour."[15]

Fortunately, medicine has always had its iconoclasts, and there were many medical men who objected to this nonsense. The entire profession was agreed about the danger from tightly laced corsets and the many layers of clothing worn by middle- and upper-class women. When the bicycle fad developed at the turn of the century and orthodox moralists railed against its moral impact upon young girls (freed them from adult supervision and turned them into tomboys and regular hoydens!), the medical profession was more sanguine. A few physicians felt the exercise was too violent for females and a few others worried about the effect of the bicycle saddle upon young girls, but most of them welcomed the bicycle as a healthy form of exercise. Clearly physicians in the late nineteenth century, like those of today, were products of their times; they accepted the prevailing moral and ethical standards and saw nothing wrong in rationalizing them in terms of their professional knowledge.

THE 20th CENTURY

The closing decade of the nineteenth century has the distinction of clearly marking the beginning of an era which brought greater changes to medicine and medical practice than any other time in history. The accumulated impact of bacteriology, pathology, and the vast developments in the basic sciences which had been going on in the previous centuries were rapidly applied to medicine in the early 1900s. Since medicine is not a science in itself but rather an art which draws upon the sciences and since the human organism is an exceedingly complex one, scientific knowledge had to reach a critical mass before it could begin to shape medical practice. By the turn of the century, this stage had been reached, and in no country was its impact greater than in the United States. American medicine had lagged behind that of Western Europe, but major reforms in medical education, combined with a series of other developments, enabled the United States to forge into a leadership role in medicine within a relatively short space of time.

Aside from the zeal and intellectual ability of its scientists, this advance was made possible largely through private philanthropy. Led by the Rockefeller and Carnegie foundations, wealthy Americans poured millions of dollars into medical schools and research institutes, and the success of these agencies in turn encouraged both the government and private corporations to follow suit. The Rockefeller Institute for Medical Research established in 1901—the first of its kind—set an exceptionally high standard and served as a model for many subsequent research institutions. Within a few years the Hooper Institute for Medical Research in San Francisco, Phipps Institute in Philadelphia, Cushing Institute in Cleveland, McCormick Institute for the Study of Infectious Diseases in Chicago, and similar institutions were all making notable contributions.[16]

Meanwhile, following the example of New York City which established a diagnostic laboratory in 1893, many states and municipalities began making practical applications of the new laboratory techniques, and the researchers in these laboratories began venturing into new areas. One of the ironies of American history is that at the Federal level the Department of Agriculture supplied most of the funds for research during the latter part of the nineteenth and the early years of the twentieth century, largely as a result of Congressional willingness to allocate money for sick hogs, cattle, and fowl. Farm animals were valuable property, whereas human life was still relatively cheap. A few crumbs were doled out to the United States Marine Hospital Service, which had established a small laboratory on Staten Island, New York, in 1888. In 1891 this laboratory was moved to Washington, D.C.

During the regime of Surgeon General Walter Wyman, 1891–1911, the Hygienic Laboratory greatly broadened its scope. In 1902, when the Marine Hospital Service was renamed the Public Health and Marine Hospital Service, the Hygienic Laboratory was enlarged to include four divisions: bacteriology and pathology, chemistry, pharmacology, and zoology. Funds were also provided for a new building, and in 1904 the Laboratory moved to a site overlooking the Potomac. The next major change came in 1912, when the Service was reorganized and given additional responsibilities. Reflecting the broadening of its purpose, the words Marine Hospital were dropped, and it became the United States Public Health Service. The law prescribing these changes authorized the Service "to study and investigate the diseases of man and propagation and spread thereof, including sanitation and sewage and the pollution either directly or indirectly of the navigable streams and lakes of the United States."

During these years of slow expansion, the Service performed very creditably with its limited funds. It assisted in the yellow fever work of the Reed Commission and performed notably in connection with the elimination of hookworm and pellagra from the United States. The outbreak of World War I greatly enlarged the operations of the Service, as the increase in its annual budget from $3,000,000 in 1917 to $50,000,000 in 1918 indicates. Concern over the rising incidence of venereal disease in the armed forces led Congress to appropriate well over $2,200,000 for venereal disease control during 1918. A Venereal Disease Division was established in the Public Health Service with a budget of $200,000 per year, and $2,000,000 was appropriated to promote state and municipal venereal disease programs. In the post-World War I period governmental activity at all levels was in the doldrums, and the temporary wartime health programs soon fell by the wayside. The Venereal Disease Division managed to survive, but at a reduced level of activity.[17]

In 1930 two measures were signed by President Hoover, one enlarging the Public Health Service by increasing the number of commissioned officers and another making the Hygienic Laboratory the National Institutes of Health. The Depression, with its demand for reduced government spending, slowed further progress in medical research until 1937, when a new era was inaugurated with the creation of the National Cancer Institute. This agency, which set the pattern for subsequent health institutes, marked the first time that the Public Health Service moved from strictly communicable disease into the area of chronic disorders. Meanwhile, early in the twentieth century other federal agencies began moving into the health field. The Food and Drug Administration and the Children's Bureau both contributed to health research in the pre-World War I era, and the Sheppard-Towner Act in 1921 did much to promote maternal and child care in the 1920s. Both the Children's Bureau and the Sheppard-Towner Act, however, were more concerned with health care than with medical research.

World War II gave a sharp impetus to applied medical research and large sums were poured into developing insecticides, chemotherapeutics, and vaccines, but basic research necessarily lagged. In the postwar years the seemingly miraculous cures effected by sulfonamides and antibiotics created a great wave of optimism and encouraged government spending for medical research on an unparalleled scale. A whole series of new institutes were added to the NIH—and all of them were generously funded. Medical schools, too, benefited from state and federal largesse. Although the funds granted to medical schools were ostensibly for medical research—and a good deal of research was accomplished—a good share of the money was used to build up teaching faculties and laboratory facilities and thus increase the number of students.

With a few exceptions, most breakthroughs in research are the result of an infinite number of small steps taken by many individuals. This has been especially true of the twentieth century, where so much of the effort is a team project. Moreover, advances in communication have enabled researchers in widely separated countries to aid in the steady accumulation of knowledge; thus, to single out a few scientists is to do injustice to the many. American researchers began by building upon a base established by Europeans, but they were soon engaged in a mutual exchange of information. Possibly as a result of frontier conditions, Americans have always been a practical people, with a facility for applied research. A fine case in point was our ability to mass produce antibiotics and DDT during World War II. Another example was the demonstration in 1900 that yellow fever was carried by a particular mosquito, the first major American medical accomplishment of the twentieth century.

Yellow fever had been a major threat to the United States for well over 100 years. Following a great epidemic in 1878 which swept far up the Mississippi Valley, the attacks appeared to be lessening, but the Spanish-American War, which involved the occupation of Cuba, raised the specter of serious losses among the armed forces. Surgeon General Sternberg, a first-rate bacteriologist, had already done considerable research on yellow fever and had encouraged Dr. Aristides Agramonte, a Cuban bacteriologist and a U.S. Army contract surgeon, to devote his time to the project. In 1900 General Sternberg decided that a full-time medical team was needed to work on the problem, and he created a special Army board headed by Major Walter Reed and including Agramonte, James Carroll, and Jesse W. Lazear. Reed was an excellent choice; he had studied under Welch at Johns Hopkins and had worked closely with Sternberg. Some nineteen years earlier, in 1881, a Cuban physician named Carlos Finlay had set forth strong evidence that a particular mosquito, the *Culex* or *Stegomyia fasciata* (presently *Aedes aegypti*), was responsible for transmitting the disease, but little attention had been paid to his theory. Shortly before the Reed Commission began work, Dr. Henry Rose Carter of the U.S. Marine Hospital Service gathered further evidence to support the Finlay thesis from an intensive study of a yellow fever outbreak in a small Mississippi town. Suffice it to say, Reed and his associates, after testing various possibilities, centered their efforts on the mosquito thesis and, with the help of Dr. Finlay, were able to demonstrate the validity of his hypothesis.

Few medical breakthroughs have had so great an impact as the work of the Reed Commission. Major William Gorgas, the chief sanitary officer in Havana, soon rid that city of yellow fever, a disease which had been endemic since the eighteenth century. It is questionable whether the Panama Canal could have been completed without the elimination of yellow fever by Gorgas. The conquest of this dramatic killer disease was of inestimable value in terms of its economic, social, and psychological impact on the southern United States, the Caribbean area, South America, and other tropical and semitropical regions.[18]

The same empirical approach which helped Reed and his associates pave the way for the conquest of yellow fever enabled Americans to make major contributions toward the elimination of two other costly disorders, hookworm and pellagra. Interestingly enough, the three diseases have little in common: yellow fever is a virus infection, hookworm is a parasitic disorder, and pellagra is a deficiency disease. In 1900 Captain Bailey K. Ashford of the United States Army noted the prevalence of hookworm in Puerto Rico, and shortly thereafter this parasite was recognized as a common disorder in the American South. A zoologist, Dr. Charles Wardell Stiles of the USPHS, in 1902 identified the American organism as a new species and began studying methods for attacking it. As the scope of the hookworm problem became evident, in October of 1909 the Rockefeller Foundation stepped into the picture and established the Rockefeller Sanitary Commission. Working closely with Stiles and the USPHS, the Rockefeller Commission began a massive educational campaign to awaken southerners to the problem. Utilizing state and local school boards, health boards, medical societies, newspapers, and so forth, a two-fold program was undertaken, consisting first of treating those infected and second of developing preventive measures to stop the dissemination of the intestinal parasite. While Stiles was concentrating on the United States, Ashford in the meantime had launched a massive campaign against hookworm in Puerto Rico. Although the program achieved notable results, hookworm is a disease of poverty, and its elimination in the United States was only made possible by the vast social and economic changes of the late 1930s and early 1940s.[19]

Like hookworm, dietetic disorders are also social diseases, and their elimination involved both medical science and socioeconomic changes. The first of the dietetic diseases to be recognized was scurvy. Although the association between it and diet had been recognized by a few perceptive individuals as early as the sixteenth century and a great deal had been learned about it in subsequent centuries, as late as the Civil War many physicians were still treating it with mercurials and other dangerous drugs. Physicians generally, however, had no illusions about the cause and cure of scurvy, but the same cannot be said for pellagra and the other diseases. The bacteriological revolution in the late nineteenth century precipitated a frantic search for the microorganisms assumed to be responsible for virtually every disorder, and pellagra was a fine case in point. When it was first found to be widespread in Europe in the eighteenth century, there was much speculation as to its cause. Hereditary factors, meteorological conditions, diet, and spoiled corn all had their advocates until early in the twentieth century when an Italian bacteriologist triumphantly announced he had isolated the bacillus causing the disease. Although his claims were soon disproved, the bacterial origin of pellagra continued to be asserted as late as the 1920s.

In 1902 a case of pellagra was diagnosed in a poor Georgia farmer and within the next three or four years the disease was found widely in the southern states. By 1908 it was clear that pellagra was a major southern problem, and newspapers and magazines began playing up the more lurid aspects of this strange

and mysterious plague, variously depicted as a hereditary, constitutional, insect-borne, bacterial, or dietetic disease. In 1909 the
USPHS began using its limited resources to look into the situation.
Dr. C. H. Lavinder was assigned to the South Carolina Hospital
for the Insane in May and provided with two bare rooms, without
water or gas, to begin his research. In 1912 two teams of scientists
began intensive study on the cause of pellagra: one was a USPHS
team and the other, the Thompson-McFadden Commission, was a
privately endowed study under the auspices of the New York
Graduate School of Medicine. Two years later, with Congressional
backing, the USPHS decided to broaden its assault upon pellagra.
Consequently, Surgeon General Rupert Blue assigned a staff of
forty-one men, provided a budget of $80,000, and—more
significant—he appointed Dr. Joseph Goldberger to head the
project.

After a quick survey of the studies already made and a field
trip into the South, Goldberger was convinced that a food deficiency was the root of the problem. He began a series of experiments in
which he first demonstrated that the disease could be cured by a
balanced food intake and culminated his work in 1915 by showing
that pellagra could be induced in humans by an inadequate diet.
The publication of his findings should have made him a popular
hero, but instead he was immediately denounced by southern
politicians, newspapers, and physicians for casting aspersions upon
their region. Despite what would appear to be indisputable evidence, Goldberger's ideas continued to be derided or dismissed by
many physicians. As late as 1918 the Pellagra Commission of the
National Medical Association declared firmly that pellagra was a
communicable disease resulting from poor sanitation.

When a depression struck following World War I, Goldberger
warned the USPHS that any decline in southern living standards
would cause a rise in the incidence of pellagra. The Health Service
decided to take action, precipitating a storm of outrage in the
South. Fortunately many southerners had no illusions about
conditions in their region, and they collaborated with the Health
Service in its fight against pellagra.

By this date, 1921, Goldberger was determined to find the
specific cause of pellagra, and he began concentrating upon amino
acids. He was working on a vitamin theory when cancer cut short

his career in 1929. In 1937 Dr. Conrad A. Elvehjem and his colleagues in the agricultural chemistry department of the University of Wisconsin reported the discovery of nicotinic acid as a cure for pellagra. The immediate result was to reduce sharply the death rate from pellagra, one which had been going down slowly, and to aid in the elimination of pellagra within the next few years.[20]

Shortly before World War I Captain Edward B. Vedder of the Army Medical Corps spent three years in the Philippine Islands studying beri-beri, a deficiency disease which arose from advancing technology. As more efficient machines for milling rice were developed, they turned out a more attractive but far less nutritious product, with the result that a new disease appeared among those populations whose food consisted largely of rice. In 1913 Vedder published his findings in a classic work entitled *Beriberi*. Meanwhile, a young agricultural chemist working for the University of Wisconsin, Elmer V. McCollum, had developed a technique for feeding rats on highly selective diets in order to determine nutritional values. His work enabled him to discover vitamin A in 1913 and vitamin D in 1922. Having discovered a substance in rice and yeast which cured beri-beri, Captain Vedder immediately began working with R. R. Williams, a chemist, trying to identify it, but the prevailing technology and scientific knowledge was not adequate for the task. Since the term "vitamin" had just been coined by Casimer Funk, McCollum called this unidentifiable nutritional agent vitamin B. Williams, who continued his research, was able in 1933 to isolate the substance which he termed thiamin, a part of the B-complex. Subsequently he was able to learn its structure and by so doing was able to synthesize it.

By the late 1930s the way was open to eliminate nearly all the nutritional diseases. Dr. Harry Steenblock of the University of Wisconsin had found a way to create vitamin D artificially in 1924, and within a few years irradiated milk and other foods were widely available. As World War II approached, interest was expressed in fortifying bread and flour with vitamins. The war itself accelerated the movement, and by 1945 pellagra and beri-beri were no longer serious problems in the United States.

The field of virology (the study of virus) began opening relatively early in the twentieth century, and American research institutes and university laboratories made significant contributions to it. Discoveries in this field were the result of scientists in many countries steadily accumulating a larger and larger body of facts. The electron microscope, an essential tool for understanding the viral structure, was a German contribution. One of the most notable American accomplishments in virology was the work with poliomyelitis. This disease was first reported in the United States by George Colmer, a Louisiana physician who presented a clear clinical picture of a polio outbreak which occurred in 1841. The disease flared up on a number of other occasions, but it did not receive much attention until the twentieth century. Even as late as 1907 an epidemic of about 2,000 cases in New York City was not discovered until the following year when the welfare department began checking on the unusual number of paralyzed individuals seeking help. A major outbreak which struck the northeastern states in 1916 caused 9,000 cases and 2,500 deaths in New York City alone.[21]

As polio and various forms of encephalitis began to strike with more frequency, American researchers increasingly turned their attention to these neurotropic viruses. In 1931 Austrian scientists discovered two strains of polio virus, paving the way for Drs. Albert B. Sabin and Peter K. Olitsky of the Rockefeller Institute in 1936 to grow polio virus in human brain cells. Progress was slow until 1949 when three Harvard professors—J. F. Enders, T. H. Weller, and F. C. Robbins—found that the virus could be cultured in monkey tissues. Four years later Jonas Salk was able to combine three strains of killed virus into one solution. Testing of this Salk vaccine began in 1953 and led to a nationwide program the following year. Meanwhile Albert Sabin was working on an attenuated virus which offered a longer period of immunity and could be taken orally. After considerable debate over the merits of the two vaccines, the Sabin vaccine finally won out and in 1961–62 it replaced that of Salk.[22]

The almost instant communication provided by radio and television in the mid-twentieth century combined with much more effective reporting of communicable diseases had made the public highly aware of the successive polio outbreaks. In consequence, the new polio vaccines were welcomed and within a few years the disease had virtually disappeared. This brief account does not do justice to the many researchers who contributed to the conquest of polio, but it does illustrate the tremendous advances in virology during the twentieth century.

Early in the 1920s Thomas M. Rivers was called to the Rockefeller Institute and assigned the task of working with viruses. While he and his associates made no major discoveries, their work helped to open the field of virology. One result of their studies was an attenuated smallpox vaccine virus which was used for vaccinating children. It eventually became too attenuated to provide complete smallpox protection, but the research was not lost. Rivers discussed it at length with Dr. Wilbur A. Sawyer of the Rockefeller Foundation Virus Laboratories, and both men agreed that it might be possible to develop a vaccine from an attenuated strain of yellow fever virus. Dr. Sawyer assigned Max Theiler to the task, and by 1937 he produced an effective vaccine for this disease, an accomplishment for which he subsequently received the Nobel Prize.[23]

The awarding of Nobel Prizes in itself gives ample proof of the development of American medical research during the twentieth century. The first American-based researcher to receive the award was Alexis Carrel, a French surgeon who joined the Rockefeller Institute in 1906. Carrel, a pioneer in blood vessel surgery and organ transplants, was given the Nobel Prize in 1918 for his work in physiology and medicine. Eighteen years elapsed before another American worker received the Nobel Prize. The recipient was Karl Landsteiner, an Austrian-born scientist who, shortly after the turn of the century, laid the basis for the classification of human blood groups. He was brought to the Rockefeller Institute in 1922 where his studies helped to establish immunochemistry as a branch of science.

As American research moved into high gear by the 1930s, several Americans won or shared Nobel Prizes: Thomas Hunt Morgan for his research in genetics; George R. Minot, William P. Murphy, and G. H. Whipple for their work on pernicious anemia; and Otto Loew for his studies in pharmacology. The 1940s demonstrated that American universities and research institutes were playing a major role in the development of medicine. Five Americans won or shared prizes in such diverse areas as sex hormones, rheumatoid arthritis, and the electrophysiology of nerves. The past twenty-five years have been equally successful ones, with Americans receiving a relatively high percentage of the awards. Among the most outstanding scientists to receive the Nobel Prize have been men such as Max Theiler, producer of the first yellow fever vaccine; Selman A. Waksman, who isolated a number of antibiotics; and John F. Enders and his associates for their work on polio viruses. Enders, who received the Nobel Prize in 1954, subsequently applied his knowledge and technique to studying the measles virus, and by 1962 produced an effective measles vaccine. A brief survey such as this necessarily overlooks a host of other leading medical scientists. Two good examples of prominent Americans falling into this category are Simon Flexner, who deserves mention for his scientific work with cerebrospinal meningitis and his effective administrative guidance of the Rockefeller Institute for over thirty years, and René Dubos for his research on antibiotics and his perceptive writings on various health topics.

Imposing as the foregoing list of American scientists may be, it should be kept in mind that a survey of major medical discoveries would accord much of the credit to scientists from other countries. Aside from those American recipients of Nobel Prizes whose outstanding work was done while in their native countries, most significant advances have not been the work of Americans. The credit for the discovery of X-rays, radium, insulin, penicillin, sulfa drugs, and a good part of the basic studies in biochemistry, endocrinology, nutrition, chemotherapy, and other areas belongs to scientists from other nations. America's vast resources and ability to mobilize large numbers of highly trained scientists and technicians have given us a leading role in medicine, but original minds are rare and are not circumscribed by national boundaries.

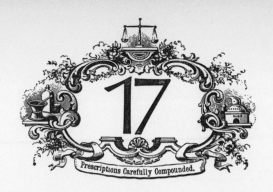

Prescriptions Carefully Compounded.

SURGERY GAINS RESPECTABILITY

By the end of the Civil War, anesthesia, the first of two discoveries which revolutionized surgery, had already gained wide acceptance. Freed of the pressure arising from agonized struggling patients, surgeons were much more willing to resort to radical treatment and were performing longer and more complex operations. The consequence, as noted in an earlier chapter, was a sharp rise in the death rate from surgical infections or the traditional gangrenes and septicemias. In 1865 an English surgeon, Joseph Lister, deduced from a study of Pasteur's work that microorganisms derived from the air must cause the septic poisoning of wounds. In 1865 he began experimenting with an operating technique which involved cleanliness and the use of weak carbolic acid as an antiseptic. His aim was to kill any pathogenic organisms in the wound and to prevent the entrance of others. He first published an account of his method in 1867 and thereby precipitated a heated controversy. The elaborate precautions required by the

Listerian method seemed ridiculous to traditional surgeons, and even under the best of circumstances the system did not always work. Skeptical surgeons who attempted antiseptic measures often applied them in so perfunctory a manner as to negate their effectiveness.

In America, Oliver Wendell Holmes's plea for cleanliness and antiseptic procedures in connection with obstetrics had won many converts, but even so the cumbersome Lister method made only slow gains. Whereas anesthesia had won almost instant acceptance, antiseptic surgery took well over twenty years to gain respectability. In 1877 Dr. Robert F. Weir, a well-known New York surgeon, declared that only recently had the teachings of Lister received any attention in American surgical practice. "In fact," he went on, "aside from an article by Schuppert in the *New Orleans Medical & Surgical Journal* little or nothing has appeared in our medical journals relative to the result of the so-called antiseptic method."[1]

Dr. Moritz Schuppert, a German physician who had settled in New Orleans in the 1850s, had heard of the remarkable results achieved by German surgeons using the Listerian technique and decided to visit Germany and see for himself. On his return to New Orleans in 1875, he immediately introduced the antiseptic method. In January 1878 he reported that he had performed 120 operations in the past two and a half years using Lister's method, and that the mortality rate had been only 4 percent, an astonishing figure for this period. Shortly thereafter Schuppert retired, and the antiseptic method fell into disuse at the New Orleans Charity Hospital. Ironically, it was not revived until a flare-up of puerperal fever in 1887 led the assistant house surgeon, Dr. Frederick W. Parham, to introduce rigorous antiseptic precautions. The success of these measures encouraged him to reintroduce the antiseptic technique into surgical service.[2]

As indicated, cleanliness in dealing with open wounds had already won some converts even before Lister, and the value of carbolic acid as an antiseptic gradually became recognized. Hence some aspects of Listerism were acceptable almost immediately, but it was the 1890s before the Lister principles carried the day. Their relatively late introduction into America meant that the aseptic procedures developed by the Germans won out over the antiseptic procedures. Rather than kill microorganisms with antiseptics, the aseptic method sought to create a sterile operating field in order to prevent the entrance of pathogenic organisms. It involved sterilizing all instruments, dressings, sponges, and the gowns and other items in the operating room. A major item which did not lend itself to sterilization was the surgeon's hands, but this problem was solved almost by inadvertence. In 1889 Dr. William S. Halsted of Johns Hopkins suggested that his surgical nurse, Miss Caroline Hampton, use rubber gloves to protect her hands from the antiseptics to which she was allergic. It was not until six years later that Dr. Joseph C. Bloodgood, one of Halsted's assistants, began using them routinely for surgery.[3]

Before discussing the remarkable advances which characterized surgery in the late nineteenth century, it is well to realize that surgery had still not cast off its former reputation as a callous and bloody business. Nor were physicians—and most surgery was still in the hands of physicians—willing to operate except in cases of dire emergency. Dr. Rudolph Matas, one of the best southern surgeons, wrote that "even in the eighties, *noli me tangere* was written large on the head, chest and abdomen, and their contained organs were still held as in sanctuaries which no one dared to open with unhallowed hands. Surgery," he went on, "was still largely restricted to such interventions in the visceral cavities . . . made compulsory by accidental injuries or imperative vital indications."[4]

Probably no better illustration of Dr. Matas's point can be found than the case of President James A. Garfield. He was shot on the morning of July 2, 1881, by a single bullet which entered his body above the third rib. Other than probing the wound with their fingers to look for the bullet—a procedure which almost guaranteed infection—his attending physicians followed a policy of watchful waiting. When inflammation was reported on July 5, one of the physicians described it as natural. On July 13 the medical report stated there were indications of a "circumscribed peritonitis in the abdominal region," but it was not considered "alarming." The wound, which was continuing to "discharge healthy pus," was doing quite satisfactorily. As the infection slowly spread, the physicians continued to stand by helplessly. Other than making incisions to permit the accumulated pus to escape, they gradually watched the President decline until his death on September 19.

As with a good many medical developments, surgery required

hospitals and a large patient population in order to become a specialty. Hence urban areas were the first to support physicians who could concentrate upon surgery. Traditionally specialization had been equated with traveling lithotomists, eye doctors, clap or venereal disease practitioners, and other quacks—and so strong was the suspicion of specialism within the medical profession that even the better surgeons maintained a private medical practice to the end of the nineteenth century. Away from the major cities, surgery did not emerge as a full-time practice until later.

Although American surgery did not measure up to that of Europe in the nineteenth century, the American aptitude for mechanics proved of value in areas such as dentistry, X-ray technology, and anesthesia. In connection with the latter, one of the most useful devices was the O'Dwyer tube, an instrument to pass air through the larynx and trachea in cases of mechanical obstruction. When Dr. George H. Fell of Buffalo, New York demonstrated an apparatus for giving artificial respiration, O'Dwyer simplified and improved Fell's device by combining it with a modified version of his own tube, and it became known as the Fell-O'Dwyer apparatus. Rudolph Matas of New Orleans was the first to recognize the potential value of the Fell-O'Dwyer apparatus for chest operations, and in 1900 he redesigned the Fell-O'Dwyer apparatus so that it could be used to maintain respiration and continuous anesthesia during chest surgery.[5]

Before leaving this subject, it may be well to mention a few of the other Americans contributing to the development of the many forms of anesthesia, remembering, of course, that a major share of the early work was performed by Europeans. In 1884 Carl Koller of Vienna publicized his pioneering work on the value of cocaine as a local anesthetic. Dr. William S. Halsted, who was then in New York, began experimenting on himself and his associates by injecting nerve trunks with a cocaine solution. These dangerous experiments opened the entire field of conduction anesthesia, and it remained for other surgeons, such as George Washington Crile of Cleveland and Harvey Cushing of Johns Hopkins, to help refine the technique.[6]

While Halsted was conducting his studies, Dr. J. Leonard Corning of New York began experimenting with spinal anesthesia, and in 1899 Dr. Rudolph Matas of New Orleans first employed it for surgical purposes. Matas also devised an improved method for massive infiltration anesthesia and pioneered in regional anesthesia.[7] The twentieth century witnessed a stream of new anesthetic agents, some for use by themselves and others in combination with established agents. It also saw vast changes in the mechanical devices used for administering anesthesia. As anesthesia emerged as a medical specialty, the modest stream of contributions by Americans in the early years turned into a flood as the United States assumed a dominant role in medicine by the mid-twentieth century.

DENTISTRY

Modern dentistry dates back to the eighteenth century when French and English surgeons, most notably Pierre Fauchard and John Hunter, removed it from a state of crude empiricism and placed it on firmer foundations. In the nineteenth and twentieth centuries the development of dentistry was largely an American accomplishment. American practicality and mechanical ingenuity are part of the explanation, but a better one may lie in the lack of discrimination toward surgeons and the higher American standard of living. Surgeons still had the aura of tradesmen in Europe and dentists ranked below surgeons. In America physicians and surgeons were one and the same, and the better dentists usually acquired medical degrees—not a hard task in nineteenth-century America. The close relationship between medicine and dentistry can be seen in the 1847 decision of the Baltimore College of Dental Surgery to form a joint committee of five physicians and three dentists to examine candidates for the degree of Doctor of Dental Surgery.[8] Since dentistry is concerned with comfort and appearance and seldom confronts the patient with a life or death situation, it flourishes best among a prosperous people—and Americans were relatively prosperous.

The French introduced the use of porcelain for teeth and gold for fillings in the eighteenth century, and by the early nineteenth century American dentists were familiar with both. For one reason or another, Americans concentrated on saving teeth instead of merely extracting them, and they made rapid progress in their gold-filling technique. At the same time dental manufacturing companies began making porcelain teeth on a large scale, and a new industry was born.

The individual generally credited with establishing American dentistry as a profession is Horace H. Hayden (1768–1844). Hayden became interested in dentistry when he encountered John Greenwood (George Washington's dentist) in New York. In 1800 he moved to Baltimore, where he continued his studies in medicine and dentistry. The Baltimore Medical and Chirurgical Society voted in 1805 to grant licenses to dentists, and Hayden was licensed to practice in 1810. Anxious to remove the stigma of traveling quacks that still hovered over dentists, in the 1820s he began lecturing on dental physiology and pathology to medical students at the University of Maryland. His efforts to improve dentistry were finally rewarded when he helped found the first national dental organization in 1839 and the first dental college in 1840.[9]

Without detracting from Hayden's contribution, a good deal of the credit for establishing dentistry as a profession belongs to the notable work of a second pioneer dentist, Dr. Chapin A. Harris (1809–60). Harris studied and practiced medicine in Greenfield, Ohio, before turning to dentistry. Subsequently he centered his activities in Baltimore, where in 1833 he was granted a medical license by the local medical society. In 1839 he published *The Dental Art*, which he later expanded and published under the title, *Principles and Practice of Dental Surgery*. This first dental textbook, periodically revised, remained a standard work for fifty years.[10]

Both Harris and Hayden were anxious to raise the level of dental education, and they first centered their efforts upon establishing a dental department in the University of Maryland School of Medicine. When their efforts failed, in part as a result of internal problems within the medical school, they turned to the state legislature and in 1840 obtained a charter for the Baltimore College of Dental Surgery, the first school of its kind. Although the University of Maryland medical faculty had voted against establishing a dental department, the dental school received strong support from the local medical profession. In fact, two thirds of the membership on the school's first advisory board were physicians. In the following years the school experienced a slow but steady increase in enrollment, and by the Civil War it was drawing students from all sections of the United States and even from the British Isles and France. Within the next few decades dental schools proliferated. By 1880 some thirteen schools were in operation. Despite the high standard set by the Baltimore school, dental colleges had no university connection until 1867 when Harvard opened a dental department, thereby giving academic respectability to dental education.[11]

Two other significant developments aided the cause of dentistry. In 1839 the *American Journal of Dental Science* began publication under the auspices of a group of New York dentists. The following year Horace Hayden and Chapin Harris founded the first national dental association, the American Society of Dental Surgeons. Thus, with a formal system of education, a national organization, and its own publications, the American dental profession was well established by the Civil War.

At the same time, several technical innovations greatly aided dental treatment. In 1838 the hand mallet was introduced, and in 1855 Charles Goodyear made the first application of vulcanized rubber as a base for false teeth. The next decade saw the development of the rubber dam to keep teeth dry during dental work and scientific dental prosthesis (artificial dentures). In the following years American dentistry continued its world leadership. In connection with the bacteriological revolution in the latter part of the century, men such as Willoughby Dayton Miller introduced antiseptic and aseptic dentistry. World War I turned dental attention to facial injuries and helped the development of maxillofacial surgery. A dental innovation which benefited surgery was the invention of the automatic electric suction pump by Dr. C. Edmund Kells of New Orleans. Originally designed to deal with saliva in dental practice, the device was modified by Kells, Joseph Hume, and Samuel Logan in 1916 so as to make it suitable for general surgery.[12]

In the postwar years state and local dental societies, working through school and health centers, promoted oral hygiene and created a public awareness of the role of the mouth in relation to general health. In this connection it was the dentists who first urged their patients to have regular checkups. In the past, individual dentists and dental associations have far outshone the medical profession in their willingness to cooperate with school and public health authorities in promoting preventive medicine and providing dental care. It will be interesting to see what effect the affluence that has come to dentists since World War II will have upon their social conscience.

X-RAY

As with anesthesia, the discovery of the X-ray was immediately seized upon by the American medical and dental professions. Wilhelm Conrad Roentgen first announced his discovery of the X-ray on December 28, 1895, and in January 1896 Professor M. I. Pupin of the Columbia University physics department made the first diagnostic radiograph in the United States. Within the next few years surgeons such as William B. Cannon of Harvard, who used X-rays to study the movements of the stomach and intestines, and dentists such as Dr. C. Edmund Kells of New Orleans began making broad-range applications of X-rays. Another American deserving mention is William Herbert Rollins, a New England physician and dentist who was among the first to recognize the danger involved in the use of X-rays. In 1901 he reported on his laboratory work with guinea pigs which demonstrated that X-rays were capable of causing death. These experiments led him to warn about the danger of overexposure and made him one of the leading advocates of X-ray housing devices.[13] The development of the X-ray and its technology was essentially an international accomplishment, but it was one in which Americans played a significant role. For example, the introduction of the Crookes tube in 1913, the work of W. D. Crookes of Detroit, opened a new era in X-ray work. Suffice it to say, the evolution of the X-ray into a major diagnostic instrument and therapeutic device was an important contribution to medical knowledge in the twentieth century.

AMERICAN SURGEONS

In the immediate post-Civil War years American surgeons made relatively few contributions to advances in surgery. The United States was still largely rural, and a good part of surgery was performed by physicians operating in private homes—either theirs or the patients'. Although a few large hospitals and urban centers provided an opportunity for surgery to develop as a specialty, America had nothing comparable to the great European medical centers. The large crowded European hospitals, however, were plagued with what was termed "hospitalism"—the rampant surgical infections which regularly swept through the wards, nullifying the best efforts of the surgeons. The dread of "hospitalism" was undoubtedly a factor in the European acceptance of the antiseptic principle, and the fact that the danger was not so acute in America may help to explain the reluctance of American surgeons to adopt the Listerian method.[14]

Two outstanding surgeons in the postwar era were Henry Jacob Bigelow (1816–90) of Boston, the first American to excise the hip joint, and Samuel David Gross (1805–84), professor of surgery at the Jefferson Medical College in Philadelphia from 1856 to 1882. Gross made many contributions to surgery but is best known for his writings on pathology, surgery, and medical history. His two-volume works, *Elements of Pathological Anatomy* (Boston, 1839) and *A System of Surgery: Pathological, Diagnostic, Therapeutic, and Operative* (Philadelphia, 1859), remained standard for many years. Another outstanding surgeon in this period was Nicholas Senn (1844–1909), a graduate of the Chicago Medical College who became professor of surgery at Rush Medical College in Chicago. His major contribution was in the area of intestinal surgery.

The 1880s were a transitional period in American surgery. Writing in 1885, Dr. Stephen Smith, a prominent New York physician, surgeon, and public health figure, emphasized that surgeons in New York's Bellevue Hospital no longer accepted suppuration as an inevitable process but rather expected primary healing. "Cleanliness is the one great object sought . . . in all operations," he wrote, for by this means the surgeon may with "absolute certainty, protect an ordinary open wound from suppuration." The significance of this statement lies in the fact that it was written only four years after President Garfield's wound had been probed by the attending surgeons' fingers.[15]

In the 1890s American surgery came of age. Aseptic techniques generally became accepted, and a new generation of surgeons appeared on the scene. These men were far better educated than their predecessors, and nearly all of them had studied in Vienna, Paris, and the other European medical centers. Not all of the prominent surgeons in this period belonged to the new generation, for William W. Keen (1837–1932) had a career spanning the entire latter part of the nineteenth century. Keen is best known for his pioneering work in abdominal and cranial surgery and for his medical textbooks. Among the new men coming to the fore at this time were Rudolph Matas of Tulane University in New Orleans, who specialized in abdominal and vascular surgery; George W. Crile (1864–1943) of Western Reserve University in Cleveland, best known for his work on surgical shock; William Stewart Halsted (1852–1922) of Johns Hopkins, a master surgeon whose work in connection with anesthesia has already been mentioned; and John Benjamin Murphy (1857–1916) of Northwestern University in Chicago. The latter contributed to end-to-end resections of arteries and veins and devised the Murphy button for use in intestinal repair work. [16]

The diagnosis and treatment of appendicitis is one area of abdominal surgery in which American surgeons took the initiative. During the nineteenth century the disorder was called typhlitis, based on the assumption that the problem lay in the cecum, the blind pouch in which the large intestine begins. Although as early as 1837 individual American physicians had diagnosed perforation of the appendix in cases of so-called typhlitis, it remained for Reginal Heber Fitz (1843–1913) of Boston to pinpoint the source of the problem. In 1886 he read a paper analyzing 466 cases involving this type of abdominal distress and showed that in the vast majority of them inflammation of the appendix was the primary cause. So convincing was his study that by the 1890s the term typhlitis was being replaced by appendicitis. The next development was the work of Charles McBurney (1845–1913) of New York, who discovered a major diagnostic aid and promoted a surgical technique. In 1889 he identified McBurney's point, the area in the abdomen in which tenderness indicated inflammation of the appendix, and in 1894 he described an operative method for removing the appendix which is still called McBurney's incision. Ironically, as McBurney himself admitted, the method was first used by Dr. L. L. McArthur of Chicago.[17]

With the twentieth century, American surgery began to

flourish, and there is scarcely any field of surgery in which Americans did not play a prominent role. Vascular surgery was literally revolutionized by Alexis Carrel of the Rockefeller Institute. He laid the basis for modern surgery of the aorta and heart, performed basic work in physiology and physiological surgery, and built the foundation for organ transplants. His work on aortic aneurysms was carried forward in the 1960s by Michael DeBakey and his associates in Houston. In 1964 DeBakey reported the successful use of Dacron vascular grafts. DeBakey's interest in the heart and great arteries led him on to heart transplants, a radical step which has yet to prove its value.

Open heart surgery and other complicated operative procedures would scarcely have been feasible without the emergence of hematology and improvements in blood transfusion techniques. Experimental work had been done with transfusions in the nineteenth century, but it was not until Karl Landsteiner of Vienna discovered blood types that the procedure became relatively safe. As transfusion techniques improved, the need arose for blood reservoirs. Chicago's Cook County Hospital established the first blood bank in 1937, where blood was stored at a temperature of from 4° to 6° centigrade. Another major step came with the discovery of heparin by Jay McClean of Johns Hopkins between 1911 and 1916. Its anticoagulant qualities have made it invaluable for both surgery and medicine.[18]

As ancillary aids to surgery became available, as better insights were gained into physiology, and, as surgical techniques improved, surgeons were emboldened to move into every part of the body. By the 1930s surgeons were widely utilizing thoracoplasty in cases of advanced tuberculosis, an operation which involved resecting the ribs to allow the lung to contract and rest. In the 1940s this procedure was supplanted by pulmonary resection, but the advent of antituberculous drugs in the postwar era virtually eliminated the need for surgery. Increased life expectancy and other factors have made cancer a major medical problem, and surgery has been the chief reliance for dealing with its various forms. Although in recent years radiation and chemotherapy have been added to our defensive weapons, it is likely that surgery will remain the major line of defense until much more is learned about this cruel and deadly disease.

The brief history of surgery in the foregoing pages necessarily emphasizes successes and thus gives a distorted picture to those accustomed to the relatively low surgical mortality rates of the present. While outstanding operators introduced new techniques and saved many lives, mortality rates for appendectomies and many other procedures considered routine today remained quite high well into the second quarter of the twentieth century. The opening of new areas not infrequently led to abuses and temporarily caused more harm than good. In 1885 a distinguished New York physician declared that "the race would be better off had gynecology never been invented," and one of his colleagues agreed with him that "the injury which bunglers, enthusiasts, and charlatans have done in this connection greatly outweighs the good which others have accomplished. . . ."[19]

While outstanding surgeons such as Halsted, Kelly, and others were achieving excellent results, the same cannot be said for the average surgeon. In 1895 Dr. Thomas E. Schumpert, house surgeon of Charity Hospital in Shreveport, Louisiana, reported that in a difficult case of parturition he had first considered a craniotomy but hesitated because the child was still living. Of the 1,718 women admitted to the obstetrical wards in Charity Hospital of New Orleans between January 1, 1916, and June 30, 1918, only 23 were delivered by a Cesarean section. Of these 23 Cesarean sections, 7 resulted in maternal deaths—a maternal death rate of 30 percent.[20]

The advent of sulfa drugs, antibiotics, and a host of other innovations have drastically altered surgery in the past fifty years. Aside from a great increase in surgical procedures and an equally great reduction in mortality, there has been a tremendous growth in the number of patients either cured or given some measure of relief. The following statistics from the Connecticut Hospital clearly show this development. Between 1878 and 1908, 100 cases of prostatism were admitted. Of these only 22 were treated surgically. Out of the entire group only 8 were relieved of obstruction and 38 died. Forty years later, in the nine months from December 1947 to September 1948, approximately 100 similar cases were admitted. Of this group 96 percent were relieved and the mortality rate was only 4 percent—and none of these deaths were directly related to prostatism.[21]

The enormous success achieved by surgeons has led one writer to call the last 100 years the century of the surgeon. The ability of the skilled surgeon to bring immediate or quick relief to patients has made him preeminent in the medical profession and brought him prestige and affluence. He is the new miracle worker, and the masked and gowned surgeon in the operating room has come to symbolize modern science. Beneficial as most of the vast increase in surgery has been, a good many of the operative procedures are not really necessary. A few surgeons are inclined to operate out of the sheer joy of craftsmanship, others are motivated either consciously or subconsciously by the prospects of a lucrative income, and undoubtedly other factors, too, contribute to the excessive surgery. The growing public awareness of this problem means that in the immediate future the medical profession must either police itself or face action by the state.

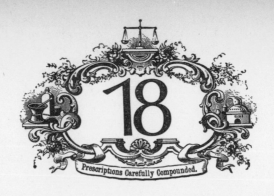

WOMEN AND MINORITIES
IN MEDICINE

MEDICAL EDUCATION

THE practicing physician in the second half of the nineteenth century continued to derive his training from a variety of sources. The old apprenticeship system still hung on, although the ease of obtaining diplomas guaranteed that most doctors had some type of medical degree. Aside from the relatively large number who bought their degrees from diploma mills, a subject which will be considered under medical licensing, the quality of medical training varied widely. The better physician obtained a bachelor's degree from a reputable school, took an M.D. in an equally good institution, and then spent one to three years studying abroad. The average physician, however, had no more than a high-school education—and frequently less—and had acquired his medical degree by attending the same four- or five-month course of medical lectures for two years in a row.

Medical schools were still proprietary institutions in which the admission of students took precedence over any entrance requirements. As late as 1887 an officer of the Maine State Board of Health had an eight-year-old girl apply in her own handwriting for admission to a number of medical schools. Although she stated that she had none of the requirements for admission, over half the schools accepted her application, several of them assuring her that the examinations for a degree were not difficult. Even in the best schools there were few obstacles to taking a degree. As of 1870, examinations at Harvard Medical School consisted of nine professors spending five minutes each questioning the candidate. To pass the examination, it was only necessary to satisfy five out of the nine professors; thus the candidate could fail four out of nine medical subjects and still obtain his degree. Dr. William Pepper pointed out in 1877 that it took at least four or five years of apprenticeship to become a craftsman, but that one could obtain a medical degree in less than one third of the time.[1]

Dr. Edward H. Dixon, a well-known New York physician, described the lecture room of the Medical Department of New York University as "an ill-constructed, dirty room, drenched with tobacco, and perfumed with vile odors." The audience, he wrote, was "utterly indescribable." At the end of the class hour a "most excruciating noise splits your ears" as "the students rush forth like mad buffaloes. . . ."[2] Charles McIntyre's statistics on the percentage of college men who entered the medical profession show that medicine held little attraction for college graduates, for he found that the percentage declined as the century advanced. He gloomily concluded in 1882 that it was a mistake to classify "the *medical business* among the learned professions. . . ."[3]

The growing awareness of the inadequacy of medical training led to the establishment of many state licensing boards during the latter part of the century. Since these boards tended to accept almost any medical degree, the net effect was to stimulate the rise of inferior schools. For example, the number of medical colleges increased from 90 in 1880 to 151 by 1900. Despite this discouraging picture, American medical schools could not help but react to the explosion of scientific knowledge which was drastically altering all aspects of Western society. Led by the Chicago Medical College and Harvard, in the 1870s a three-year graded curriculum was introduced, the school year was lengthened, and written examinations were required. President Eliot of Harvard, who introduced these reforms in 1871 over the opposition of the older members of the medical faculty, was informed by Professor Henry Bigelow that half the medical students could barely write and that it was ridiculous to expect them to pass written examinations. Eliot was also warned, correctly as it turned out, that the effect would be to reduce the number of students. As was predicted, Eliot's reforms reduced the medical school's enrollment by 43 percent between 1870 and 1872. Nonetheless, Eliot persisted, and when the universities of Pennsylvania, Syracuse, and Michigan followed suit, the three-year graded curriculum was established in the leading schools.[4]

The example set by these institutions eventually influenced the entire course of American medical education, but the process was a slow one. When the American Medical College Association was organized in 1876, it sought to establish a three-year course as standard, but its efforts proved abortive and the Association soon disappeared. It was revived in 1890 as the National Association of Medical Colleges (later the Association of American Medical Colleges), and this time it became a successful force for reform. Member schools were expected to require entrance examinations and to offer a three-year course of instruction, a six-month academic year, written and oral exams, and laboratory work in chemistry, histology, and pathology. Three years later the Association voted to increase the course of study to four years. Although membership fell from 71 in 1894 to 54 in 1897, the Association held firm to its requirement for a four-year course.[5]

While the medical colleges were striving to raise their standards, the appearance of the Johns Hopkins University profoundly affected all American education. Established in 1876 under the inspired leadership of Daniel Colt Gilman, it quickly set new standards for graduate education and brought a radical change in medical training. Gilman, with the help of John Shaw Billings, the founder of the Army Medical Library, began searching for a medical faculty in the early 1880s and his first choice was Dr. William H. Welch, a bright young man who had gone to Europe to complete his medical education and had studied with two great scientific leaders, the pathologist Julius Cohenheim, and the physiologist Willy Kuhne. Gilman heard Welch highly recommended by both Cohenheim and Billings and in 1884 appointed him professor of pathology. With the assistance of Welch and Billings, Gilman gradually recruited a faculty representing the best physician-scientists and clinicians available. In short order he brought in William S. Halsted to head surgery, William Osler as professor of medicine, Howard A. Kelly as associate professor of gynecology and obstetrics, Franklin P. Mall as professor of anatomy, and Henry M. Hurd as superintendent of the University Hospital.

While helping to recruit a staff for the Hospital and School and engaging in his own laboratory studies, Welch was in close contact with the regular academic faculty and learned to appreciate the role of research in connection with teaching. This conditioning accorded with his own bent, and Welch deserves much of the credit for making American medical schools centers for research and teaching. Johns Hopkins was not the first school to build a teaching hospital; this honor goes to the University of Pennsylvania, which opened its University Hospital in 1874. What Johns Hopkins did, however, was to make the hospital an integral part of a research-oriented medical institution. It also provided a permanent clinical staff for the hospital and established a nurses' training school in close conjunction with it.[6]

The opening of the Johns Hopkins School of Medicine in 1893 marked the first time in America that a bachelor's degree and a knowledge of French and German were required for admission. The emphasis upon laboratory and clinical research which characterized the school and hospital soon won for Hopkins a reputation for preeminence in medical education. Within a few years the school's graduates and younger faculty members were spreading the Hopkins system throughout the United States.

Meanwhile the American Medical Association was belatedly reentering the picture. Throughout the first fifty years of its existence it had been preoccupied with fighting the irregulars, most notably the homeopaths, but early in the twentieth century it turned its attention once more to the training of physicians. In 1904 the Association voted to make its committee on education a permanent one, and the following year the AMA Council on Medical Education came into existence. This latter body began meeting regularly, and initially its annual reports presented a discouraging picture. In 1906 it named five states in which the medical schools were notoriously poor, and the following year it reported that only half of the 160 medical schools were equipped to "teach modern medicine," that 30 percent were doing a poor job, and that the other 20 percent were "unworthy of recognition."[7]

In 1907 the Council asked the Carnegie Foundation to take a look at medical education. The Foundation acceded and turned the job over to Abraham Flexner, a layman who had already published one study on American colleges. Flexner had taken a bachelor's degree at Hopkins and was an admirer of William Welch. He first studied the Hopkins Medical School and then decided to use it as a model. Flexner's study was completed in 1909 and published in 1910.[8] It came at a time when the AMA's Council had made the medical profession acutely aware of the inadequacies of medical training, and the *Report* proved a bombshell.

Flexner made a complete and detailed analysis of each school and passed judgment on it in firm and decisive prose. Speaking of the Atlantic Medical College and the Maryland Medical College, Flexner declared: "That such unconscionable concerns should at this day continue to flourish is a blot upon the state of Maryland and the city of Baltimore." Of the South he wrote that it "is generally overcrowded with schools with which nothing can be done; for they are conducted by old-time practitioners, who could not use improved teaching facilities if they were provided."[9] While the Flexner *Report* would undoubtedly have created a stir, it might well have aroused a brief flurry of attention and then faded away had it not been that Flexner was able to persuade the Rockefeller family to make grants which eventually amounted to almost $50,000,000 to those schools which Flexner considered worthwhile. Rockefeller's contributions in turn stimulated other philanthropists to support medical education, with most of the money going to those institutions designated by Flexner as worthy of support. The result was to widen the gap between the better and poorer schools, causing the latter gradually to fall by the wayside. By 1930 the number of medical schools in America had dropped from 148 to 66.[10]

In 1924 Flexner evaluated the changes which had taken place in medical education and rejoiced that almost half the schools in existence in 1910 had closed their doors, including nearly all the weakest ones found in the South and West. Virtually all schools, he added, were now equipped with laboratory and clinical facilities and the basic courses were being taught by qualified faculty members on a full-time basis. By this date, too, the four-year graded curriculum had become standard.[11] While Flexner could take justifiable pride in these changes, much of the credit belongs to the AMA's Council on Medical Education, which, through its annual rating system, exerted continuous pressure to raise educational standards. The work of the Association of American Medical Colleges (1890) and the rising standards required by state licensing boards, which formed a strong national body in 1912, the Federation of State Medical Boards, also contributed to the general advance in medical education.

By 1920, aided by the spread of Hopkins graduates who held positions in nearly every medical school, the Hopkins system was well established in American medical education. An undergraduate degree was generally a prerequisite to medical training, and a three- or four-year graded curriculum was standard. Nearly all schools provided hospital facilities and clinical instruction and required their graduates to take a year's internship. The curriculum consisted of two years of basic sciences, including laboratory work, and two years clinical training in hospitals and outpatient clinics. The constant pressure exerted by the AMA's Council on Medical Education not only weeded out the weaker schools but helped to strengthen the better ones, with the result that the average medical graduate in the 1920s was far better trained than his predecessor of thirty years previously.

Without disparaging the excellent work of Johns Hopkins, Abraham Flexner, and the AMA's Council on Medical Education, it is clear that by the beginning of the twentieth century social and scientific changes were undermining the proprietary medical schools. Expensive laboratories and medical equipment were becoming essential to medical training and the limited income of proprietary schools could neither build nor maintain these facilities. Medical education was moving into a new era, and even without Flexner, Welch, and the others the change would have come.

On the face of it, the movement to improve medical education was an intelligent and progressive step; better-trained physicians clearly meant better medicine. Yet it is evident from any perusal of medical journals in the late nineteenth and early twentieth centuries that economic and class motives provided much of the impetus for reform. The ineffectiveness of the licensing laws prior to 1900 and the ease with which one could acquire a nominal medical degree guaranteed a plethora of doctors. It also insured a relatively low financial status for those in the profession. Obviously, raising entrance standards into medicine was a prime means of reducing the number of physicians, and an effective way to increase the social and economic status of the profession. This argument was set forth frequently in medical journals and may well have had more influence than the more idealistic appeals. The question of social status was almost as important as the economic one in the drive to raise standards. The better-trained physicians with college and university backgrounds were almost exclusively products of the middle and upper class, while the proprietary schools tended to recruit more from the lower economic groups. With some justice, university-trained physicians could complain about their poorly educated colleagues, but a class bias shows through many of the diatribes against doctors from the lower classes.

Whether or not physicians intended to keep members of the lower economic groups out of medicine, this was the result of the reformed medical schools. The prerequisite of a bachelor's degree fifty years ago automatically excluded a major part of the public from medical education, and, as medical training became longer and more costly, the net effect was to make medicine more and more exclusive. The selection of elitist schools by Rockefeller and other foundations added still further to the exclusiveness of medicine. The well-established eastern schools were the chief recipients of foundation largesse, along with a handful of leading schools in the South, the Midwest, and the West. Since medical schools for women and blacks were generally among the weaker institutions, they were swept away.

In the case of women, token acceptance of female students by many leading medical schools seemingly eliminated the need for separate women's medical colleges. Unfortunately, biased entrance requirements and a deliberate policy by most faculty members of discouraging women students resulted in a steady drop in the number of women M.D.'s during the early years of the twentieth century. One last point worth noting in this connection is that, as the medical profession drew its membership increasingly from the upper class, it became more and more conservative. The leadership which medicine had shown in the public health movement and other progressive reforms of the late nineteenth century was no longer in evidence by the 1920s.[12]

The basic pattern of modern American medical education was well established by 1920, and it continued relatively unaltered for the next forty years. The only changes of consequence were a gradual lessening in the time devoted to anatomy and a corresponding increase in the hours devoted to physiology and biochemistry. Along with this, the original Hopkins curriculum which assigned third-year students to outpatient clinics and fourth-year students to hospitals was reversed, with the students first entering the hospital wards and then attending outpatient clinics, a change which gave them a chance to see more serious cases with well-developed symptoms before working in the outpatient clinics. While the basic curriculum remained the same, the content of courses changed drastically with the expansion of medical knowledge, a situation which held true for virtually every course.[13] This same information explosion was also responsible for a proliferation of courses in specialty areas and a tendency to increase the number of class and laboratory hours.

As indicated earlier, the internship was firmly established by the 1920s and became a standard part of medical education by the 1930s. At the same time residency programs expanded and multiplied. Specialty training, however, took two main directions: one under the auspices of schools and universities and another in connection with hospitals having no medical school connections. This seeming divergence of training created some difficulty in determining how to regulate specialty training, but the issue was solved by the emergence of specialty boards.[14] The snowballing effect of medical research raised yet another problem which had not beset earlier physicians—the need to keep abreast of new developments. In response medical schools began offering postgraduate education: short courses, clinics, and seminars designed to keep practicing physicians aware of the latest findings in their particular areas.

World War II brought few immediate changes. Insofar as medical education was concerned, the only direct impact of the war was to speed up medical training. The prerequisite of a bachelor's degree for admission to medical school was reduced in some cases to two years, and the four-year medical curriculum was concentrated into three years of intensive study. From a long-range standpoint, the war brought a renewed interest in medical research, a development which was to have a profound impact on medical schools in the succeeding years. The wartime gains made by the National Research Defense Council and its successor, the Office of Scientific Research and Development, convinced Congress and the public that money spent for research was a sound investment. The development of atomic energy was the most striking success of government-sponsored research, but the appearance of a veritable host of miracle drugs, led by the sulfa compounds and antibiotics, encouraged the belief that with sufficient funds American medical scientists could create a brave new healthy world.

The enthusiasm for medical research in the postwar years led to a massive increase in government funding. According to J. A. Shannon, a former director of the National Institutes of Health, spending for medical research rose from $87 million in 1947 to over $2 billion in 1966. In this same period the federal government's share of this money rose from 31 percent to 68 percent. While the National Institutes of Health and other agencies conducted a good part of the research, the tradition of research-oriented medical schools started by Johns Hopkins meant that university medical centers played a major role in the expanding research. They not only supplied most of the manpower, but with federal help they greatly enlarged their own facilities. The effect was to strengthen medical school faculties and to make possible a sharp increase in the number of medical graduates. In the fifteen years from 1951 to 1966 the annual number of medical degrees awarded increased by 25 percent.[15]

Although medical education was receiving indirect benefits from the funds voted for medical research, Congress, while willing to vote money for cancer or heart research, was reluctant to provide appropriations for the more prosaic task of medical education. Hence medical deans and administrators were compelled to shuffle research funds around in order to provide for their teaching faculties. It was not until 1965 when the Health Professions Educational Assistance Act was passed that any significant money was appropriated for medical education *per se*. Even today medical administrators are compelled to give a broad definition to what constitutes research in an effort to balance teaching and research responsibilities. Another beneficial side effect of the availability of Federal and state funding has been a proliferation of medical schools. From a low point of sixty-six institutions in 1933, the number of medical schools moved up to eighty-seven by 1967 and is now approaching the 100 mark.

The large sums available for medical research, however, made medical schools even more research-oriented and turned them away from the equally fundamental task of teaching. Grant money was given to institutions on the basis of the research abilities of individual faculty members. Understandably medical schools recruited new professors and evaluated the existing ones on their ability to attract research grants. Nor did the infusion of huge sums of research money bring any significant change in medical education. Schools grew larger and new ones were established, but the basic pattern set by Johns Hopkins remained unchanged. The one significant contribution to medical education in the postwar years was a major curriculum revision undertaken by Western Reserve Medical School in 1952. This institution sought to break away from the traditional disciplines or departments and utilize interdepartmental committees for teaching purposes. While considerable interest was expressed in the experiment, the majority of medical schools, preoccupied in part with acquiring and spending research funds, continued their time-tested teaching methods, and at least ten years or more elapsed before the Western Reserve system had any appreciable effect on medical education.

In glancing back over medical education for the past eighty years, one cannot help being impressed with the vast improvement in the training provided for young physicians. A good share of the credit for this can be ascribed to fundamental changes in medicine itself. The bacteriological revolution was only one of a series of advances which drastically altered the practice of medicine. The image of the physician at the bedside of the patient has been replaced by the white-coated surgeon in the operating room or the research man in his laboratory. Encouraged by television and by the medical profession itself, the public considers medicine a science and expects precise diagnoses and quick cures. In the first flush of enthusiasm arising from the discovery of bacteria and the development of antitoxins, physicians forgot that patients were complex human organisms, and they concentrated upon fighting germs or viruses. As laboratories and technology began playing a greater part in medicine, it was inevitable that medical training tended more and more toward science and technology; and, as the curricula became overcrowded with laboratory and technique courses, it was perhaps also inevitable that humanistic training would be pushed into the background.

It was an awareness of this and the need for a thorough curriculum revision which in the 1960s led a number of medical schools to undertake considerable soul-searching. These faculty self-evaluations, which are still continuing, have led to sharp reductions in the core curriculum and a corresponding increase in the hours available for electives. In a number of schools more time is now assigned to such topics as community medicine, social medicine, medical ethics, and the history of medicine. The number of hours allocated to and the form of these courses varies widely. Medicine, by its very nature, must be conservative, and many institutions are content to pay lip service to the humanities and the rubric of social medicine. Yet the omens are promising, and medical education may be returning again to the Hippocratic concept of dealing with the whole patient.

WOMEN IN MEDICINE

The United States has the distinction of giving the first medical degree to a woman, yet, far more than most countries, it has continually discriminated against females in medicine. The awarding of the first medical degree came during the 1830s and 1840s, an age of great social ferment in which zealous advocates of many reforms were attracting followers. The dominant reform movement was the abolition of slavery, but reformers were fighting against tobacco and alcohol, urging women's rights, and seeking reforms in clothing, diet, and many other aspects of American life. The health crusade of the 1840s fought for fresh air, exercise, comfortable clothing, and moderate diet, and sought to give some understanding of physiology. Of particular concern to intelligent women reformers was the effort to give females some understanding of their anatomy and physiology, subjects which were taboo in polite society.

One development in British and American medicine in the late eighteenth and early nineteenth centuries was the substitution of the physician for the midwife in obstetrical care. How this came about in a society which rated modesty as a prime womanly virtue and in which a respectable female carefully covered herself from head to toe is difficult to explain. It is even harder to understand when one realizes that physicians in the early nineteenth century were not allowed visually to examine females with gynecological problems and were compelled to assist in deliveries with their hands under a sheet or some other cover. As this form of prudery gained wide acceptance, many "modest" women with serious female problems were reluctant to call in a physician. An obvious solution was to train women physicians to deal with obstetrics and gynecology, but the idea was not considered seriously until women began seeking entrance into the medical profession.

The chief impetus leading women into medicine was the movement for women's rights. The majority of women who pioneered in medicine were active in the reform movements of the day, and their interest in medicine reflected their liberal outlook. The widespread belief that women were sickly and frail, periodically incapacitated by menstruation and subject to "female complaints," led to the rise of "Ladies Physiological Reform Societies," which in turn brought a demand for women teachers versed in anatomy and physiology. Ironically, the state of medicine in America in the midcentury both facilitated the entrance of women into it and at the same time aroused opposition to lady doctors. The emergence of irregular medical schools—eclectic, homeopathic, and so forth—was an advantage, since these institutions were willing to accept women in an effort to gain support for their particular school of medical thought. Moreover, the excessive number of proprietary medical schools anxiously trying to build their enrollments insured that women would be accepted, and the elementary academic requirements guaranteed them a degree. In the majority of states, possession of a medical degree was an automatic license to practice. Against these advantages, the ease with which an individual could enter the profession meant an excess of practitioners, and the fear of additional competition in an already overcrowded profession undoubtedly accounted for some of the opposition encountered by women.[16]

The first woman to obtain a medical degree was Elizabeth Blackwell. The product of a liberal English background, she came with her family to America at the age of eleven. She began her career as a teacher, but, motivated at least in part by her zeal for women's rights, decided to study medicine. She found a friend and guide in Dr. Samuel H. Dickson of the Charleston Medical School who helped her to "read" medicine. She tried unsuccessfully to gain entrance to various medical schools and was delighted when in 1847 Geneva Medical School of Western New York accepted her application. In a masculine-dominated atmosphere, only an attractive and strong personality enabled her to overcome the suspicions, resentment, and ridicule of her professors and fellow students. A correspondent to one of the medical journals reported in December that Miss Blackwell "comes into class with great composure, takes off her bonnet and puts it under the seat (exposing a fine phrenology), takes notes constantly, and maintains, throughout, an unchanged countenance. The effect on the class has been good, and great decorum is preserved when she is present."[17] Upon obtaining her degree in 1849, she was unable to find a hospital which would admit her for clinical training, so she set off for England and the Continent to continue her studies. On her return in 1850, she began practicing in New York, where she encountered considerable opposition. Excluded from hospitals, she opened a private dispensary for women and children.

A major hurdle preventing women from obtaining medical training was the refusal of hospitals to accept them. To help remedy this situation, Dr. Blackwell, along with her sister Emily and Marie Zakrzewska, both of whom had earned medical degrees from the Cleveland Medical College (Western Reserve), founded the New York Infirmary for Women and Children. Despite initial difficulties, the Infirmary flourished, and in 1868 the three women opened the Woman's Medical College of the New York Infirmary. Shortly thereafter, Dr. Blackwell, who had been commuting between England and America, returned to England to carry on the fight for various health causes.

Once Dr. Blackwell had broken the barrier, women began making rapid progress in medicine. The women's rights movement was gaining strength, and Geneva Medical College gained a historical first by sheer chance. The year Dr. Blackwell graduated, 1849, Central Medical College of New York, an eclectic school located in Syracuse, admitted three women. The Eclectics school opened all of their schools to women in 1855, and fifteen years later admitted women to membership in their national association.

Reflecting the general ferment of the 1840s, a group of physicians, including several Quakers, began planning for a women's medical school in Philadelphia. After some preliminary steps, the Female Medical College of Pennsylvania was chartered in 1850. The majority of students during the first year were females interested in learning something about their own anatomy and physiology, but eight of them sought medical degrees. Opposition from conservative male practitioners and suspicions that the school was tinged with Eclecticism made the first few years difficult. The outbreak of war in 1861 closed its doors, but at the end of hostilities, the institution reopened as the Woman's Medical College of Pennsylvania under the able leadership of one of its first graduates, Ann Preston. It still survives today as the last of the female medical schools.

Meanwhile, in 1848 a group of enlightened Boston physicians interested primarily in teaching midwifery opened the Boston Female Medical College. The chief founder, Dr. Samuel Gregory, two years later secured a charter for the Female Medical Education Society to promote the cause of women's medical education in Boston. In 1856 the original school was rechartered as the New England Female Medical College. It struggled along for a few years and finally merged in 1874 with the Medical Department of Boston University, at that time a homeopathic institution.[18]

By the Civil War at least three medical schools for women were granting degrees (the third one was Penn Medical University, an offshoot of the Woman's Medical College of Pennsylvania), and a number of schools, largely irregular ones, had gone coeducational. Even Harvard, affected by the liberal atmosphere, in 1850 accepted a female and three black students. When their fellow students rioted in protest, the four individuals withdrew their applications. In consequence Harvard Medical School waited almost 100 years, until 1945, before finally admitting women.[19]

While the majority of physicians opposed the entrance of

women, a highly articulate minority actively supported the women's cause. The *Boston Medical and Surgical Journal* took a moderately favorable stance at first. It published letters and articles on both sides of the issue, including one from Mrs. Paulina Wright Davis, a leading exponent of women's rights. A later change in the editorship, however, subsequently altered the *Journal*'s viewpoint, for the new editor strongly opposed women in any area of medicine—even midwifery.[20] An Atlanta physician in 1854 argued that female physicians were essential to "the safety and happiness" of a large portion "of the most refined and lovely women. . . ." Every practitioner, he wrote, almost daily saw cases which had "become incurable on account of the reluctance of females to submit" to examination. Most female diseases, he asserted, could not be cured because of "the almost insuperable objections of the fair sufferers, to the inevitable exposure of their sexual secrets to a male physician."[21]

Unfortunately, the voices raised in opposition to women were far more numerous and strident. They repeated and embellished all the traditional arguments. Women were too frail, too sensitive, too emotional, and too lacking in rational ability. Physicians asked what would happen to female modesty and chastity if women medical students were exposed to the details of their own anatomy— and, inconceivable as it seemed, to male anatomy. Even as the diehards fought for morality and decency, some opponents of women's rights manfully faced reality, for, as the editor of the *Medical and Surgical Reporter* conceded, "in some degenerate age of the world women may be received into favor as practitioners of medicine."[22]

While women were gaining acceptance into medical schools, they were not so successful with respect to hospitals and medical societies. As part of their fight to raise professional standards, the AMA and local medical societies tried to prevent their members from consulting with irregular practitioners. They also used this weapon against women physicians. In 1859 the Philadelphia County Medical Society forbade its members to consult with the professors and graduates of female medical schools, and the State Society concurred in the action. All was not harmony, however, for the Montgomery County Society protested the decision. When the issue was raised again in 1866–67, the Montgomery County

Society resolved that females were as well fitted for medicine as males and instructed its delegates to vote in favor of consultations with females.[23]

Although the tide was gradually turning in favor of women, the conservatives gave ground only grudgingly. When the council of the Massachusetts Medical Society voted to admit women in 1879, the editor of the *Boston Medical and Surgical Journal* commented in sorrow: "The Society [has taken] a long step downward from the dignified attitude which it has hitherto assumed, and its moral tone will have been perceptibly lowered." Yet four years later, when the Society polled its members on the question of admitting women to full membership, 706 responded favorably and only 400 opposed it. Moreover, 931 of the members expressed a willingness to consult with female physicians.

At the national level, the AMA first took up the question of female membership in 1868, but a resolution in favor of it was tabled. The question continued to pop up in the succeeding years, and always a substantial minority could be counted on to support the admission of women. For example, the vote on a resolution in 1871 was eighty opposed and twenty-five in favor. In 1876 the Illinois Society sent a female delegate, Dr. Sarah Hackett Stevenson, who was received with a few misgivings. Despite consistent support within the AMA and slow but steady gains at the local and state levels, the national society did not admit women until 1915.[24]

Despite conservative opposition and the reluctance of the AMA to admit them, a limited survey in 1881 demonstrated that women medical graduates were generally accepted by the public and by most members of the profession. Dean Rachel Bodley of the Woman's Medical College of Pennsylvania sent questionnaires to 244 of the school's graduates and received answers from 189. Of the 189, 166 were actively engaged in medical practice, most of whom concentrated largely or in part on gynecology and obstetrics. A total of 150 of the 189 considered that they received "cordial social recognition" and only 7 reported negatively. Approximately one third, 68, were members of a state, county, or local medical society. The average income for the entire group was around $3,000, with four of them reporting annual earnings of between $15,000 and $20,000 a year.[25] In terms of income and membership in medical societies, female medical graduates would appear to have been doing better than their male counterparts. This success probably speaks more for their middle- or upper-class background than any other factor. The semiliterate lower-class males who had access to the medical profession at that time were not too likely to build a profitable middle-class practice.

In the post-Civil War years a number of women's medical schools appeared, although most of them were short-lived. Altogether nineteen schools were established between 1850 and 1895, including the Chicago Women's Hospital College organized in 1870, the New York Free Medical College for Women in 1871, and the Woman's Medical College of Baltimore founded in 1882. By this latter year women's position in the medical profession was steadily improving. For example, the *Journal of the American Medical Association* in 1882 carried a favorable account of the graduation ceremonies at the Women's Hospital Medical College of Chicago, adding: "The institution is enjoying a fair degree of prosperity, and we are informed that a new college building will be erected during the present season."

Meanwhile many established institutions and newly formed schools were becoming coeducational. Medical departments were opened to women at the University of California in 1869, Syracuse University in 1870, and the University of Michigan in 1871. While state universities and schools west of the Appalachians were liberalizing their admissions, the old and well-established schools in the Northeast continued to resist. Harvard, which had shown a brief sign of weakness in 1850, was sorely tempted in 1879. The offer of a gift from the estate of Mr. George O. Hovey amounting to $10,000 was made contingent upon the admission of women to the Medical School. A committee appointed to look into the matter divided, with the majority favoring acceptance of the gift and the minority recommending the establishment of a separate medical school for women. Subsequently, the faculty met and voted thirteen to five that it was "detrimental to the school to enter upon the experiment of admitting female students." The overseers concurred with the faculty, voting seventeen to seven to reject the Hovey offer, although they did vote sixteen to ten to admit women for medical studies "under suitable restrictions."[26] The faculty, however, remained adamant, and the admission of women awaited another sixty-odd years.

The first major eastern school to make a concession was Johns Hopkins, a relatively new institution. Having made the decision to establish a medical school and appointed a faculty, the University in 1892 was unable to raise enough money to begin operations. A group of able and wealthy women, led by Misses M. Carey Thomas, Mary Garrett, Elizabeth King, and Mary Gwinn, the organizers of Bryn Mawr, decided to take advantage of this financial crisis to further the course of women's rights. They raised $100,000 and offered it to Johns Hopkins on condition that women be admitted to the medical school on an equal basis with men. The reluctant administrators and trustees agreed to accept the offer providing the women raised a total of $500,000, expecting that this would end the matter. When a national appeal brought only about $200,000, Miss Garrett personally offered over $300,000 to complete the requisite half-million dollars, but she also insisted that all students must have as prerequisites a B.A. degree or its equivalent, a knowledge of French and German, and some premedical studies. The trustees and faculty were horrified, but Miss Garrett and her cohorts were insistent and finally won the day. The victory gained by this determined group of intelligent women was not only an advance for women's rights, but it profoundly affected the entire course of American medical education.[27]

The decision by Johns Hopkins was a straw in the wind, and other schools soon began modifying their admission policies. Tulane University was authorized by the state legislature in 1894 to grant diplomas in law, medicine, and pharmacy to women, while Cornell University, a combination private–land grant institution, opened its medical school on a coeducational basis in 1898. As more and more schools accepted female students, the *raison d'être* for separate women's schools ceased to exist, and they soon began closing their doors. By 1909 only three were still operating: the Woman's Medical College of Pennsylvania, the Woman's Medical College of Baltimore, and the New York Medical College and Hospital for Women.

Ironically, as Abraham Flexner observed, women's interest in medical education appeared to decline in a direct ratio to their ability to obtain it. Between 1904 and 1909 both the number of women medical students and those graduating showed a steady decline. Whereas a total of 254 women received medical degrees in 1904, only 162 were granted them in 1909. On a percentage basis, women represented 4 percent of all medical graduates in 1905, but by 1915 this figure was down to 2.6 percent. The percentage climbed to 5.4 in 1927 and then dropped below 5 until 1940. The enrollment of women in medical schools began rising again in 1945, peaked in 1948, and then declined until 1952. It held steady until 1960, when it again took a slight upward trend. In consequence, the percentage of women graduates reached a high point of 12.1 in 1949—only to decline to below 5 percent in 1955. In the 1960s another slow upward movement took place in the number of women enrolled in medical schools, but in the early 1970s the relative percentage of women students moved sharply higher. By 1972–73 they represented 16.7 percent of medical students, and the following year the figure rose to 19.8 percent.[28]

Obviously many factors were at work limiting the entrance of women into medicine in the twentieth century. The tendency for medical schools to require a bachelor's degree as a prerequisite and the increasing cost of medical school education itself undoubtedly prevented many girls from entering medicine. Most parents were reluctant to spend a relatively large sum to give their daughters a professional education when they hoped and expected that she would make a "good" marriage and become a mother and house-wife. Furthermore, graduate education for women was thought to reduce their chances for marriage—a belief with a sound basis in reality.

Over and above social and economic factors were deliberate efforts by medical school faculty members and administrators to discourage women students. Unofficial quotas played some role in this, but probably more important was the attitude of many professors who openly proclaimed and demonstrated their distaste for teaching women. Medicine for many was still considered a masculine domain, in which coarse and sometimes macabre humor was used to relieve the tension and grimness of anatomy and related fields. A not uncommon practice in medical and dental schools to awaken drowsy students, stupified by four consecutive hours—or even as many as seven or eight—of lecture and laboratory during the day, was (and still is) to flash pictures of nude women in the midst of a serious slide presentation. Obviously "humor" of this sort was poorly suited for coeducational classes. More important, it bespoke the attitude of many instructors. Happily, many women no longer feel compelled to accept slights and disparagement, and the rise of a new generation of faculty members is contributing to an improved atmosphere. If one can extrapolate the present trend, women are destined to play a larger and larger role in medicine.

NURSING

Women have nursed the sick since time immemorial, but, as an organized profession, nursing is less than 100 years old. The best nursing care for most of the Christian era was provided by religious orders, both Catholic and Protestant. The Ursulines who came to manage the Royal Hospital in New Orleans in 1727 were the first nursing group within the present United States, although Catholic religious orders had played an important role in Canadian hospitals since the establishment of Hôtel Dieu in Quebec in 1639.[29] Another important Catholic nursing order was the Sisters of Charity, whose American branch dates back to Mother Seton and the founding of the Sisterhood of St. Joseph in 1809 at Emittsburg, Maryland. In the nineteenth century Protestant nursing orders representing the Episcopalian, Lutheran, and Methodist churches began work in America.

Secular nursing dates back only to the mid-nineteenth century and owes much to the great English personality, Florence Nightingale. Her example helped make American women aware of the atrocious conditions which characterized most hospitals and inspired them to rectify these conditions. Hospitals in the nineteenth century, as noted earlier, were charitable institutions, designed to care for the sick poor. With a few exceptions all of them were crowded and underfinanced. Such nursing as was given was provided by ignorant, impoverished women, frequently of dubious moral character. Until better women could be attracted to nursing, there was little hope for improving hospitals.

The first who attempted this were the Friends in Philadelphia, who during the 1850s appealed to young women to enter nursing. With the help of a local physician, they also offered some practical training. A few years later, just before the outbreak of the Civil War, the Woman's Hospital in Philadelphia and the New England Female Medical College began giving some elementary instruction in nursing. The war halted further progress in nursing education, but it brought large numbers of women into hospitals, most of whom received their only training in the field. Dr. Elizabeth Blackwell, who was an intimate of Florence Nightingale, at once began organizing women volunteers in New York for wartime nursing, and she was the logical choice to head the Union Army nurses. The Army surgeons, however, were too dubious of a "female doctor," and the choice fell upon Dorothea Dix, a great personality and promoter whose major field of activities, care of the insane, did not intrude upon the medical profession. As superintendent of nurses in the Union Army, Dix performed quite well, despite the rigidity, incompetence, and resentment of women evidenced by many Army physicians. She was able to provide a limited training for some of her nurses, but her work resulted in neither a nurses' training school nor in a permanent Army nursing corps. In the Confederacy nursing was performed largely by individual volunteers.[30]

Following the war, the AMA appointed a Committee on the Training of Nurses headed by Dr. Samuel Gross, and in 1869 the Committee advocated the establishment of a nurses' training program under the direction of the medical profession. Nothing came of the report, but it did show a developing interest in the subject.[31] In 1872 the New England Hospital for Women and Children began giving a graded course in nursing and graduated its first class in 1873. In this same year three other hospitals established nurses' training schools: Bellevue in New York; Massachusetts General in Boston; and the New Haven Hospital in Connecticut. The Bellevue school resulted from the discovery by a group of women visitors of the atrocious conditions in the Hospital. The school was modeled on the Nightingale pattern with an emphasis upon uniforms and military discipline. Unlike the English system which accepted class distinctions, Bellevue sought, through its educational requirements, to attract middle-class students.[32]

The post-Civil War years saw a proliferation of hospitals, a growth resulting from urbanism and from improvements in medicine and surgery. As the curative power of medicine increased, treatment for serious cases began moving from the home to the hospital, and private patients began to occupy more hospital beds; hence it was no coincidence that nursing schools multiplied in these years. By 1880 the number of nurses' training schools had increased to fifteen and by 1900 the figure had jumped to 432.[33] Hospital administrators quickly recognized the value of trained nurses—and even more quickly recognized that nursing schools provided a cheap form of labor. Whereas the original concept of the nurse training school had been one in which systematic classroom and practical instruction would be given, most hospitals provided little or no formal teaching and relied largely upon what was in essence an apprenticeship. By merely providing room and board, hospitals were gaining the services of young women for incredibly long hours per day. Moreover the products of these "schools" were lowering the general educational, social, and economic status of nurses in general.

The establishment of a nursing school at the Johns Hopkins Hospital in 1889 helped to raise educational standards in the field and also provided three outstanding leaders in the nursing profession—Isabel A. Hampton (Mrs. Hunter Robb), Mary Adelaide Nutting, and Lavinia L. Dock. Although Johns Hopkins rated as one of the best schools, the usual rigid discipline and rigorous routine were observed. Students had to be up for breakfast and morning prayers and be ready for duty by 7 A.M. to begin a twelve-hour day, with one hour off for "lunch, rest, and study." The only relief from nursing duty were the twice-weekly classes held from 5 to 6 P.M. In addition, staff physicians gave lectures from 8 to 9 P.M. The first lesson students were taught was "absolute and unquestioning obedience" to their superiors and complete deference to physicians.[34] This tradition, which survives in a modified form today, has hindered the development of nursing and has not been necessarily productive of sound medical care.

The Johns Hopkins nurses took the initiative in establishing the first national nursing association in 1894. It was designed to improve educational standards and to raise nursing to a professional status. The next step was a journal, a course advocated by Mary Adelaide Nutting in 1893. By valiant efforts, in 1900 the *American Journal of Nursing* appeared to begin a long and successful career. As nurses began to organize, they recognized the need to distinguish between the graduates of good nursing schools and self-trained practitioners. State nursing groups organized to pressure legislatures, and by 1915 virtually all states had nurse registration laws.

Recognizing that university training was essential if nursing was to achieve professional status, Mary Adelaide Nutting and Isabel Hampton Robb in 1899 persuaded Dean James Earl Russell of Teachers College, Columbia University, to institute a course in hospital economics. In the course of negotiations Nutting made an excellent impression upon Dean Russell, and in 1907 she was appointed to the newly established professorship of nursing at Teachers College, the first of its kind in the United States. In the ensuing years nursing schools steadily raised their academic standards. The University of Minnesota in 1909 established a nursing school as part of the university, and by 1920 nearly 200 nursing schools had some university connection.[35]

The emergence of public health nurses in the early twentieth century greatly helped the public image of the profession. These nurses were employed in schools, child health centers, settlement houses, and a variety of other positions which brought them into wide contact with the public. The early nurse pioneers, such as S. Josephine Baker and Lillian D. Wald, were middle-class women whose devotion to the cause of infant welfare in the tenement and slum areas won them widespread recognition and reflected credit upon the entire nursing profession.

Another impetus was given to nursing by America's involvement in various wars. The excellent work performed by female volunteers in the Spanish-American War had led to the creation of a small permanent Army Nursing Corps. This corps was expanded to a total of 22,000 during World War I and was supplemented by another 11,000 nurses in the Red Cross.[36] In the immediate postwar years interest in nursing waned and the number of students in nursing schools fell sharply. World War II provided still another stimulus to nursing. Recognizing that nurses had achieved professional status, the armed forces granted commissions to female graduate nurses.

Although the sharp decline in the number of nursing students following World War I brought pressure to relax educational standards, nurse organizations continued the fight for professional status, and they made slow progress in the ensuing years. The expanding demand for medical services following World War II, however, created another nurse shortage, one which came about despite the rising number of graduate nurses. Nursing education was now making rapid progress. The Public Health Service during

World War II had organized a program of nursing education in conjunction with junior or community colleges. In addition, by 1946 many of the better hospital nursing schools had strengthened their ties with universities, and over ninety of these institutions had developed five-year nursing programs leading toward a bachelor's degree. More significant, several universities had established separate schools of nursing which offered a choice of a four- or five-year curriculum.

Along with requiring a better educational background for nurses, the professionalization of nursing carried with it a high degree of specialization. Increasingly nurses were performing functions formerly handled by physicians, and, as medicine specialized, it brought with it a corresponding movement in nursing services. Surgical, pediatric, obstetrical, and psychiatric nurses, to name a few, now began working with physicians. The need for trained nurses in psychiatric wards and institutions pointed up the shortage of males in the nursing field. The domination of nursing by women is reflected in the relative percentages of male and female graduate nurses. As of 1940 males represented only 2.3 percent of the total number of graduate nurses. In the postwar years the emergence of professional schools for nursing encouraged the entrance of males into the profession, but progress has been far too slow.[37]

As the level of their skill and knowledge has advanced, the autocratic and hierarchical tradition in nursing introduced by the early British nurses and reinforced by the efforts of the pioneer nurses to gain acceptance by male physicians gradually declined. Increasingly nurses are beginning to assume broader responsibilities, and they are becoming less subservient to physicians. The growing use of paramedical personnel, a direct result of the complexity of medicine, undoubtedly will help nurses to achieve, at least within their own specific domains, coequal status with the physicians.

BLACKS IN MEDICINE

An area of history which has been sadly neglected is the role of blacks in medicine prior to the late nineteenth century. Since no sound historical research has been done, the resulting vacuum has been filled by an extensive semifictional literature produced by sympathetic white and black historians who have joined in an effort to build a black tradition in medicine. No better illustration of this can be found than in the case of "Dr. James Derham" or "Durham." Derham, who is firmly enshrined in such reputable historical journals as the *Bulletin of the History of Medicine* and the *Journal of Negro History*—and a great many other historical works—is a nebulous figure to say the least. The original account of his career as a prominent New Orleans physician in the late eighteenth and early nineteenth centuries was published in 1916 in the *Journal of Negro History*. This article, which describes Derham as "the most distinguished physician in New Orleans," was based upon a eulogistic quotation attributed to Dr. Benjamin Rush, an account published by a Pennsylvania society for the advancement of blacks, and a brief mention in H. Gregoire, *De la Littérature des nègres* (Paris, 1808).[38]

Over the years Dr. Derham has steadily increased in stature. A recent study of blacks in medicine states that he had an extensive practice among whites and blacks and describes him as "a man of liberal education," "a superb linguist," and "an authority on the relationship of disease to climate." Derham, according to the standard version, was born in Philadelphia and, through the vicissitudes of the Revolutionary War, finally ended up in the hands of a "Dr. Robert Dove" of New Orleans. The latter, according to the traditional story, was so impressed with Derham's intelligence and knowledge of medicine that he completed Derham's medical training and freed him to practice in the city.[39]

Having lived in New Orleans and spent some years examining nearly all existing records for the period when Derham is supposed to have practiced, I can say that these versions are all nonsense. This illustrious black physician may have practiced in Philadelphia or in some other city—but not in New Orleans. There are ample historical sources for Louisiana. The Spanish authorities required all physicians and surgeons to submit to an examination and to obtain a license before engaging in practice. These records are fairly complete and the names of virtually every medical practitioner in Louisiana can be found in them.

Only two blacks are mentioned in these early years—a black

phlebotomist named Domingo and a free black called "Derum." In 1801 the Cabildo, noting that five practitioners were practicing medicine without a license, ordered them to cease and desist until they had passed the required examination. Mention was also made of "a free negro Derum . . . having the right only to cure throat disease and no other." Nothing further was said about licensing Derum, and presumably he was allowed to carry on with his limited practice.

The "Dr. Robert Dove" mentioned in connection with Derham was undoubtedly Dr. Robert Dow, a Scottish physician who was a leading practitioner in the city. New Orleans had a good many Spanish, French, and American visitors in these years, many of whom discussed health conditions and the state of medical practice. A former slave with an extensive practice among whites would certainly have aroused their interest, and it is inconceivable that Derham, had he been a prominent physician, would not have been mentioned in the official records, newspapers, travel accounts, or descriptions of Louisiana. Obviously the story of James Derham is a myth based upon garbled versions of the activities of the free black Derum. Unfortunately, so many historians have quoted each other about Dr. James Derham that now he is firmly established as an historical "fact."[40]

The tragedy is that the accomplishments of blacks in the face of enormous handicaps during the nineteenth century are real and so do not need to be bolstered artificially. A number of free blacks in the years prior to the Civil War did manage to acquire medical skills and engage in practice. Some were self-taught, others learned medicine through an apprenticeship, and a few were able to earn medical degrees in American schools in the decade or so before the Civil War. Several of the most fortunate ones studied abroad. Dr. James McCune Smith, who took a medical degree from the University of Glasgow in 1837, was probably the first of these. It is likely that some of the free black men in New Orleans may have acquired medical degrees in France. An editorial in a New Orleans newspaper on the death of Dr. L. C. Roudanez (1826–90) described him as a "worthy and intelligent representative of the colored element that was free before the war—a man of undoubted skill in his profession and great popularity in this city."[41] In the North the abolition movement led several medical schools to open their doors to blacks, but only a handful of degrees were awarded before the Civil War.

Despite the widespread racial prejudice, which was particularly strong in the armed forces, eight black physicians were appointed to the Army Medical Corps. In light of the very limited number of qualified black practitioners, this figure is all the more surprising. The highest-ranking black medical officer was Dr. Alexander T. Augusta, a graduate of Trinity Medical College in Toronto, Canada, who was raised to a lieutenant-colonel in March, 1865. The most beneficial effect of the war, however, was to eliminate slavery and thus enhance opportunities for blacks in all areas.[42]

The work of the Freedman's Bureau, limited though it was, and the actions of liberal individuals in promoting black education encouraged blacks to enter the professions. As was the case with women, the best hope for progress lay in the establishment of special medical schools for blacks. The first of these was Howard University, an institution established under the auspices of the first Congregational Church of Washington, D.C., to educate both whites and blacks, males and females. With the help of General Oliver Otis Howard of the Freedman's Bureau, the school opened in 1867, and its medical department was established the following year. Despite many difficulties, including active opposition from the faculty of the Medical College of Georgetown, Howard managed to survive. The second black medical school, Meharry Medical College of Nashville, was founded by the Methodist Episcopal Church in 1876, and, like Howard, continues to make a significant contribution to medical education. Other black schools came into existence in the succeeding years but all had relatively brief careers. By the time Flexner made his celebrated survey, only seven medical schools for blacks existed: Flint Medical College (New Orleans), Howard (Washington, D.C.), Knoxville (Tennessee), Leonard (Raleigh, North Carolina), Louisville (Kentucky), Meharry (Nashville), and the University of West Tennessee Medical Department in Memphis. All but two of these, Howard and Meharry, soon disappeared.[43]

Although those institutions accepting black students were willing to accept women, few black females acquired medical degrees. According to M. O. Bousfield, only about ninety had graduated from American medical schools up to 1923, and sixty-four of these were products of Meharry and Howard.[44]

While medical schools for blacks were designed to facilitate entrance into medicine, black medical societies arose out of sheer necessity. For example, when three able black physicians, two of whom were members of the Howard faculty, were proposed for membership in the Medical Society of the District of Columbia in 1869, all three applications were rejected. In consequence, the following year Howard faculty members founded the National Medical Society of the District of Columbia, an organization of both white and black physicians. Since the American Medical Association, on one pretext or another, refused to support membership for blacks in its constituent societies, local black medical associations gradually evolved as the century drew on. By 1895 these organizations were able to fuse into the National Medical Association. Shortly before this, in 1892, Dr. Miles Vandahurst Lynk of Jackson, Tennessee founded the first Negro medical journal, the *Medical and Surgical Observer*. This was followed in 1909 by the appearance of the *Journal of the National Medical Association* under the editorship of Dr. Charles V. Roman.[45]

The late nineteenth century also witnessed the growth of black hospitals. Here again they arose out of necessity, since the vast majority of hospitals either refused to accept blacks or else provided them with miserable accommodations. The need for hospitals was even worse in the case of black physicians, who were rigidly excluded from practicing in most institutions. By 1910 almost 100 black hospitals were in existence. Aside from providing better care for patients and facilities for black physicians, these hospitals contributed to medical education by increasing the number of internships and residencies open to blacks.

Although a small number of black physicians and surgeons have been able to overcome the direct and subtle handicaps facing them because of their race, on a proportionate basis blacks have never had adequate representation in the medical profession. As medical education became more difficult and expensive, blacks, whose collective economic status was well below that of the whites, were caught in an economic squeeze. The Great Depression aggravated the situation, and the number of black medical graduates declined to around seventy per year by the late 1930s. In the years from 1910 to 1942, despite a considerable increase in population, the number of black physicians in the country increased by only 400, from 3,409 to 3,810.[46]

The World War II era, however, marked the beginning of a renewed effort by blacks to gain their rightful place in society. Whereas only 356 blacks were commissioned as medical officers during World War I, in the Second World War the figure was around 600. A mere token of black nurses was allowed to enlist in World War I, but about 500 were accepted in World War II. In the postwar years blacks steadily pressured for entrance into white medical societies and hospitals and, with the help of the government, were able to force southern and border-state medical schools to admit them.[47]

Nonetheless, segregation barriers were still impeding the entrance of blacks into the medical profession and their progress within them when the advent of the 1960s signaled a renewed drive for equal rights. Aided by the formation of the biracial Medical Committee for Civil Rights and its successor, the Medical Committee for Human Rights, black physicians and other medical personnel began a more militant quest for justice. One of their chief objectives was to amend the Hill-Burton Act of 1946 which had permitted federal funds to subsidize the building of 104 segregated hospitals by 1964. The first victory came in the courts in 1964 when the Supreme Court held that the "separate-but-equal" clause in the Hill-Burton Act was unconstitutional. In August of this same year Congress backed up this action by requiring equal health opportunities in all federally aided hospitals.

Although the Nixon administration, which took over in 1968, was scarcely enthusiastic about minority rights, the momentum from the sixties carried over for several years. The early 1970s have seen a determined effort by the Federal government and many responsible citizens to guarantee that blacks and other minorities have an equal opportunity to enter professional schools. The number of blacks in medical and paramedical fields today is still not representative of the total black population, but the gap is closing.

OTHER MINORITIES

Discrimination in medical schools has not been restricted to women and blacks. Two other groups have also experienced difficulties in gaining entrance to the medical profession—Jews and

Catholics. For Catholics the problem has never been acute since the existence of their own schools and hospitals guaranteed them access to medical training and clinical experience. Yet in certain geographic areas a subtle discrimination is practiced between Catholics and Protestants. For example, a five-year study by the Philadelphia Fellowship Commission published in 1957 showed that Protestant premedical students from Temple and the University of Pennsylvania had a better chance for acceptance into medical schools than Catholics, who, in turn, fared better than Jews.[48]

Insofar as Jews are concerned, little discrimination existed in medicine prior to about 1920, but the next thirty-odd years witnessed both official and unofficial discrimination against Jewish applicants to medical schools. So long as medical schools were largely proprietary institutions vying with each other for students, white males had little difficulty in gaining acceptance. Moreover, Jews constituted a relatively small percentage of the population and as such they represented no economic threat to practicing physicians. By the 1920s both of these factors had altered radically. The efforts of organized medicine to raise educational standards and to limit entrance into the profession greatly reduced the available places for medical students. At the same time, the children of the relatively large numbers of Eastern European Jews who had entered America around the turn of the century were beginning to move into the professions. In a day and age when college, particularly in the East, was still largely a gentleman's prerogative, these highly motivated and intelligent young Jews in the eastern cities represented a serious threat to the relaxed "gentlemanly" college way of life. Shortly after World War I, Harvard University established a "Sifting Committee," which placed a quota on Jews in order to maintain what it felt was a proper balance within the student body. Whereas Harvard openly limited Jewish students, most other institutions used subterfuge to achieve the same ends. An article in the *Nation* in June 1922 pointed out that Columbia and New York University within a short period had reduced the percentage of Jewish students by over 50 percent.[49]

In most schools, admissions committees and officers quietly and unofficially limited the entrance of Jewish applicants. Where quota systems were more or less official, it was argued that admitting students on a competitive basis into the private eastern schools might result in a 50 percent Jewish enrollment, a situation thought to be socially unacceptable.[50] Although periodic protests led to occasional investigations, discrimination with respect to Jewish students continued at all college levels during the 1920s and 1930s. It was particularly acute in medicine, since the AMA's fight to reduce the number of doctors was proving all too successful.

In 1930 Dr. Frank Gavin of the General Theological Seminary asserted that it was three times as hard for a Jewish male student to enter medical school as for other male applicants, and he denounced the application of a quota system in an area "where the best competence and ability must be secured for the public good." In response, an article in the *Literary Digest* maintained that there was little point to admitting Jewish students since non-Jews would not consult with Jewish physicians. Four years later, in 1934, *School and Society*, citing the high percentage of Jewish applicants to medical schools and the restrictions placed upon them by foreign governments and state legislatures, advised Jewish premedical students to seek fields other than medicine.[51]

The rise of Hitler, rather than shocking Americans into an awareness of the full implications of anti-Semitism, gave an added stimulus to it. Since Jews were concentrated in the northeastern cities, policies which restricted the number of admissions from large cities, geographic areas, or out of state all served to keep the number of Jewish medical students to a minimum. School officials who disclaimed the anti-Semitism implicit in their actions resorted to sophistry by arguing that a disproportionate number of Jews in medicine and law would breed resentment; thus the quota system was in the best interest of the Jews.[52]

As the full horror of the consequences of anti-Semitism in Germany was revealed in the late 1940s, overt discrimination began to fade. Nonetheless, studies conducted by the New York State Department of Education and the State Board of Regents in 1950 and 1952 still showed some discrimination. By the late 1950s, however, almost 50 percent of the students in the state's nine medical schools were Jewish.[53] By the 1960s the quota system had generally been abandoned throughout America, and, although a small measure of anti-Semitism still remained, discrimination among applicants to medical schools had been reduced to a minimum.

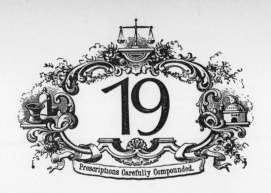

Prescriptions Carefully Compounded.

MEDICAL LICENSURE, FEES, AND SOCIETIES

I N glancing back over the history of American medical licensure, it is clear that from the Revolution to about 1830 the licensing of physicians was done by a variety of means—state boards of examiners, medical schools, and medical societies. In the succeeding years, until about 1875, licensure laws were virtually eliminated and possession of a medical degree from any college was an automatic qualification to practice. As colleges vied with each other for medical students and medical degrees became successively easier to acquire, the practice of medicine was opened to everyone. Beginning in the 1870s stronger state medical societies emerged, and they helped to reform medical education and to revive state medical examining boards. The process, however, was long and complicated.[1]

In North Carolina a State Board of Medical Examiners had been created in 1859, but to all intents and purposes it was powerless, for one clause in the enabling act specified that no one practicing in violation of the law should be guilty of a misdemeanor. In 1885 this provision was eliminated, but the new measure included a "grandfather clause"—one which declared that the law would not apply to anyone who had acquired a diploma from any regular medical college prior to 1880. Four years later all physicians were required to register with the clerk of the Superior Court in the county in which they practiced. The term "physician" encompassed almost every practitioner in the state, since the law described three classes of doctors: those licensed by the Board of Medical Examiners, those with medical degrees dated before March 7, 1885, and those taking an oath that they had practiced medicine in the state prior to March 7, 1885. No further changes were made in the law until 1899 when an amendment prohibited anyone from applying to the Examining Board who was not a medical graduate. In the succeeding years the licensing law was gradually strengthened, although it was not until 1921 that the grandfather clause was eliminated.[2]

In South Carolina the first licensing law in the postwar era was passed in 1869. As with all early laws, it was a weak measure with enough loopholes to include anyone wishing to practice. In 1881 a new act enabled county boards of health to license physicians. Seven years later prospective doctors were given the choice of obtaining their license from the state examining board, the Medical College faculty, or the local county board of health. Other modifications followed, but it was not until 1897 that a reasonably effective law was passed. [3]

Louisiana, which had one of the best licensing systems in the early nineteenth century, enacted a law in 1862 requiring physicians to make an affidavit stating that they possessed a medical degree from a reputable school. Ten years later the penalties for making a false affidavit were increased—a futile gesture, since few physicians bothered to file one in the first place. In 1882 responsibility for licensing was transferred to the state board of health. As might be expected, a grandfather clause was included. Although a few minor changes were made subsequently, when the state medical society pushed for a stronger law in 1890 its efforts were defeated in the legislature, in part due to the objection of the homeopaths. After several unsuccessful tries, in 1894 the medical society joined with the homeopaths and secured the establishment of two state boards, one appointed from the ranks of the regular state medical society and another from the homeopathic society. Although the usual grandfather clause blanketed all existing practitioners, the law guaranteed that henceforth those entering the profession had at least minimum qualifications.[4]

The divisions within the medical profession which delayed passage of Louisiana's first good licensing law are even more evident in the case of New York. This state's first postwar law, passed in 1874, was a compromise between the factions within the regular medical profession and the many irregular practitioners. So many compromises were made that the law was meaningless. The main issue dividing the State Medical Association was the AMA's code of ethics, which prohibited its members from consulting with homeopaths and other irregulars.

As was true in some other states, the orthodox physicians in New York finally succeeded in passing a sound licensing law in 1891 by collaborating with the homeopaths and eclectics. Under the terms of the 1891 act each of the three groups was given its own board. This development led the osteopaths and Christian Scientists to make a similar demand. In the face of this challenge, the allopaths (regulars), homeopaths, and eclectics united in support of a single board. The result was a new law in 1907 creating a single board with the three groups equally represented. By this date the osteopaths had raised their educational standards and were permitted to take the examination.[5]

The process by which the foregoing states achieved some measure of medical regulation shows the major problems encountered. Of the four, Louisiana's progress toward medical licensure best typifies the path followed by most states. First, a weak law requiring registration with local officials, medical societies, or some type of examining board; second, a measure authorizing either the state health board or local health boards to issue licenses; and finally, the creation of a relatively effective state licensing system. Frequently this final step was made possible only when the state medical society joined with the homeopaths or eclectic practitioners. This is the supreme irony, since the AMA and state medical societies had devoted their major efforts during the second half of the nineteenth century to fighting irregular practitioners. Their acceptance of the old adage—"if you can't beat them, join them"—

was made easier, however, by the willingness of the two irregular medical sects to modify their theories and accept the new developments in medicine.

By 1900 every state had some type of medical registration law, although six of them still granted a license to anyone holding a medical diploma. More significant, about half the states required both a medical degree and an examination before granting a license. In North Carolina, Louisiana, and some eighteen other states midwives were partially or totally exempted from the licensure laws, and few if any states closely regulated them. The 1894 Louisiana law, which stated that the act was not "to apply to the so-called midwife of the rural districts and plantation practice," clearly shows a class bias.[6] Midwives practiced largely among the blacks and poor whites, and neither the medical profession nor the legislature were concerned with such unprofitable patients.

As part of the general effort to raise professional standards in the late nineteenth century, in 1891 certain medical examining boards organized the National Confederation of State Medical Examining and Licensing Boards. The aim of the group was to help standardize testing programs and to encourage medical schools in their efforts to improve education. Despite this step toward standardizing licensing procedures, the qualifications required by the state boards varied widely, and the problem of reciprocity soon came to the fore. A Confederation of Reciprocity was established in Chicago in 1902 to promote inter-board acceptance of each other's licenses. After achieving only limited success, in 1912 this body merged with the National Confederation of State Boards to form the present Federation of State Medical Boards.[7]

While the quality of medical practice was rapidly improving in the first quarter of the twentieth century, grandfather clauses in the licensing acts guaranteed that thousands of poorly trained and semiliterate physicians would continue to practice. Moreover, the enforcement of the licensing acts required public support, and a good many Americans were still dubious of laws which seemingly gave a monopoly to physicians or lawyers. A "Dr. Allen" who began practicing in rural Louisiana sometime prior to 1894 is a good case in point. He had no medical degree and never bothered to register as a physician, but he was apparently well liked. When a grand jury brought charges against him for practicing without a license, he simply decided to leave medicine. Faced with this prospect, the grand jury withdrew the indictment, and he continued to practice until his death in 1920.[8]

Reflecting improvements in medical education, licensure laws were gradually tightened as the twentieth century advanced. One area in which medical licensing boards failed to meet a new challenge was that of specialties. Fortunately, specialists, led by the ophthalmologists, had started organizing on a national basis in the 1860s, and they took the initiative. The ophthalmologists established a national examining board in 1916, and other specialist boards soon began certifying those qualified to practice. The state boards also neglected still another important consideration: the need for busy practitioners to keep abreast of the rapid developments in medicine. In this instance medical schools stepped in by providing refresher courses. Since these courses are optional, they provide only a partial answer. In the past—and even today—those physicians most in need of additional training are frequently the ones least interested and least willing to spare the time.[9]

The problem of quackery has been and still is a difficult one for medical licensing boards to solve. Prosecution depends upon the willingness of patients, local authorities, or district attorneys to press charges, and even when charges are brought, a complicated legal fight often ensues. In the 1920s the *Literary Digest*, the *Ladies' Home Journal*, and other magazines and newspapers ran exposés on diploma mills which revealed the weaknesses of the licensing boards at that time. Two states, Connecticut and Missouri, were notorious for issuing bogus medical degrees and licenses. A reporter for the St. Louis *Star* in 1923 applied to a diploma mill posing as a coal salesman looking for an easier job. For $25 he obtained a high-school diploma and for $1,200 he was given a medical diploma. Missouri, which had a long history of disreputable medical colleges, as late as the 1920s had a large number of institutions rated among the worst in the country by the AMA's Council on Medical Education.

While journals and newspapers contributed to the fight, the major battle against quacks and abuses in the drug field was fought by the AMA. Its first victory came in 1906, when it joined with Harvey W. Wiley, Samuel Hopkins Adams, and the Progressives to secure passage of the Pure Food and Drug Act of that year, a relatively weak measure but one which initiated some federal action. Assisted by state and Federal drug officials, the AMA continued the struggle to expose quackery and to strengthen the drug laws. Although some progress was made, it took a national drug scandal in the 1930s over "Elixir Sulfanilamide," a drug which brought a horrible death to at least 107 individuals, to bring about a major revision in the 1906 act. This tragedy, in conjunction with agitation by the AMA, the FDA, and other interested individuals and groups, resulted in passage of the Food, Drug, and Cosmetic Act of 1938, a much stronger law.[10]

In the late 1950s Senator Estes Kefauver of Tennessee began hearings on the drug industry. He was concerned largely with the excessive profits of the drug industry, but he was also interested in the danger inherent in the distribution of new and powerful drugs. His campaign for stronger control over drugs was strengthened by another major tragedy, the thalidomide affair. This drug was submitted to the Federal Drug Administration for clearance as a sleeping tablet, sedative, and anti-emetic in pregnancy. Dr. Frances O. Kelsey of the FDA was dubious and refused to give it clearance until she had made a thorough check. In the meantime the drug company distributed thousands of free samples to physicians. On hearing of the birth of a number of deformed babies to English and German mothers who had taken thalidomide, Dr. Kelsey began a public campaign against the drug. Although never officially placed on the market, thanks to Dr. Kelsey, the samples which had already been distributed resulted in a number of deformed infants. At a time when Kefauver's campaign against the drug industry was losing headway, the thalidomide incident revived public interest, and on October 10, 1962 the Kefauver-Harris Drug Amendments unanimously passed both Houses of Congress. The result was to strengthen the Federal Drug Administration's control over the licensing of new drugs and to aid in its fight against quackery.[11]

A major weakness of the American medical licensing laws has always been their diversity. Even today licensing is handled by fifty-five separate jurisdictions. The AMA sought to deal with this problem early in the century and in 1915 established a National Board of Medical Examiners. The Board, which included representatives of the AMA, the Association of American Medical Colleges, the American College of Surgeons, and the Federation of State

Medical Boards, began giving examinations on a voluntary basis the following year. In the first five years the examinations were taken by only 325 students, of whom 269 passed. In 1922 the examinations were divided into three parts, with medical students taking the examinations at three intervals. As the better schools and state boards recognized the value of the program, more students applied. By 1940 about one fourth of all medical students were taking the examinations, and the concept of national board examinations was gradually gaining acceptance.[12]

The licensing of physicians is far better today than it was seventy-five years ago, but much remains to be done. The standards applied by the various state licensing boards still vary widely. Some boards apparently pass every applicant, while others use the examinations as a means of limiting the number of practitioners. In a mobile society, American physicians cannot move freely around the country because of the barriers created by the variations in state licensing requirements.[13] Until standardized state licensing laws are enacted or a national qualifying board is created, these problems will remain with us.

As indicated earlier, the immediate post-Civil War years brought little improvement, if any, in the financial status of the average physician. While a few outstanding individuals were able to acquire considerable wealth—usually as a result of a combination of skill and social position—the average practitioner continued to earn a minimum living from his practice. And, as they had done since the founding of America, many doctors continued to supplement their incomes by operating small businesses and farms. The large number of medical schools actively competing for students and the lax licensure laws gave even the lowest income groups access to the profession, thus swelling its ranks. Nonetheless, sharp social and financial barriers separated the elite physicians with their European training and well-to-do patients from the average practitioner whose academic background before entering medical school often did not include even a high school diploma.

As might be expected, medical fees were highest in urban areas, but this advantage was offset by keener competition among doctors. Charles Rosenberg estimated that physicians starting their careers in New York City in the 1860s probably earned about $400 per year.[14] Despite a general rise in living standards, the income of physicians improved little by the end of the century. In 1898 a Dr. Sexton, addressing the local medical society in New Orleans, asserted that seven-eighths of the city's 358 physicians made less than $1,000 per year. The situation was worse in rural areas. A physician practicing in New Paltz, Ulster County, New York, a village of about 500 to 600 inhabitants, claimed that his patients were indignant if he charged more than 50 cents for a housecall and 35 cents for an office visit. For this munificent sum, the doctor was also expected to supply them with medicine. For an out-of-town call involving a distance of up to six miles, the fee was $1. To add to Dr. Sexton's woes, patients often took from one to five years to pay their bills. He mentioned in passing that this small village had two practitioners, a fact which in itself helps to explain the relatively impoverished status of the profession.[15]

A financial problem besetting doctors which is as old as medicine itself has been their inability to collect fees. In the colonial period it was not unusual for a medical bill to be carried for many years, occasionally remaining unpaid until the settlement of the patient's estate. Ancient medical authors often warned the physician to collect his bill before the patient was fully recovered. In the modern period economic depressions always aggravated this problem, and the late nineteenth century was no exception. During the depressed years of the 1870s, about seventy New Orleans doctors formed a Medical Protection Association to assist them in collecting their fees. These same physicians also denounced the contract practice of medicine as demoralizing to "the profession of medicine, and ruinous to the financial welfare of us all."[16]

Contract medicine—an agreement by which physicians provided complete medical care for an annual fee—had long been traditional in the South. With the growth of unions, large-scale industries, and business and social organizations throughout the country, the contract method gradually spread. Sharp competition among physicians not only insured their availability for such contracts, but it also kept contract fees to a minimum. As state and local medical societies gained strength, they prohibited their members from engaging in contract medicine. In the twentieth century the AMA, too, threw its weight into the balance and by the 1920s reduced this form of practice to negligible proportions. Nonetheless, fear of the contract system continued to condition the attitude of organized medicine for many years, and it was used as a major argument against much of the proposed federal health legislation in the 1930s and 1940s.

Another financial complaint of the medical profession arose with the appearance of free dispensaries and clinics. The impetus for these institutions came from two sources: one was simple philanthropy; the second was the specialists' need for clinical subjects. Specialists seeking to improve their skills and train their students needed access to relatively large numbers of patients. General practitioners in the late nineteenth century, however, were resentful of competition from colleagues who set themselves up as specialists, considering them a threat to an already limited practice; thus the specialists sought to avoid conflict by establishing dispensaries for the poor. Since many workers lived at a poverty level, it was not easy to determine where the line should be drawn between those who could afford to pay and those who could not. This same situation held true for the general dispensaries and public hospitals. Understandably, physicians whose own incomes placed them in the category of genteel poverty argued that the dispensaries were depriving them of paying patients.

In the twentieth century, the developments largely responsible for increasing the income of physicians were the successful drives to improve the quality of medical education and to limit entrance into the profession. Physicians were fortunate that, in the fight to upgrade the quality of medical training, virtue and self-interest went hand in hand. As the medical school curriculum was extended and entrance requirements were raised, first to a high-school diploma and subsequently to a minimum of one or two years of college, increasingly entrance to medicine was restricted to the middle and upper classes. While more rigid educational and licensing requirements clearly benefited the patient, the physicians who fought for them were not unaware of the value of limiting competition. Even a cursory reading of medical journals and transactions at the turn of the century will turn up many editorials and articles appealing for medical regulation purely on financial grounds.

Beneficial as higher professional standards were in the long run, their immediate effect was limited. Although stricter licensure laws curtailed the number entering the profession, thousands of poorly trained doctors continued to practice. Richard H. Shryock (1893–1972) who spent a good part of his life studying the history of

American medicine, estimated that the number of physicians was excessive at least until 1910.[17] Ironically, as lessening competition enabled physicians to raise their fees, they automatically cut down on the demand for their services by the lower-income groups. The depressed years of the earlier 1930s affected all economic levels, and it was not until late in the decade that a noticeable improvement occurred in the economic position of physicians.

By World War II the success of the AMA and the Flexner Report in eliminating over 50 percent of existing medical schools and raising the academic level of the remaining ones had greatly improved the quality of medical graduates—and at the same time had brought the physician population ratio to a minimal level. Meanwhile, economic prosperity accruing from wartime conditions steadily increased the demand for medical services. The families of factory workers, clerks, and other lower-income groups who had formerly seen doctors only under emergency conditions were now beginning to visit physicians for checkups, preventive vaccines, and minor ailments. By the late 1930s physicians' incomes began to rise at a rate well in excess of rising prices. By the 1950s medicine was at least one of the highest paid professions, and despite the current inflation it has more than held its own. For the immediate future the high cost of building and operating medical schools and the time lag before they can produce medical graduates insures that there is little danger of competition limiting the physician's income. Moreover, volunteer and government health insurance agencies virtually guarantee a relatively high level of income.

By the mid-nineteenth century local and state medical societies began appearing on a fairly wide scale. In most states medical societies centered around the major cities, and, even when state societies were organized, they tended to be dominated by physicians in the largest city. For example, Blanton states that the "Medical Society of Virginia for the first thirty years of its existence was in reality Richmond's local association."[18] Certainly this was true in Louisiana, where New Orleans tended to dominate. Within the major cities, medical organizations often competed with each other for members, and on occasions denounced opposing organizations. The rise of medical sects increased the number of societies, for homeopaths, eclectics, osteopaths, and other irregulars found it necessary to organize in self-defense.

Many of the local societies were short-lived, and not infrequently bitter quarrels within a society led to the founding of a competing organization. In the meantime, state societies, too, were experiencing a renewal and strengthening. In 1878, when Louisiana established its state society, every state in the Union possessed some type of state organization. The strength of these societies varied widely, but the general trend was upward. Yet nothing bespeaks the weakness of these societies better than their failure to establish official journals. Not until 1899 did the first state medical society journal appear.[19]

While local and state societies were building their membership rolls, several regional associations came into existence, and at the national level some fifteen specialty groups were established between 1864 and 1902. During these years the AMA, organized in 1846, was struggling for survival and having little success in meeting its original objective of improving medical education and raising professional standards. The sheer size of America and the transportation difficulties tended to restrict membership to the Middle Atlantic and Midwestern states, and the AMA's attempt to become an effective national organization was further hindered by a cumbersome and ineffectual structure. The Association's lack of success in promoting higher educational standards was discouraging. Some of its members fought valiantly for this reform, but the gains which had come by 1900 can scarcely be credited to the AMA. It had consistently supported public health measures at the national level, but the American Public Health Association, established in 1872, quickly became the chief spokesman in this field. The AMA, however, did continue to fight for a national health department, and many of its members were active in promoting state and municipal health laws. Nonetheless, President Charles A. L. Reed declared in an address to the Association in 1901 that, during the first years of its life, the Association had "exerted relatively little influence on legislation, either state or national."[20]

The year 1901 marked the second of two developments which put the AMA into the forefront of the medical profession. The first had been the appearance of *The Journal of the American Medical Association* in 1883. This publication gave the Association an effective voice and generally enhanced its status within the profession. The second was a constitutional reorganization in 1901 which made the Association both more representative and at the same time more effective as a national body.[21] The first product of these changes was the creation of the Council on Medical Education in 1904, the active educational reform group which prepared the way for the Flexner Report. Through its annual reports and classification system for medical colleges, this council continued to exert a strong beneficial influence upon medical schools in the succeeding years. In addition, a growing membership and an improving financial state enabled the AMA to strengthen its committees and councils by the creation of bureaus with permanent staffs. While the AMA did not actively participate in most of the reform movements of the Progressive era—child labor, occupational health, tenement reform, and so forth—it was influenced by the movement in matters directly relating to health. Hence it energetically promoted a Federal health agency, maternal and child health, health education, pure food and drug laws, and better-kept vital statistics.[22]

The major piece of Progressive social legislation which aroused the interest of the AMA was health insurance. The Progressive Party in 1912 espoused the concept of compulsory health insurance, and, despite the disappearance of the party after the election, health insurance became a significant political issue. Although apprehensive that health insurance might revive contract practice, the Association through its *Journal* and national officers expressed considerable interest in the subject. Precisely what happened to change this favorable climate of opinion within the next two years is not clear. James G. Burrow, in his history of the AMA, attributes it to the end of Progressivism, the preoccupation with World War I and the League of Nations, and the general conservative reaction which followed. Whatever the case, the majority of physicians rejected compulsory insurance, and their views were soon reflected by the AMA and its *Journal*. In 1920 the Association officially went on record as opposing any plan of compulsory health insurance—a view which it maintains today.[23]

A medical profession by its nature must be conservative. In dealing with life and death, one can scarcely undertake experiments lightly. Yet in health matters organized medicine in the nineteenth and early twentieth centuries had generally supported the liberal viewpoint. Physicians individually and collectively advocated sanitary measures, public health laws, regulation of food and drugs, and the collection of vital statistics. In addition, they had helped establish and support hospitals, clinics, and dispensaries—nearly all of which provided free medical care for the lower-income groups in the nineteenth century. Toward the end of the century, however, physicians began to have doubts about making medical care too easily available to the working poor. In the twentieth century, as licensure laws and higher educational standards began limiting entrance into medicine and more physicians moved into the middle and upper classes, the profession gradually turned against all forms of social legislation and firmly supported the status quo. Following World War I the AMA consistently took a conservative stand on social issues—except for those relating to food, drugs, and matters which directly concerned the quality of medical care. At the same time, they strenuously opposed all proposals to provide medical care by any method other than the fee system.

In the 1920s the AMA fought against the Sheppard-Towner Act, which provided Federal subsidies to encourage states to establish maternal and child health programs. The Association also opposed the law establishing Veterans Hospitals in 1924 because it proposed to offer medical care for non-service-connected disabilities. As group hospitalization plans developed in the 1920s, the AMA first expressed qualms about them, and, as they grew stronger, by 1930 was denouncing them as socialistic and unworkable.[24]

The Great Depression forced the AMA to modify its views somewhat. While accepting most of the principles embodied in the social security legislation of the 1930s, it constantly warned about the danger of the government encroaching upon medical care. It also deplored the relatively large sums voted for maternal and child care and for aid to dependent children. The social and economic problems of the Depression created a public awareness of health, since welfare and health are inextricably entwined. As public interest in national health insurance programs became widespread, the AMA launched a counterattack. One of its main themes was the purported failure of the British system. In publishing its misleading reports about the British health plan, the Association paid no attention to independent surveys by the American College of

Dentists and the Michigan State Medical Society which showed the program strongly supported by prominent British physicians.[25]

In response to accumulating evidence that a high percentage of Americans received little or no medical care, the AMA conducted its own survey and declared that the only citizens receiving inferior care were those under the jurisdiction of governmental agencies. In 1938 the AMA's Council on Medical Education and Hospitals surveyed Mississippi and concluded "that there is practically no one in Mississippi who cannot secure medical care regardless of his ability to pay." At this time the state's physician-to-population ratio was about half the national average, the per capita income was about $200, and the Council itself conceded that hospital facilities for blacks were exceedingly limited.[26] As political pressure began to build in support of a national health bill in the late 1930s, the AMA modified its earlier opposition to voluntary health insurance programs, recognizing that these voluntary programs offered the only alternative to a compulsory one.

By this time the United States was involved in World War II, and the AMA performed highly creditably in helping to mobilize medical resources. Among one of its major contributions was its insistence upon deferments for medical students. At the end of the war it advocated refresher courses and other means to assist physicians returning to civilian practice. While dubious of proposals to increase sharply the number of medical schools, it did support passage of the Hill-Burton Act in 1946, which provided Federal subsidies for hospital construction. When the Cold War raised prospects of atomic bombing, the Association played a significant role in organizing an emergency medical service program. The Veterans Administration after the war suffered considerable corruption and inefficiency, and the AMA's efforts to eliminate waste and make the program more effective were highly beneficial—yet at the same time it fought against care for veterans with non-service-connected medical problems. However, the AMA also deserves credit for a major contribution to the World Medical Association and for its active support of the World Health Organization.

Starting with the Wagner-Murray-Dingell Bill in 1943, national health legislation was pushed strongly for the next few years, particularly during President Truman's administrations. Matters came to a head with Truman's unexpected election victory in 1948.

He immediately proposed a comprehensive national health program. The AMA's Board of Trustees promptly employed a public relations agency and began a full-scale campaign involving speakers' bureaus, pamphlets, press and radio releases, and a variety of other methods against the Truman proposal. The Association's House of Delegates in December of 1948 gave full backing and undoubtedly contributed to the defeat of the program.

The Republican victory in the presidential election of 1952 eased the pressure for compulsory national health insurance, and the AMA was given time to rest on its laurels. In the ensuing years, however, it kept close watch on any proposals threatening the fee-for-service system. For example, it fought against proposals such as those of Representative Aime J. Forand of Rhode Island in 1959 and others to incorporate hospitalization and medical benefits for the aged into a social security system, but it did support the Kerr-Mills bill providing Federal funds to help states deal with medical costs for the aged.

The relatively peaceful years of the Eisenhower administration ended abruptly with the Democratic victory in 1960, for it presaged a renewed drive for a national health program. The AMA once again issued a call to arms and fought a rearguard struggle against rising public support for a Federal program to provide medical care for the aged. While unsuccessful in stopping the proposed legislation, the AMA did manage to modify the laws in accordance with its own views. In 1965 the Social Security laws were amended to include the programs known as Medicare and Medicaid. The Medicare program, which became effective July 1, 1966, provided a Federally financed insurance system for paying hospital, doctor, and other medical bills covering all individuals eligible for Social Security benefits. Members starting at the age of 65 pay a small monthly premium ($6.70 as of 1976) which insures them against most hospital and doctors' bills. Medicaid provides Federal assistance to state medical programs. These programs may include a broad range of medical services: family planning, nursing homes, screening and diagnostic programs, laboratory and X-ray services, and so forth.

In glancing back over the twentieth century, the medical profession has made remarkable gains. From an impoverished and scarcely respectable group, it has moved to preeminence among the professions in terms of affluence and prestige. This success has tended to make it politically and socially conservative, and for the past half century the organized profession has a record of opposing virtually every piece of progressive legislation. Since the word "progressive" tends to connote the assumption of governmental responsibility for health, education, and welfare, one can argue that the medical profession may well be fighting for traditional American values with their emphasis upon individual responsibility and initiative. Historically, as societies become more complex, life has tended to become more regulated. Every new development spawns a multitude of laws, regulations, ordinances, and administrative rulings, and health is too fundamental to society to escape such effects.

Although a good many health measures opposed by organized medicine have been enacted in the past forty years, the AMA has played a decisive role in shaping them. Throughout these changes it has successfully preserved a measure of private practice and the fee system, yet it has not been able to prevent encroachments by both governmental and private agencies. Members of the armed services, millions of veterans, and other groups are already receiving medical care under government auspices, and the number of health maintenance organizations—such as the Health Insurance Plan of Greater New York and the Kaiser Foundation Health Plan in California—is growing. The decision for organized medicine is whether it can successfully fight this growing trend, or whether it would be best to accept a basic change in the health delivery system and concentrate on making it more effective.

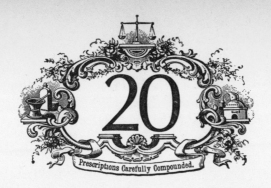

Prescriptions Carefully Compounded.

THE PUBLIC'S HEALTH

T HE rapid growth of urban areas in the nineteenth century had as its corollary a comparable increase in human misery. The current phrase "flight to the suburbs" describes a traditional pattern in city life. With the exception of a few fashionable areas which tend to remain stable, the well-to-do have always moved out of their old homes into new ones on the outskirts of the town or city, leaving the former residences to be occupied by the influx of workers seeking employment in the city. As these overflowed, newcomers were forced to move into barns, stables, old factory buildings, and any available type of shelter. In the second half of the century entrepreneurs began building multistory tenements, most of which had neither water nor any other amenities, and in which windows and ventilation were sadly deficient. It is a commentary on such conditions that New York, a relatively progressive city, passed a law in 1887 requiring new tenements to have one water closet or privy for every fifteen persons.[1]

There is scarcely an American city that does not have its horror stories depicting the squalid circumstances under which a good share of its inhabitants lived in the late nineteenth century. In one small area of Chicago in the 1890s there were 811 sleeping rooms without outside windows and less than 3 percent of families had their own bathrooms. The *Weekly Medical Review* reported that industrial workers were compelled to live in tainted tenements or "low fetid hovels, amidst poverty, hunger and dirt," where "in foulness, want and crime, crowded humanity suffers, and sickens, and perishes." Dr. Joseph Jones, President of the Louisiana Board of Health, declared in 1881: "One-third of those dying in New Orleans die in poverty, and are buried at the public expense. One sixth of those who die in New Orleans, perish in silence and misery, with no kind companion, no efficient medicine, and no generous physician." New Orleans at this date had no sewerage system, a completely inadequate water system, and an inefficient city government.[2]

New York City, which established the best municipal health board in the country in 1866, had only limited success in dealing with the health and social problems of its residents. Its teeming tenements produced so much garbage and human wastes that even under the best of conditions horses and wagons would have had difficulty removing them. The situation was compounded by inefficiency and corruption. Street cleaning and the removal of garbage and the contents of privies was still a lucrative form of political patronage in American cities; and the resultant corruption and inefficiency guaranteed that the streets and gutters of New York were constantly filled with piles of garbage and the overflow from privies. To add to the distinctive urban atmosphere, dairy barns and stables accumulated huge manure piles, slaughterers let blood drain into street gutters and dumped offal outside their doors, and a host of other so-called "nuisance" industries befouled the atmosphere and created breeding grounds for myriad flies.

Life was not only grim for lower-income groups in the cities, but it was also short. After studying the 1880 census report, Dr. Stanford E. Chaillé of New Orleans calculated that life expectancy for a white baby born in the city in 1880 was 38.1 years and that of a black child 25.56.[3] While New Orleans deservedly had a reputation as a pesthole, the figures for a good many other major cities are not much better. Understandably, among the impoverished masses jammed into slum areas the infant mortality rate was exceedingly high. In this connection it is well to bear in mind that a good part of the increased life expectancy during the first half of the twentieth century arose from the reduction in infant mortality.

Nothing indicates human degradation and the wastage of infant life better than the large numbers of foundlings picked off the streets of major cities. The outlook for these infants was almost hopeless. Prior to 1866 foundlings in New York City were cared for by the female inmates of the almshouses and few lived beyond a year. Public exposure of these conditions led to the opening of a special Infant Hospital in 1866, complete with wet-nurses, a paid nursing staff, and a physician. Even with these measures the death rate remained close to 60 percent. After the public furor died down, the situation returned to normal and the mortality rate once again shot up. In 1897, when the hospital was again under attack, the Commissioner of Charities blandly stated that the 96 percent mortality rate was "not as bad as it looks," since many children were sick on arrival and others had been sent there to spare the parents the cost of a funeral. He further explained that limited funds compelled the institution to use women from the workhouse who mistreated the babies.[4]

In rural areas and small towns, health conditions were better for the lower-income groups than in the cities. The environment could absorb the limited quantities of garbage and wastes, the water supply was usually safer, fresh air and sunshine were plentiful, and the food supply was generally—although not always—better. In the South, for example, the one-crop system tended to discourage vegetable gardens, and tenant and small farmers who did raise chickens and vegetables often sold them for cash. While escaping some of the endemic disorders of the cities— smallpox, measles, mumps, scarlet fever, diphtheria, whooping cough, typhoid and other enteric infections, rural areas were subject to fatal and debilitating forms of malaria. Scarcely any section of America avoided malaria at some time in history, and the disease moved westward with the frontier all the way to California. It was 1890 before northern Illinois was free from it. New York City was recording about 100 deaths annually from malaria as late as 1900, although the disease was usually contracted outside the city, and in 1874 the New Jersey State Health Commission declared that malaria was the state's principal medical problem.[5] Not until the New Deal in the 1930s brought better housing, screening, improved medical care, and a higher standard of living was malaria brought under control.

As a familiar endemic disease, malaria did not receive nearly the attention given to the more dramatic epidemic contagions such as yellow fever and Asiatic cholera in the late nineteenth century, and Spanish influenza and poliomyelitis in the twentieth. Another even more familiar—and more deadly—disorder was tuberculosis. The pulmonary form, known as consumption, was the leading cause of death in every section of the United States. A diagnosis of consumption was tantamount to a death sentence, and about the only hope was to move to a different climate. Koch's discovery of the tubercle bacillus in 1882 opened the way for effective treatment in the twentieth century, but as late as the 1930s pulmonary tuberculosis was a serious problem, and its diagnosis aroused grave apprehensions in the patient and his family.

Asiatic cholera, which had swept through the country twice in the antebellum years, returned in 1866–67, but on a much reduced scale. Scattered outbreaks may have occurred in the early 1870s, although the diagnosis could well be suspect. While relatively insignificant in terms of morbidity and mortality, the threat of cholera played a major role in building up the quarantine system and developing public health agencies. Fear of cholera helped establish New York's Metropolitan Board of Health in 1866 and was responsible for the creation of the city's diagnostic laboratory as late as 1892.

The second of the great epidemic diseases, yellow fever, represented a real danger to the southern states throughout the century and was widely feared in every port as far north as Boston. The disease had peaked in the 1850s, but it continued to strike, although less intensely, at the southern ports. The last great outbreak occurred in 1878 when New Orleans suffered over 4,000 deaths and the contagion swept up the Mississippi Valley as far north as Cairo, St. Louis, Chattanooga, and Louisville. This epidemic aroused such a public outcry that it led directly to the establishment of the first federal public health agency, the National Board of Health, and the first national quarantine system. The final yellow fever epidemic in the United States struck New Orleans in

1905. By this date it was no longer a strange and mysterious disease. Federal, state, and local health officials collaborated in a massive antimosquito campaign, one which involved draining pools and low-lying areas, screening homes and cisterns, and the use of oil to kill mosquito larvae in open waters. By eliminating the vector, the epidemic was cut short at the beginning of September—but not before the city had lost 452 of the 3,402 residents who contracted the disease.[6]

Throughout the nineteenth century and continuing into the early twentieth, a host of serious diseases continued to take a heavy toll among young and old alike. Smallpox, which had been reduced by vaccination to minor proportions in the early nineteenth century, began to flare up anew—for, as the memory of the dreadful epidemics of earlier years receded, the public grew careless about vaccination, until renewed drives for vaccination gradually brought the disease under control. Throughout these years, diphtheria, scarlet fever, measles, and whooping cough constantly winnowed the ranks of infants and children. The most fatal one, diphtheria, showed a rising incidence in the late nineteenth century. Fortunately, just as it reached a peak in the 1890s, advances in bacteriology made it possible to diagnose, treat, and finally to prevent this fearful children's disease. The same advances also made possible a sharp reduction in the other major children's diseases during the first three decades of the twentieth century.

Although health conditions generally left much to be desired, for blacks and other minority groups the situation was even worse. The Indians were still fighting a hopeless battle to maintain their way of life. Those tribes who had given up the struggle found themselves in a netherland. The old values were gone, but they could not accept those of the whites; hence they eked out a bare living on reservations, beset by disease and alcohol. The case of the blacks was little better. The freedom they had gained by the Civil War was minimized for most of them by their economic dependence. Without capital or resources and with few skills, the majority gradually were forced into economic peonage, either as free laborers or through the sharecropping system. Whereas most planters had felt some responsibility for the health and welfare of their slaves, they quickly shucked off this responsibility with emancipation.

Freedmen, who had spent their entire lives on a single

plantation, took liberty to mean they could freely move on. Slavery at least had kept the blacks relatively isolated, enabling them to avoid most of the crowd diseases. Once they started moving in the thousands, many of them pushing into towns and cities, they encountered all of the prevailing diseases. To compound the situation, their economic position was almost hopeless. With the South in a state of virtual collapse after the War, there was little work available. The North, having freed the slaves, promptly disclaimed responsibility for them except for some limited help from the Army and the Freedman's Bureau. Although new evidence is gradually coming to light, the exact health condition of the blacks is still not clear. The indications are, however, that poverty, malnutrition, and disease killed thousands of them in the immediate postwar years. As the blacks perforce returned to the plantations, the owners employed only the healthy ones and quickly discharged those too sick to work. State and local authorities were unwilling to assume responsibility for social welfare, and one can only speculate about the fate of the aged and sick.[7]

A recent study of the blacks in Kentucky in the immediate postwar years clearly shows their desperate situation—and blacks constituted only about one fifth of the state's population, a much lower figure than in the deep South states. Despite the fact that there were over 200,000 freedmen in Kentucky, the Freedman's Bureau never employed more than five physicians to care for them. With a few exceptions private physicians refused to treat those who could not pay, automatically excluding the majority of blacks. Dr. J. G. Temple of Covington estimated that no more than one fourth of blacks were able to pay even small medical bills. The chief of the medical division in Kentucky for the Freedman's Bureau, Dr. Robin A. Bell, found the blacks in a deplorable state in every city he visited. In Covington he found them living in "wretched, old dilapidated warehouses, cellars, garrets and miserable shanties, crowded with half starved, half clad and squallid [sic] looking men, women and children with well marked disease depicted in their countenances. . . ."[8]

In the northern cities discrimination forced blacks into the lowest-paying jobs and compelled them to live in the worst slums. While many were able to fight their way out of the poverty cycle, the majority shared the abject misery of the poorest whites. Their depressed economic condition was faithfully reflected in vital statistics—everywhere their morbidity and mortality rates were far in excess of that of the general population.

The traditional viewpoint holds that the sanitary movement, which helped to institutionalize public health, was essentially a reformist engineering accomplishment. The two classic illustrations cited are Sir Edwin Chadwick in England and Lemuel Shattuck in Massachusetts, neither of whom was a physician. Whatever may have been the case in England, the public health movement in America was led by physicians and was strongly supported by medical associations at all levels until World War I. True, the medical profession was divided for a good part of the century as to whether sanitation or quarantine was the answer to preventing epidemic diseases, but the leadership was supplied by physicians. The early presidents of the American Public Health Association were all prominent physicians, active in the profession and its associations. Their names include Dr. Stephen Smith of New York, Joseph M. Toner of Washington, D.C., Edwin Snow of Providence, Elisha Harris of New York, James L. Cabell of Virginia, and John Shaw Billings of Washington, D.C. Moreover, an equally impressive list of outstanding physicians and surgeons can be found on municipal and state health boards.

An intriguing question is why organized medicine, which had stoutly supported all public health measures earlier, began to oppose a good many of them after World War I. One of the first developments which may help to explain this shift was the reorganization of the AMA in 1901, which altered the power base and made it more responsive to general practitioners. Formerly public health departments and medical schools had played an important role in the Association's policy-making. Second, the emergence of organized public health tended to draw the more socially conscious physicians out of private practice and lessen their influence in the AMA precisely at a time when medical school professors, too, were losing ground in the Association. Thus the two groups which had supplied a leavening to the profession were relegated to minor roles. A third factor was the success of the AMA in raising the profession's standards and economic status. With the improved financial position of physicians, they were inclined to support the status quo at a time when there was a major shift in public health policy. Communicable diseases could be dealt with by the application of scientific principles and laboratory work, but the noncommunicable disorders forced public health to return to its original concern with the entire social and cultural environment. Still later, public health began moving toward health care, thus coming into direct conflict with the AMA, the chief spokesman for private medicine.

By consistently opposing social legislation, the AMA has diminished some of the luster it has acquired in the past seventy-five years. By its refusal to concede that there are inadequacies in our medical care system, the profession has weakened its case. In a democracy there are certain social and political realities; by facing up to them, physicians may well be able to write safeguards into new legislation, whereas blind opposition may bring on precisely what they most fear.

The role of physicians, reformers, and progressives in the public health movement is common knowledge, but what is not so well known is the extent to which individual businessmen and commercial organizations in the late nineteenth century mobilized the political and economic power necessary to bring about major sanitary reforms. Health reformers from earliest times have argued that health is wealth and that an unhealthy population is an unproductive one. In New Orleans, which depended upon trade and commerce, intelligent businessmen in the 1880s and 1890s realized that the city's reputation for disease and pestilence was scarcely conducive to encouraging the influx of new capital or business enterprises. In consequence, the more enlightened ones began to support the local sanitary association, pushed for expensive water and sewerage systems, and generally advocated public health measures. In Memphis, which was devastated by the 1878 yellow fever epidemic and in which health conditions may have been even worse than in New Orleans, the business community initiated a complete overhaul of the municipal government and instituted major public health reforms. Enlightened self-interest did not characterize all of the business community, but members of the community did contribute to public health reform.[9]

The organization of temporary health boards dates back to the colonial period. Under the impact of yellow fever and Asiatic cholera, their numbers multiplied in the early nineteenth century, but it was not until after the Civil War that permanent health agencies began to appear on a large scale. The creation of the Metropolitan Board of Health (later the New York City Department of Health) in 1866 marks the beginning of effective municipal health departments. Within a few years most major cities had some sort of health board or health department, although they functioned with widely varying degrees of effectiveness. The next step was the formation of state health boards, most of which arose as a result of successful municipal health agencies. The same individuals who led in municipal health were usually responsible for the organization of state boards.

The first two state boards of health, those of Louisiana and Massachusetts, however, were an exception to this rule. Louisiana can rightly claim priority, since, as a result of two major yellow fever epidemics, in 1855 it established the first state board of health. Although a state health agency, the Louisiana board concentrated its attention largely on New Orleans until the end of the century, and Massachusetts can claim credit for establishing in 1869 the first board of health to function on a statewide basis as part of a general movement to strengthen the structure of state governments. New Orleans, which could claim neither good government nor a reputation for healthfulness, did not establish a city health department until 1898.[10]

Shortly after Massachusetts took action in 1869, Virginia, California, and Minnesota followed suit, and by 1883 some twenty-seven states were operating health departments. Encouraging as were these developments, the existence of laws and formal institutions was no guarantee of adequate public health programs. City councils and state legislatures were far more willing to create agencies than they were to finance them. Tennessee established a state board in 1877, but made no appropriation for it until 1879. In 1883 Dr. F. D. Cunningham reported to the AMA that the Virginia legislature had appointed a state board several years earlier "but gave it no funds and assigned no specific duties, so that its existence, if any, is only nominal."

By 1900 virtually every major city and state had a health department, and in most urban areas health officials, aided by laboratories, were beginning to gain ground in the battle against communicable diseases and the omnipresent pollution of air, water, and food. Although public health programs were restricted primarily to cities and towns, many good local and state health agencies were operating, and there was a growing public awareness of the need for governmental action. The extension of public health programs into rural areas and small communities, however, was a slow process, one which awaited the extension of electric and telephone lines, improved roads, and better transportation.[11] The movement to improve rural health did not really accelerate until the New Deal in the 1930s. One of the agencies which had the greatest impact was the Tennessee Valley Authority. This comprehensive social and economic program brought major changes in rural life not only in the Tennessee Valley and border states but throughout the entire South as far as Louisiana and Mississippi. As the TVA illustrates, the initiative for changes in public health in the twentieth century, increasingly moved from the local to the federal level.

As was true of medical research, the Federal government contributed relatively little to public health in the nineteenth century. The care of sick and disabled seamen through the United States Marine Hospital Service and medical services for those in the armed forces represented the main focus of the government's attention until the great yellow fever epidemic of 1878 terrorized the entire Mississippi Valley and brought both a national quarantine law and a National Board of Health. The Board, which functioned from 1879 to 1883, envisioned a fairly large role for itself, but Congress, viewing it primarily as a quarantine agency, gave only limited support. It struggled along for four years, bedeviled by meager appropriations, a weak organization, and strong opposition from certain state health boards, most notably that of Louisiana, and from the Marine Hospital Service which viewed it as a bureaucratic rival. The Board's appropriation was cut off after 1883, and ten years later a new law transferred federal quarantine responsibility over to the Marine Hospital Service.[12]

The establishment of the Hygiene Laboratory in Washington in 1901 and the Pure Food and Drug Law of 1906 have been touched upon in another connection. The next Federal action came in 1912 with the creation of the United States Children's Bureau and the transformation of the Marine Hospital Service into the Public Health Service. The Children's Bureau was a coordinating and informational agency to assist state and local programs. The Public Health Service was the old Marine Hospital Service with additional responsibility for research and investigation on communicable diseases. World War I drew attention to venereal diseases, and a Federal Division of Venereal Diseases was established to assist cities and states in dealing with these infections. The first significant move by the Federal government into the health care field came with the Sheppard-Towner Act of 1921. This measure broke new ground by providing grants-in-aid to states instituting maternal and child care programs. As mentioned before, in part due to opposition from the AMA, this program was allowed to lapse in 1929.[13]

The New Deal marked the first attempts to provide a national health program. Almost every New Deal agency, temporary or permanent, made some contribution to health. As early as June 1933 the Federal Emergency Relief Administration authorized the use of its funds for medical care, nursing, and emergency dental work; Civilian Conservation Corps workers received medical care; the Civil Works Administration promoted rural sanitation and helped to control malaria and other diseases; and both the Works Progress Administration and the Public Works Administration built hospitals and sewerage plants and contributed to other public health projects. In 1935 Titles V and VI of the Social Security Act authorized the use of federal funds for crippled children, maternal and child care, and the promotion of state and local public health agencies. As Roy Lubove has pointed out, the Social Security Act is of special significance, since it established a permanent machinery for distributing Federal funds for health purposes and recognized special needs in allocating these funds.

The appropriations for health under the Social Security Administration grew rapidly in the late 1930s, aided by the results of a National Health Survey undertaken in 1935–36. This survey confirmed what earlier ones had shown: that the lowest economic groups suffered the greatest amount of sickness and disability and received the least medical care. It also showed that the average expenditures by states for public health amounted to only 11 cents per capita, and that municipal expenditures were not much better. This survey further provided ammunition for those seeking to arouse a public awareness of health problems. As health became a major issue, in 1939 the Wagner bill was introduced into Congress to establish a national health program. As indicated earlier, President Roosevelt's preoccupation with the war, the opposition of organized medicine, and other factors prevented its passage.[14]

The decade of the 1940s saw limited progress in the public

health field, although general health conditions improved steadily, largely as a result of the wartime prosperity. For example, the billions of dollars spent on military camps and industries in the South raised the economic standard and the health level of the entire region. Efforts to promote a national health program proved abortive, and the only significant step by the Federal government was the Hill-Burton Act of 1946 to promote the construction of hospitals. The tremendous expansion of the armed forces, however, meant that millions of Americans received medical and dental care—for many of them a relatively new experience. In addition, as veterans they were henceforth eligible for health benefits.

The 1950s saw the Federal government support the construction of medical and public health schools, appropriate large sums for health research, and in 1953 establish a Department of Health, Education and Welfare. The fight for direct health care remained in abeyance during the Republican years, 1952–1960 and was not revived until the 1960s. The opening wedge was a bill to provide medical care for the aged—a group whose emotional appeal, while not quite on a par with motherhood, was still high—and, what was possibly more important, a group whose numbers and voting power were increasing. The Kerr-Mills bill, passed in 1962, was a very limited act which provided medical assistance to those aged sick who were not eligible for the old age assistance program and whose income was below the state-prescribed minimum level. The fight to extend these medical benefits, as noted previously, culminated in the Medicare and Medicaid amendments to the Social Security laws in 1965. Essentially these amendments provide low-cost government-subsidized medical insurance for Social Security recipients.

The concept of health insurance in America dates back to the contract practice of medicine in the nineteenth century, but its present form is of more recent origin. In 1929 a group of school teachers in Dallas, Texas, contracted with Baylor University Hospital to provide service benefits at a fixed fee per semester. The idea was picked up by the American Hospital Association in the early 1930s and led directly to the Blue Cross (hospital) and Blue Shield (medical and surgical) programs. The AMA was somewhat dubious of these at first, but gave in when faced with more radical alternatives. As unions and corporations began negotiating health benefits, private corporations moved into the health insurance business. In the twenty years from 1940 to 1960 voluntary health insurance experienced an explosive growth, encouraged in part by the medical profession's acceptance of it.

Growing alongside health insurance came another form of medical care somewhat akin to the former contract practice, the prepaid group practice. The most successful of these are the Kaiser Foundation Health Plan organized in California in 1942 and the Health Insurance Plan of Greater New York dating back to 1947. By 1960 each of these plans was providing complete medical care to over half a million subscribers. Physicians participating in these programs and similar ones have been subjected to considerable pressure both from the AMA and local medical societies, but health maintenance organizations (HMO) such as these have continued to grow.[15]

American medical care today is provided by and paid for through a variety of methods and agencies—private medicine, prepaid group practice, Blue Cross and Blue Shield, commercial insurance, government-subsidized health insurance, and so forth. In addition, the government provides direct medical care to millions of individuals through the Armed Services, Veterans Administration, and other agencies. The net effect of the government participation in health care has been to make this service available to millions of Americans who formerly seldom visited a physician except in dire emergencies. An incidental result of the government's action has been to increase the demand for medical services, resulting in increasing affluence for the medical profession and an even greater increase in governmental expenditures for health services. These rising costs have led to an examination of the distribution of health manpower and resources, and it is clear that the availability of physicians and hospitals varies widely between geographic regions and income groups. How to use the available medical resources most effectively and to channel medical personnel into those areas where they are most needed is a serious problem, since national planning has never appealed to Americans. Health, however, is a matter of vital concern to everyone, and the trend is in the direction of governmental action. Whether or not America follows the British and European pathway to nationalized medicine will depend upon the willingness of the American medical profession to admit inequities and to propose a sound alternative.

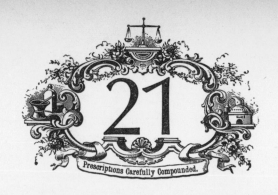

Prescriptions Carefully Compounded.

MEDICINE TODAY

THROUGHOUT its history medicine has been subject to fads and
fashions and has seen its public image range from poor to excellent.
Medical ethics are a reflection of public morality, and the profession must constantly redefine its ethical code to meet societal
changes. In the twentieth century medical science and technology
have made enormous strides, but in the process they have raised
new ethical issues and have enormously increased medical costs.
The multiplying cost of medical care in turn has drawn attention to
the cumbersome, expensive, and inefficient method of health care
delivery in the United States. The duplication of health care
services, maldistribution of physicians, and lack of standardized
licensing procedures are well documented; and the multiplicity of
licensing agencies bears a good part of the responsibility for the
current crisis over malpractice insurance. The public attitude
toward the medical profession is one of ambivalence, characterized
on one hand by a profound faith in scientific medicine and

individual practitioners, and on the other by a skepticism about the profession as a whole.

Health is too important a matter to be left exclusively to doctors, and American laymen have always engaged in do-it-yourself medicine, resorted to irregulars and quacks, and supported health movements. As a result of the current fad for physical fitness, our streets are beset by sweat-suited individuals of all ages and sex doggedly jogging their way to health and long life. In addition, stores selling "natural" foods are flourishing, physical fitness salons have become a major business, and antismoking and weight-losing clinics and workshops are attracting thousands of individuals bent on leading cleaner and leaner lives. And those for whom physical activity in itself is not enough are seeking physical and mental well-being through Christian faith healing, yoga, Transcendental Meditation, and a host of major and minor gurus.

When neither mental effort nor physical exercise can solve medical problems, the skeptics of modern medicine can always turn to the irregulars. A few homeopaths still practice, although their numbers are rapidly dwindling. Osteopathy is flourishing, but, as with homeopathy, it was absorbed into regular medicine at the turn of the century and no longer can be classified as an irregular medical group. The chiropractors, whose early success was predicated on the inability of the orthodox profession to deal with spinal problems, have lost much of their *raison d'être* with the advance of medical knowledge, but they have survived strong attacks by organized medicine, and, aided by the high cost of orthodoxy, are reviving. After having been driven out of business in many areas, by 1975 they had regained the right to practice in every state in the Union.

The latest medical fad to intrigue the public and the medical profession is acupuncture, an age-old Chinese technique. Chinese medicine and philosophy are inextricable, since both are dominated by the concept of dualism: the two forces, principles, or essences known as yin (female) and yang (male). Health represents the successful interaction of these two principles via a complicated system of channels. When one or more of these channels is blocked, ill health ensues, and the aim of the acupuncturist with his needles is to restore the normal flow and reestablish bodily balance. This technique is based on the assumption that the body has six major channels or meridians each of yin and yang, with many subsidiary channels branching off. This network connects 365 points on the skin to the internal organs. A few Western physicians, surgeons, and laymen have visited China and brought back glowing accounts of the achievements of acupuncturists in the realm of anesthesia and in relieving chronic pain. Feature stories in newspapers and magazines have further stimulated public interest, but until more concrete evidence can be found to justify acupuncture it must be considered another form of faith healing.

If the history of medicine proves anything, it does demonstrate that faith healing, by whatever name, plays a significant role in physical well-being. A major aspect of the doctor-patient relationship is a feeling of confidence or faith on the part of the patient, and whether this faith is placed in a witch-doctor, medicine man, guru, or Christian faith-healer it can have beneficial effects. Yoga has long demonstrated, and recent studies have given further proof, that with training an individual can control at least some of the involuntary muscles. Moreover, as Hippocrates recognized five centuries before Christ, worry and anxiety do cause disease; hence the success of the most recent fad, Transcendental Meditation. Whatever its rationale or philosophic merits, it probably does offer a measure of peace and tranquility to the faithful and by so doing promotes their physical well-being. On the basis of past experience, we can reasonably assume that Transcendental Meditation, except for a few devotees, will fade away like all other fads and fashions.

Far more important than these minor aberrations from orthodox medicine are the fundamental problems raised by the advancing frontiers of medicine. The relatively recent breaking of the genetic code has opened the way to various forms of bioengineering. Whether these research programs involve creating new types of bacteria or experimenting with in vitro fertilization of human ova, they raise basic ethical questions. For example, do we have the right to create new forms of bacteria which may pose a threat to human existence? Or should we fertilize human ova and grow test-tube babies for experimental purposes? At the same time the rapid technological developments in the last fifty years which now permit heart, kidney, and other transplants, which provide electric pacemakers for the heart, the mechanical filtration of blood for kidney patients, and mechanical feeding and elimination have all accentuated old moral questions and created new ones. Transplants, by creating a need for living tissue, have forced a redefinition of death. At what point can an individual be considered beyond hope? The traditional view that cessation of heart action and respiration constitute death no longer suffices in a day when cardiac arrest is not necessarily fatal. Nor is major brain damage sufficient in itself to proclaim death when modern technology can maintain individuals in a vegetablelike existence for many years.

Transplants have also raised the question of priorities—where available organs are limited, who gets them? The issue is particularly acute in the case of kidney patients where the expense of kidney machines is great enough to preclude their ready accessibility. Should a patient suffering from a terminal illness be taken off a kidney machine to make way for one with a better chance for survival? And this brings up the whole issue of euthanasia. Since euthanasia involves killing individuals suffering from terminal illnesses or hopeless injuries as an act of mercy, it was relatively simple for a Christian society to apply the commandment, "Thou shalt not kill," and condemn the practice. Euthanasia under such circumstances was an act of commission and as such was forbidden by medical ethics and society's moral code. With medical technology able to provide substitutes for the heart, kidneys, lungs, and other organs, the distinction between life and death has become blurred. The physician's obligation to preserve life was predicated on the assumption that his efforts were largely supportive. Today it is possible to prolong life in elderly senile patients long after their existence as thinking conscious human beings has disappeared, or to preserve life in the bodies of younger patients for years after irreversible brain damage has guaranteed that they will never again be aware of the world around them. Euthanasia can now result from an act of omission. By simply cutting off the power supply to a mechanical respirator or some other device or by deciding not to use a life-preserving piece of equipment the attending physician makes the decision for life or death.

The problem is not a new one, for physicians have always had to make arbitrary decisions about prolonging the life of suffering, terminally ill patients. These decisions are generally made either in conference with the patient's family or else the physician, often in concurrence with his associates, makes a professional judgment as to what is best for the patient. In the past this was largely a matter of concern to the individual physician or to the physician and the patient's family, but in today's world these decisions have become public record. Seriously ill patients almost invariably end up in a hospital where their medical care involves a large number of professionals and paraprofessionals. Decisions by attending physicians are subject to hospital review boards, and the existence of detailed case records, which can be made available for a malpractice suit, necessarily makes doctors reluctant to withhold any form of life-preserving technology. The advent of life-supportive mechanical devices which have a viability of their own has thrown the whole problem into sharper focus. Where these devices are in use, euthanasia is no longer the result of an act of omission but rather one of commission or direct action. Conflicting court actions to force physicians and hospitals to maintain life in hopeless cases— even over the objection of the patient's family—indicate that the public is no longer willing to leave these decisions to the medical profession. If this situation continues, then society must redefine the ground rules.

Just as medical advances have complicated the question of euthanasia, they have also raised new questions in connection with contraception and abortion. Dating back to primitive societies in which fertility rates were low and infant mortality high, abortion has rarely received social sanction, although it appears to have been practiced to some extent even by early civilizations. The emergence of gynecology and obstetrics as a specialty and a vastly improved understanding of the physiology involved from conception to birth has made abortion a much simpler and safer form of medical intervention. In consequence, abortions to save the life or health of the mother have gradually gained social acceptance, but the effect was also to make abortion available to all who could afford it. Physicians who believe in a woman's right to make her own decision and doctors attracted by the relatively large fees are all willing to perform abortions. Regardless of the legal aspects, middle- and upper-class women seeking abortions can have them performed under safe medical supervision. The only effect of legal restrictions has been to raise the cost and effectively exclude poor and lower-income women from resorting to physicians. The result is that these women have had to turn to empirics, quacks, and folk practitioners, subjecting themselves to the possibility of serious pelvic infections and other complications, including death.

There is a measure of irony in the fact that the research directed toward helping women conceive has also contributed to more effective birth control and contraception. One might well ask whether facilitating conception and birth is any more of an interference with nature than preventing them. The present abortion controversy raises still another interesting point. Recently a movement has developed calling for a moratorium on in vitro fertilization of human ova. Proponents of this type of research argue that it is essential if we are to understand gestation and make progress toward the elimination of birth defects. If abortions can be performed legally up to the twenty-fourth week of gestation for the convenience or welfare of the mother, than in vitro fertilization for scientific purposes has a far more legitimate claim, providing that the fetus is destroyed before the twenty-fourth week.[1] Assuming that genetic engineering does make it possible to manipulate the genetic code, we may well open a Pandora's box. Man is infinitely more than the sum total of his parts, and, while we can and have improved upon his physical makeup, the realm of the spirit or intelligence is still beyond our comprehension.

Whatever the truth of the foregoing statement, the fact remains that man has been interfering with nature and assuming the role of God from early times. As soon as he began curing and preventing illness, domesticating his food supply, and modifying his environment, he was altering nature's way. If bioengineering constitutes man playing God, then it is a role he assumed long ago. Individuals in advanced countries today mature earlier and are taller, heavier, and healthier than their forebears. When medicine resorts to vaccinations to provide immunity, cosmetic surgery, or radical surgery to remove pathological conditions, it is remaking man. The question as to whether or not man should play God has already been answered; the real issue is how well we do it. Expanding knowledge has gradually obliterated the sharp distinctions between scientific fields, and it is becoming clear that medicine and the biological sciences cannot go blindly along without considering the implications of their work in terms of human values. One hundred years ago Rudolph Virchow declared that medicine is a social science; we are only beginning to appreciate this fact.

Aside from the ethical questions raised by current developments in medicine, there is an equally grave question as to what direction medical research should take. In a recent thoughtful analysis, Dean Lewis Thomas of the Yale School of Medicine defined three categories of medical technology, suggesting that society needs to establish priorities among them.[2] The first and highest level is the one seeking to understand disease processes and to find relatively simple and easy ways to prevent or alleviate them. Prime examples of this type of research are the development of vaccines to prevent a wide variety of bacterial and virus diseases and the use of hormones to treat endocrine disorders. The cost of this basic research is often high, but the payoff is much greater. Aside from the loss of human life, the expense of caring for thousands of cases of tuberculosis, poliomyelitis, and a host of other diseases now virtually banished would be prohibitive at today's medical costs. Nothing illustrates the huge savings arising from basic research better than the hundreds of iron lungs relegated to storage now that poliomyelitis is no longer a serious threat.

Dean Thomas's second category, which he calls "halfway technology," concerns itself precisely with the development and operation of iron lungs—and with kidney machines, pacemakers, and all other medical devices or procedures designed to alleviate or compensate for damage caused by little understood disease processes. If we can discover the factors responsible for the destruction of the capillaries in the kidneys and prevent this process, then the intelligence, creativity, and material resources devoted to devising kidney machines and improving transplant techniques can be turned to more productive purposes and the highly skilled manpower and equipment used to support these halfway measures can be released for other services. The same situation holds true in the case of atherosclerosis and cancer. The elimination or reduction of costly coronary care units and complicated cardiac surgical procedures would make a wide range of medical resources available for other uses. Aside from the human suffering and death caused by cancer, its victims often require exceedingly expensive care. Radical surgery, irradiation, and chemotherapy have proved effective in dealing with many forms of cancer, but the real solution lies in preventing the formation of cancerous cells. Once an understanding of cancer can be found through basic research, these costly, painful, and mutilating methods for dealing with cancer will be relegated to a minor role.

The third category, which Dean Thomas calls "nontechnology," is the supportive care provided for patients with terminal or incurable diseases for which little can be done other than to alleviate pain and discomfort and provide reassurance. While not requiring as great an expenditure as "halfway technology," this care does take a great deal of valuable time on the part of physicians and other medical personnel. These last two categories are largely responsible for the soaring cost of American health care. While medicine must take responsibility for the sick, the increasing cost of medical care makes it essential that medical research be concentrated on disease causation rather than mitigating or relieving the results of disease. Artificial hearts are an intriguing prospect for a gadget-minded civilization, but a better understanding of irreversible muscle or valve diseases might well make them unnecessary.

The problem of understanding disease processes is an exceedingly difficult one, since the pathway to the solution often includes many blind alleys. Cancer research is a fine example. Vast sums have been invested in cancer research, yet the survival rate for the major forms of the disease, such as cancer of the lung, colon, stomach, rectum, and pancreas, have improved only slightly—and even this improvement has not come from any significant breakthrough in treatment. Antibiotics, transfusion techniques, and other aids to surgery may well be responsible for the improved cancer survival rates, *i.e.*, more people are surviving cancer operations than cancer itself. In the late eighteenth and nineteenth centuries physicians were generally convinced that disease arose from climate and environmental conditions, and the medical journals were filled with meteorological studies seeking to tie temperature, humidity, and other factors to epidemic disease. In recent years virologists have successfully claimed a major share of cancer research funds, although the answer to cancer may lie in nutrition, environmental, or immunological factors. Health authorities are increasingly coming to believe that cigarette smoking, industrial chemicals, and natural agents such as solar and cosmic radiation are largely responsible for inducing cancers. Research, too, has its vested interests, and the line between innovative ideas and absurd theories is ill defined. Virology, which holds the possibility of a quick, simple answer and possibly a Nobel Prize, is much more attractive than the slow, dogged hard work necessary to identify a wide variety of environmental factors.[3]

Mental health is another area where progress has been slow.

The United States lags behind other countries in accepting mental illness on a par with physical ailments, in part because a measure of stigma is still attached to mental disorders. As already noted, the emergence of state mental institutions in the mid-nineteenth century offered little help to the mentally ill, for these institutions merely provided custodial care. Despite a few experiments such as shock therapy and prefrontal lobotomy, virtually nothing was done for the vast majority of inmates in state and local institutions until the 1950s. The advent of tranquilizers, by relieving symptoms and enabling patients to function more or less normally, drastically reduced the population of mental institutions. Buoyed by the prospect of saving tax money, mental institutions began a wholesale discharge of patients, many of whom were absolutely incapable of surviving in the everyday world.

Ideally these discharged patients should have received counseling and help from psychiatric social workers and nurses and other trained professionals, and they should have had access to halfway houses and community mental health centers. In a few areas this sort of assistance was available, but the majority of patients were shown how to get on welfare and then left to sink or swim. The Joint Commission on Mental Illness, a group of interested professionals and laymen, issued a report in 1961 urging a national system of community mental health centers. Congress responded in 1963 by providing matching funds on a limited basis for the development of these centers. Their creation, however, depended upon the willingness of local authorities to support the program. Often poorer areas where the centers were most needed showed little interest and in those areas where local authorities did cooperate, they have had to pay an increasing share of the costs, since the past two Federal administrations have opposed continuing Federal support. This factor, combined with the financial stringencies of the past two years, has nullified many of the gains resulting from the 1963 measure. To make matters worse, Blue Cross–Blue Shield has provided only minimal coverage for mental illness, and even these benefits apply largely to institutionalized individuals. Consequently, relatively little insurance money is available for patients utilizing community mental health centers.[4]

We still know relatively little about the major forms of psychosis, but we have learned to prevent or cure those diseases such as syphilis that formerly caused many mental disorders. We also have the knowledge to deal with many minor disorders and to alleviate symptoms in more serious cases. The major problem today is a matter of delivering health services, and, short of a national health system, the present prospects are not too promising.

The foregoing issues represent only a part of the current difficulties confronting the American medical profession. Equally important are those problems relating directly to medical practice. The specific issue arousing the greatest public attention today, although not necessarily the most serious, is the rapidly increasing number of malpractice suits and the corresponding increase in malpractice insurance rates. To the average American, insurance companies are vague conglomerations of wealth; and he has little compunction about distributing this wealth to individual citizens. The increasing affluence of physicians and the steady rise in medical fees undoubtedly contribute to the ordinary juryman's inclination to favor the plaintiff in malpractice cases. Insurance companies, too, may have contributed to the rash of suits by their willingness to settle many unjustifiable ones out of court, thus encouraging the filing of so-called "nuisance" suits. Moreover, since insurance companies traditionally have passed on additional costs to their customers, they have had little incentive to minimize either the cost or number of suits.

While insurance companies share part of the blame, an even greater share can be attributed to the legal profession. The contingency fee system, which allows lawyers to collect as much as 50 percent of the settlement, has encouraged a small number of lawyers to institute many unnecessary and unwarranted suits.

The fundamental reason for the growth of malpractice cases, however, probably results from basic changes in health delivery. Despite the medical profession's constant emphasis upon the doctor-patient relationship, the close personal contact between the doctor and the patient is steadily diminishing. Urban society by its nature is impersonal, and the patient who sees his physician periodically in the course of an office visit scarcely has the same relationship that obtained when the family doctor regularly visited the homes of his patients. Moreover, heavy case loads, combined with the use of laboratory tests and paramedical personnel, have tended to make office visits merely brief encounters. The high degree of specialization has also furthered the impersonalization of medicine. The dermatologist, urologist, or other specialist who constantly sees new patients can scarcely develop a close personal identification with them. The nature of specialists' training, too, tends to make them see cases rather than individuals.

The multiplicity of specialists may have increased the possibility for discovering cases of malpractice. In the days when the family physician took major responsibility for medical care, if a patient died or suffered complications it was assumed the physician had done all that was possible and the matter rested. Today the patient or his family might secure the opinions of one or more specialists, any one of whom might cast doubt on the original diagnosis or therapy. Whereas the family doctor was a close friend and advisor, the practitioner today is more apt to be simply another professional for whom the patient has limited regard. The emergence of group practice in one form or another has also contributed to the impersonalization of medicine, and this trend has been furthered by the increasing use of hospital facilities. Many forms of surgical intervention are performed in hospitals by specialists, a situation giving little opportunity for a close interaction between patient and surgeon.

Had the medical societies been more zealous in policing their membership, the malpractice situation might not have arisen—but one might also apply the same reasoning to Watergate and the legal profession. The American Association of University Professors has never dropped anyone from membership because of bad teaching, nor, judging by the many stock frauds, have the accountants paid much attention to the ethics of their fellow professionals. Despite all scientific developments and the use of sophisticated instruments and laboratory techniques, medicine is still an art, and much of what the physician does is a matter of judgment. While cases of gross negligence or flagrant incompetence are fairly clear cut, defining the line between good and bad judgment is a matter of judgment itself. Precisely because physicians are constantly making judgments themselves, they hesitate to question those of their fellow practitioners. This reluctance to testify against each other, however justifiable, has only increased public suspicion of the profession.

The failure of medical societies to guard professional standards would not have been so bad had the state licensing agencies properly performed their task. As indicated in a previous chapter, the multiplicity of these licensing boards and the wide difference in standards have greatly limited their value. Instances in which medical licenses have been revoked are rare and these usually have involved only the most flagrant of cases. Unscrupulous and incompetent individuals exist in every profession, but the nature of medicine requires that this number be kept to an absolute minimum. Unfortunately, by permitting the existence of a few incompetents, the profession has opened the way for legitimate malpractice suits which have besmirched all physicians and encouraged the present flood of cases.

Aside from increasing medical fees, since the cost of malpractice insurance must be passed on to the patient, malpractice suits have forced physicians into practicing defensive medicine. Expensive biopsies and other laboratory tests are frequently ordered by physicians in routine cases simply as a matter of protection. The net effect is that malpractice suits have raised the cost of medicine far beyond the actual money involved in the court cases.

It is possible that the present flurry of court activity may die down or fall to a manageable level. In the event it does not, one solution would be a reform of the entire legal system, scarcely a likely prospect in view of the enormous vested interests in it and the preponderance of lawyers in elected offices. A more promising solution would be to raise professional standards in medicine by working through the licensing boards or professional review agencies. Licensing requirements could be standardized, incompetent physicians weeded out, and all practitioners forced to participate in refresher courses and continuing education. By keeping the number of legitimate malpractice suits to a minimum, public opinion itself would discourage flimsy and dubious ones.

A much more serious problem than malpractice suits is the enormous general increase in the cost of medical care. Whereas patients formerly worried about the loss of income from a serious illness, today the economic impact of medical bills for even a short stay in hospital can be devastating. The development of sophisticated diagnostic, supportive, and therapeutic devices is an expensive process, and their operation and maintenance necessitates highly specialized technicians and paraprofessionals. Delicate and elaborate surgical procedures require not only years of training on the part of the surgeons but also a large supportive cast of surgical nurses, anesthetists, and so forth, and the present radiation and chemotherapy procedures are far removed from the simple prescriptions of fifty years ago. Thus, the medical advances which have done so much to improve health and extend life have also raised the cost of medical care.

A factor seldom recognized in the growth of medical costs has been the steady upward movement of wages and salaries for ancillary workers. Hospital and clinic employees, nurses and receptionists, and many other individuals involved in medical or medically related fields were for many years among the lowest paid of workers. The $10 to $20 daily hospital charges of former years were predicated on virtual starvation wages for orderlies, nurses, and other staff employees, while interns and residents were expected to put in six or seven long days a week for room, board, and a nominal cash income. Minimum wage laws, stronger nursing associations, and rebellions by interns and residents have rectified a good share of these abuses, but the consequence has been a major increase in hospital and clinic budgets. The improved standard of living for hospital workers was part of a general rise in living standards which has dramatically raised the demand for medical services. This increased demand, combined with the growth of private and nonprofit health insurance associations, enables hospitals to accede to the wage demands of their employees by simply raising their charges.

Hospital trustees and administrators, however, do share some responsibility for making medical care almost prohibitive. Since they manage nonprofit institutions, many of them have made little effort to watch expenses, contenting themselves with meeting their growing budgets by increasing rates. Not infrequently hospitals have added expensive units such as kidney machines and coronary care centers simply as prestige items—and in many cases duplicating similar facilities in adjacent institutions. In some instances these installations are acquired purely for the convenience of attending physicians or as a matter of local pride. All too often new hospitals are built when existing ones have far more capacity than the community needs. Widespread recognition of the problem of excessive hospital capacity and duplication has led to the creation of regional health planning boards, but since virtually all plans to date have depended largely upon voluntary compliance they have had limited success.

The rising cost of medicine takes on even more significance in view of the fact that health care has become a major industry in America, with an estimated 4.5 million employees or almost 5 percent of our total labor force. Of these, less than 300,000 are practicing physicians.[5] The sheer numbers of those employed in health fields guarantee that health care cannot be inexpensive, but, as indicated in the case of hospitals, a great deal of inefficiency and duplication characterizes the delivery of medical care. Private medicine, voluntary associations and institutions, state and local governments, and Federal agencies all provide some measure of medical care. The Federal government alone offers complete medical services to millions of Americans. The approximately 2 million men in the armed services and their dependents constitute one large group in this category. An even larger group are the 30 million veterans from past wars who are eligible for inpatient and outpatient services at the Veterans Administration Hospitals and Clinics. The Public Health Service, the Indian Health Service, and a wide range of other governmental agencies all provide health services of one sort or another. In addition, through outright grants and matching funds the Federal government subsidizes medical care for millions of other Americans.

Every major city has at least one municipal hospital and various clinics, dispensaries, and health centers offering outpatient and inpatient services to those who cannot afford private medicine, and state and county agencies supplement these services with a wide range of medical institutions and programs. These governmental services, which vary widely in quality, include diagnostic and treatment facilities for venereal disease and tuberculosis, maternal and child centers, mental health programs, and so forth. Paralleling the state and local government services are those offered by voluntary associations which concentrate upon specific medical problems or problem areas such as cancer, heart, mental health, and birth defects. While voluntary groups often place their major efforts upon health education and collecting money for research, they also provide some diagnostic and treatment facilities.

Private practice, as it has in the past, still dominates the delivery of medical care, although the emergence of specialists and group medical practice have drastically reduced the number of general physicians with family practices. Private group practice enables physicians to share the cost and make more effective use of expensive equipment. It also gives individual members of the group more freedom to engage in leisure activities or to advance their professional knowledge, confident that their patients will not lack for attention.

The existence of many methods for providing health care in itself assures some measure of duplication and wasted effort, but in addition it intensifies two other basic problems affecting our medical care system, the shortage of physicians and the maldistribution of health services. Although the number of medical schools has increased from seventy-seven in 1945–46 to 114 today, the demand for physicians' services has increased at an even greater rate. The primary cause for this increased demand lies, as already noted, in improving living standards, but it has been affected also by the growth of and alteration in the composition of the population. For example, a higher life expectancy has increased the relative percentages of older people and the movement from rural to urban areas has added to those sections of the population which demand more medical services. To further complicate the difficulties, the relative percentage of physicians entering private practice has fallen during the past 30 years. A higher percentage of young physicians today are drawn into research, teaching, administration, and related areas. To some extent the relative loss of private practice physicians has been compensated for by advances in preventive medicine and therapy (antibiotics, for example), the efficiencies of group practice, conditioning patients to office visits rather than house calls, and the wider use of medical technology and paramedical personnel.

Aside from the disparity in medical care between income levels inherent in any system of private medicine based on fees, the distribution of physicians among the population is another cause for the varying quality of medical care. Ironically the excellent training given to physicians is one of the factors in bringing about their maldistribution. After spending at least four years as undergraduates, four more in medical school, and one or more as interns and residents, young physicians have little desire to practice in an area which has neither cultural advantages, first-rate hospitals, nor an opportunity for professional contacts. One consequence is that the physician-to-population ratio varies directly with the population density—urban and suburban areas tend to have more physicians relatively than rural settings.

A second factor has been the growth of specialties. While a few individuals specialize for reasons other than economic, specialty training offers much in the way of economic and social advantages. Most specialists can expect to keep reasonable office hours, earn more money, and achieve greater professional and social recognition than is true of the general practitioner. Earning a lucrative living by catering to the neuroses of middle-class patients gives the psychiatrist a far more pleasant way of life than conducting a busy general practice. In fact, it has far more appeal than treating psychotics in an underfinanced state institution. While the majority of specialists do treat the sick—and not all can be sure of reasonable office hours—their professional life ordinarily can be conducted at a smoother and easier pace. This attractiveness of specialty work is a significant reason for the shortage of general practitioners. It has also intensified the problem of maldistribution, since most specialties require the high population density and first-class medical facilities characteristic of urban centers.

Attempts have been made to attack the problems of physician shortages and the irregular distribution of physicians among the population. Within the past thirty years the number of medical schools has more than doubled, but medical schools are costly and one that can graduate 200 physicians per year is large indeed. Moreover, the need for extensive laboratory and clinical experience makes it almost impossible to increase the size of existing medical school classes without major capital expenditures. Following World War II the Federal government began pouring large amounts of money into medical research, a good part of which was used indirectly to subsidize medical education. In the 1960s Federal appropriations were made directly to medical education and these tentative measures finally crystallized into the Comprehensive Health Manpower Training Act of 1971. This measure provided capital funds for research and training institutions and authorized loans for scholarships.

With a growing population and the public demanding a higher

level of medical care, it is clear that the shortage of physicians will be with us for some time. Probably the best immediate solution is to increase the number of allied health professionals, since the time and expense involved in training medical technicians and paraprofessionals is far less than that for physicians. One of the most innovative programs in recent years is the creation of a new category of health professionals, the physician's assistant. Based on the role of medical corpsmen in the military services, individuals with a high-school education are admitted to a training course that includes both basic sciences and clinical experience. Since first introduced by Duke University in 1965, programs for training physician's assistants have increased in number, and they offer one of the most hopeful solutions to the physician shortage. The programs vary considerably and the work of these assistants depends in part upon the nature of their training and in part on the willingness of the supervising physicians to give them responsibility for dealing with minor ailments and a part of routine physical examinations. By relieving the physician of much of this type of work, however, the assistants can free his time for more serious cases and enable him to increase his patient load.

Another step in this direction has been to expand the responsibilities of graduate nurses by giving them postgraduate training. Public health nurses have done notable work in maternal and child care since the beginning of the century, and, particularly in isolated areas, have provided a good deal of medical care. A good example of this is a new four-month program that leads to certification as a pediatric nurse practitioner. The graduates of this program are qualified to handle the routine problems affecting infants and children and to advise the mother on child care. Those graduate nurses willing to assume even greater responsibility can take a longer and more intensive training course which qualifies them as primary-care nurses. As such, they are qualified to take medical histories, give physicals, provide prenatal care in normal situations, and handle the routine medical problems of children and adults. Both pediatric nurse practitioners and primary-care nurses ordinarily work under the supervision of physicians, although they are capable of working with a high degree of independence.

While there is some reluctance, especially by older physicians, to make use of physicians' assistants, pediatric nurse practitioners, and other categories of health manpower, the most serious hindrance to making fuller use of their services is the multiplicity of licensing agencies already noted, and the legal status of these paramedics vis-à-vis the supervising physicians. Variations in training programs and state licensing requirements often restrict nurse practitioners and others to the state in which they received their training. In addition, the recent flood of malpractice suits has raised such questions as the right of a physician to delegate responsibility to an assistant. If these difficulties can be cleared away the use of medical auxiliaries should play an important role in solving the physician shortage.

How to deal with the maldistribution of physicians is a more difficult issue, and it is one that may not be rectified short of a national system of medicine. So far the Federal government operating through the states has offered scholarship loans to medical students with the proviso that most of the loan will be canceled if the recipient practices in a specified area for a limited time. The National Health Service Corps, designed to enroll 600 members, permitted physicians to substitute regular practice in an underserved region in place of military duty. From an immediate standpoint both of these programs are of help, but the same factors which draw physicians into affluent urban and suburban centers will still operate once these physicians have served their time. A better alternative is a current program to encourage the establishment of Area Health Education Centers. These Centers, it is hoped, will attract young physicians into areas where they are needed and at the same time provide continuing education for local health professionals. Through the Centers, resident physicians could maintain contact with medical schools and other educational institutions and thus would no longer feel isolated from professional developments.

Had the private fee-for-service medical system worked as effectively as its staunchest advocates insist, it is likely that the hodgepodge of government and private agencies involved in the delivery of medical care would not have come into existence. Yet, even with the best efforts of private medicine and the multiplicity of agencies and institutions, the fact remains that a good many Americans receive virtually no medical care—and that at least 20 percent of the population receive an inadequate amount. In addition, the threat of economic disaster resulting from a major illness still hovers over many families, particularly those in the lower-income groups, and even the majority of Americans, for whom the best medical care in the world is available, have become increasingly uneasy about the meteoric rise in medical costs. The growing involvement by the government in medicine reflects in part this unease and dissatisfaction, and on the basis of the past thirty years it is logical to assume that the future holds more, and not less, government intervention.

Granting that the present trend does continue, what can Americans expect in the future? One possibility is a comprehensive system of national health care on the order of the British system. The present British health care program began in 1912 with the National Health Insurance Act, which provided that all individuals earning less than a certain minimum wage were entitled to join approved insurance associations. For a small regular payment by employees and employers, members are entitled to the services of a general practitioner. Those physicians participating in the program are paid a capitation fee or regular fixed amount for each individual or family signing with them. In the succeeding years the British health program was broadened as government and volunteer agencies gradually expanded hospital facilities, school health programs, maternal and child health care, and other forms of health services.

Nonetheless, the uneven distribution of these services led to agitation for a comprehensive system in the 1930s, but it took the drastic mobilization of all medical and health resources during the heavy bombings and other exigencies of World War II to clarify the picture and demonstrate the advantages of a national system. In 1941 a committee was established under Sir William Beveridge to study the existing health program and recommend improvements. Five years later, after a great deal of investigation and debate, the National Health Service Act of 1946, which created the National Health Service, was passed. In 1948 the Service began providing complete physician and hospital service for every resident plus a wide range of environmental and community health services. Public reception was enthusiastic and the vast majority of physicians accepted the change and cooperated fully.

As with any new and elaborate system, certain weaknesses soon became apparent. One major problem was the accumulated medical backlog resulting from the relatively poor medical care so many Britons had received prior to World War II. In part this situation arose from the tremendous capital losses suffered by England in the First World War and the rising competition from the United States and other industrial powers, which weakened her economic position and brought a relatively lower standard of living. In addition, a large number of British hospitals, like many of her industrial plants, had been built in the nineteenth century and needed to be replaced or renovated. Thus, a private medical system designed to provide good care for middle- and upper-class patients and minimal services for the rest of the population was suddenly faced with providing adequate care for the entire population. For example, the new health service was almost overwhelmed by an immediate demand for glasses and false teeth.

In these same years the income of American physicians and surgeons was rising sharply, and the economic opportunities in the United States attracted a good many British physicians, thus further straining the limited British resources. Ironically, the improvement in American physicians' income is directly related to the growing expenditure of public funds in the health area. Despite a large backlog of medical problems, the need to invest a great deal of capital in hospitals and health centers, and manpower shortages, the British National Health Service is still in operation after almost thirty years. A reorganization act in 1973 altered the structure of the central and regional administration and remedied the major complaints of the general practitioners, but it brought no basic change. Parenthetically, the strong support by the public and medical profession for the British system is strangely at odds with the recurrent horror stories about British socialized medicine in American journals and newspapers.

Under the British system, general practitioners are independent professionals who contract with a Family Practitioner Committee. Once authorized to practice in a community, a physician is free to choose his patients. He receives a capitation fee for each one accepted plus certain extras, depending upon the age of the patient, the location of the practice, and so forth. He is free to start a new practice or apply for a vacant practice in any area, but, to prevent an excessive concentration of doctors, he first must apply to the Family Practitioner Committee which may decide that the number of doctors is already sufficient. While having the right to select his patients, a physician is required to treat emergency cases and the patients of other physicians who are away. Patients, too, have freedom of choice and the right to transfer from one physician to another.

If specialist care is needed, the general practitioner refers the patient to the area hospital. Prescriptions for medicines or appliances are provided at a nominal charge, except in the case of certain categories of patients who receive them free. Glasses are supplied at cost, although the patient may buy a more expensive frame if he wishes. In the event home nurses, midwives, or health visitors are needed, these, too, are provided by the local authorities. The British system has the advantage of placing the major emphasis upon preventive medicine, since it is to the physician's advantage to keep his patient healthy. Moreover, it frees the conscientious physician from worrying as to whether or not his patient can afford an expensive diagnostic procedure when the medical indications are not too clear.

Whatever the merits of the British system, Americans have been conditioned to react adversely to the word "socialist," and this makes it unlikely that we will follow the British example in the immediate future. Our bountiful resources and higher standard of living have guaranteed that most Americans can obtain reasonably good medical care—although not nearly as good as our resources and knowledge might indicate. War has never come directly to our shores, bringing injury and death to thousands of civilians and requiring the complete mobilization of our medical resources. Philanthropy and volunteerism are more firmly embedded in the American tradition, as can be seen in our medical organization. Whereas the British government initiated health insurance, in America the major breakthrough came with the emergence of voluntary Blue Cross–Blue Shield plans.

Equally important has been the role of organized medicine in fighting any effort by public authorities to provide direct medical care. Public health leaders are always careful to avoid antagonizing local medical societies, even when advocating programs which by their nature require health authorities to deliver medical care. Wise health advocates emphasize the diagnostic role of their programs and stress that only the most impoverished will be treated. All too frequently when a county or municipal health department begins a campaign to inoculate all children against routine diseases, the local medical society raises objections and forces curtailment of the program. The result is that lower-income workers with large families often neglect these elementary precautions.

Yet the United States is moving toward the more systematic delivery of health care. Solo practice is steadily declining as more physicians enter into group practice, and group practice, whether private or nonprofit, lends itself to a more rational system of health delivery. One of the more promising developments at present are Health Maintenance Organizations or HMOs. A fine example of these is the nonprofit Kaiser-Permanente program based in Oakland, California. HMOs require a relatively large amount of capital in the initial stages, and the funding for the Kaiser-Permanente plan came from the late industrialist, Henry J. Kaiser, and the Kaiser family foundation. Today the Kaiser HMO is a financial self-sustaining organization employing 2,500 physicians and operating fifty-eight clinics and twenty-three hospitals. Subscribers pay monthly dues which entitle them to complete medical care, and the steady growth in membership suggests that an HMO can maintain a reasonable doctor-patient relationship. Under the Kaiser program contracts are made with groups of physicians. The physicians receive a good salary plus a percentage of any profit accruing after all expenses for their particular group are paid. This form of remuneration encourages keeping costs to a minimum and has eliminated a good deal of unnecessary surgery and hospitalization.[6] It also provides an economic incentive to practice preventive rather than curative medicine. It is a commentary on current medical practice that, in all cases where HMOs or insurance programs include a measure of supervision over practitioners, the number of surgical operations and the amount of hospitalization ranges from 20 to 50 percent below that in private practice.

Although HMOs did not become significant until after World War II, today they provide medical care for about 8 million Americans. Their sponsors include nonprofit organizations, such as foundations and unions, and private groups of medical professionals and insurance companies. Congress has already indicated its support for HMOs, and insurance companies, recognizing that a comprehensive national program would eliminate billions of dollars of health insurance money, are beginning to move into the area. Organized medicine is scarcely enthusiastic, but, as pressure grows for Federal action, the medical profession will probably espouse HMOs as the lesser of the available evils.

The major problem with HMOs is the high start-up costs. Large amounts of capital are needed for clinical and hospital facilities and to pay operating expenses until the number of subscribers reaches a sustaining basis. If HMOs are to cover an appreciable segment of the population, large-scale governmental assistance may be necessary. Granting that private and foundation capital may supply part of the needed funds, HMOs can scarcely operate in low-income areas without substantial subsidies; hence government support will be essential. If HMOs continue to gain ground, they are likely to consolidate, and this action would facilitate a national organization.

Another pathway America may follow is to adopt some form of national health insurance based upon joint contributions from employers and employees and federal subsidies for the poor. While a health insurance program need not eliminate private medical practice, its cost would almost guarantee the development of Professional Standards Review Organizations (PSRO). This concept, presently under attack by many physicians, is likely to become a part of our medical system regardless of what changes occur. By defining quality standards in medicine, PSROs can provide an answer to the present rash of malpractice suits and insure better care for patients. They also offer the patient a measure of protection against unnecessary or exorbitant charges. A national health insurance program could be imposed upon the present system, leaving the individual free to select a private physician, an HMO, or some other form of medical care. Nonetheless, the possibility for abuse will require its administrators to see that full value is received for all payments—and this means precisely the sort of supervision which the medical profession is currently opposing so bitterly.

No one can predict what the future holds, but the present trend is clearly toward more government involvement in medical care. While many physicians still feel that medical care is a privilege, public opinion is beginning to consider it a right. Congress seldom provides leadership, but it does respond to public pressure. A national health law seems almost inevitable; whether or not it is a sound one will depend upon the willingness of the medical profession to face up to social and political realities and assist in writing a good measure.

NOTES

CHAPTER 1

1. John Duffy, "Medicine and Medical Practices Among Aboriginal American Indians," *History of American Medicine: A Symposium*, edited by Felix Marti-Ibañez (New York, 1959), 15–33.
2. *The Journal of Lewis and Clarke, to the Mouth of the Columbia River beyond the Rocky Mountains in the Years, 1804–5 and 6* (Dayton, Ohio, 1840), 40.
3. P. M. Ashburn, *The Ranks of Death* (New York, 1947), 18–27.
4. Count Frontenac to the King, Quebec, November 6, 1679, in E. B. O'Callaghan, ed., *Documents Relative to the Colonial History of New York*, IX (Albany, New York, 1855), 129; Mrs. Afra Coming to Sister, March 6, 1699, quoted in Edward McCurdy, *The History of South Carolina Under the Proprietary Government, 1670–1719* (New York, 1897), 308.
5. John Duffy, *Epidemics in Colonial America* (Baton Rouge, 1953), 69ff.
6. "Communications," *Mississippi Valley Historical Review* (now *Journal of American History*), XLI (1954–55), 762.

CHAPTER 2

1. John Duffy, "The Passage to the Colonies," *Mississippi Valley Historical Review*, XXXVIII (1951–52), 21–38.

2. Henry R. Viets, *A Brief History of Medicine in Massachusetts* (Boston, 1930), 13–14; Duffy, *Epidemics in Colonial America*, 13.

3. Wyndham B. Blanton, *Medicine in Virginia in the Seventeenth Century* (Richmond, 1930), 14.

4. Blanton, *Medicine in Virginia in the Seventeenth Century*, 62–68, 75.

5. John Winthrop, *The History of New England from 1630 to 1650*, 2 vols. (Boston, 1825–26), II, 310; Frances R. Packard, *History of Medicine in the United States*, 2 vols. (New York, 1931), I, 96.

6. Thomas Hassell to Secretary, St. Thomas, South Carolina, March 12, 1712, in Society for the Propagation of the Gospel in Foreign Parts Mss., Library of Congress Phototranscripts, London Letters, A7, pp. 498–501 (hereinafter cited as S.P.G. Mss. with appropriate designation of letters); William Byrd to Sir Hans Sloane, Virginia, May 31, 1737, transcript in Sloane Mss., no. 4055, Library of Congress.

7. William Douglass, *A Summary, historical and political, of the first planting, progressive improvements, and present state of the British Settlements in North America*, 2 vols. (London, 1760), I, 530–31.

8. *Pennsylvania Gazette*, April 10, 1760.

9. President Rip Van Dam to the Lords of Trade, New York, November 2, 1731, in O'Callaghan, *Documents Relative to Colonial History of New York*, V (1855), 929; New York *Gazette*, November 8–15, 1731.

10. Letter from Hugh Adams, Charleston, South Carolina, February 25, 1700, in *Diary of Samuel Sewall, 1700–1714*, Massachusetts Historical Society *Collections*, ser. 5, VI (1879), 11–12.

11. Ernest Caulfield, *The Throat Distemper of 1735–1740* (New Haven, Connecticut, 1939), 103.

12. William Douglass to Cadwallader Colden, Boston, Massachusetts, November 12, 1739, in *The Letters and Papers of Cadwallader Colden*, 9 vols. (New York, 1918–37), II, 196–200.

CHAPTER 3

1. James J. Walsh, *History of Medicine in New York, Three Centuries of Medical Progress*, 3 vols. (New York, 1919), I, 11, 18; Isaac N. Stokes, *The Iconography of Manhattan Island*, 6 vols. (New York, 1915–28), IV, 206.

2. Blanton, *Medicine in Virginia in the Seventeenth Century*, 8–24.

3. Viets, *A Brief History of Medicine in Massachusetts*, 8–17.

4. *Ibid.*, 36–37; Samuel A. Green, *History of Medicine in Massachusetts* (Boston, 1881), 30–31.

5. Joseph M. Toner, *Contributions to the Annals of Medical Progress and Medical Education* . . . (Washington, D.C., 1874), 19–21.
6. Samuel E. Morison, *Harvard College in the Seventeenth Century*, 2 vols. (Cambridge, Massachusetts, 1936), I, 281–84, 339fn.; Viets, *A Brief History of Medicine in Massachusetts*, 40–41.
7. Walsh, *History of Medicine in New York*, I, 18, 31.
8. *Ibid.*, 23, 25, 35–36; Adriaen van der Donck, *Remonstrance of New Netherland, and the Occurrences There, Addressed to the High and Mighty Lord States General of the United Netherlands, on the 28th July, 1649*, E. B. O'Callaghan, trans. (Albany, 1856), 7–8.
9. Walsh, *History of Medicine in New York*, I. 35–36.
10. John B. Blake, *Public Health in the Town of Boston*, 1630–1822 (Cambridge, 1959), 8–9; Stokes, *The Iconography of Manhattan Island*, IV, 280.

CHAPTER 4

1. David Ramsay, *The History of South Carolina . . . 1670 to the Year 1808* (Charleston, 1809), II, 116–20; William S. Middleton, "John Redman," *Annals of Medical History*, VIII (1924), 213–23.
2. Joseph Ioor Waring, M.D., *A History of Medicine in South Carolina, 1670–1825* (Charleston, South Carolina, 1964), 39; Cotton Mather, *The Angel of Bethesda*, introduction by Gordon W. Jones (Barre, Massachusetts, 1972), 250; *Papers of the Lloyd Family of the Manor of Queens Village, Lloyd's Neck, Long Island, New York, 1654–1826*, I, 309–10, in New-York Historical Society *Collections*, 1926, LIX (New York, 1927), I, 309–10.
3. Mr. Bradford to Secretary, New York, September 12, 1709, S.P.G. Mss., A5, fpp. 141–50; New York *Gazette*, January 7–14, 1733; Douglass, *A Summary . . . of the British Settlements in North America*, II, 351–52.
4. Waring, *History of Medicine in South Carolina, 1670–1825*. p. 83.
5. *Ibid.*, 36; David L. Cowen, *Medicine and Health in New Jersey: A History* (Princeton and New York, 1964), 11, 21.
6. Wyndham B. Blanton, *Medicine in Virginia in the Eighteenth Century* (Richmond, 1931), 19.
7. Whitfield J. Bell, Jr., "A Portrait of the Colonial Physician," *Bulletin of the History of Medicine*, XLIV (1970), 501–2. (Hereinafter cited as *Bull. of Hist. of Med.*)
8. New York *Gazette*, May 20, 1751.
9. Whitfield J. Bell, Jr., "Medical Practice in Colonial America," *Bull. of Hist. of Med.*, XXXI (1957), 445; William Smith, *The History of the Province of New York* (London, 1776), 272–73.
10. Arthur J. Viseltear, "Joanna Stephens and the Eighteenth Century Lithontriptics; A Misplaced Chapter in the History of Therapeutics," *Bull. of Hist. of Med.*, XLII (1968), 199–220; Blake, *Public Health in the Town of Boston*, 42.

11. Henry Lucas to Secretary, Newbury, New England, July 24, 1716, in S.P.G. Mss., A11–12, fp. 311.

12. Cotton Mather, *A Letter About Good Management Under the Distemper of the Measles, etc.* (Boston, 1739).

13. Worthington C. Ford, ed., *Diary of Cotton Mather*, 2 vols. (Boston, 1911–12), II, 634, 657–59, in Massachusetts Historical Society *Collections*, ser. 7, VIII; William Douglass to Cadwallader Colden, Boston, May 1, 1722, in Jared Sparks, ed., "Letters from Dr. William Douglas[s] to Dr. Cadwallader Colden of New York," *ibid.*, ser. 4, II (1854), 170; Edmund Massey, *A Sermon Against the Dangerous and Sinful Practice of Inoculation . . .* (London, 1722), 24; Colin Campbell to Secretary, Burlington, New Jersey, December 20, 1759, in S.P.G. Mss., B24, fpp. 151–53.

14. Blake, *Public Health in the Town of Boston*, 69–70.

15. Henry Newman, "The Way of Proceeding in the Small Pox Inoculation in New England," *Philosophical Transactions*, XXXII (1722–23), 33–34. See also Solomon Drown, "A Long Journal of a Short Voyage from Providence to N. York. With an Account of my having the Small-Pox by Inoculation in that City . . . from September 10th to October 12th, 1772," in New-York Historical Society mss.

16. Otho T. Beall, Jr., and Richard H. Shryock, *Cotton Mather, First Significant Figure in American Medicine* (Baltimore, 1954), 87–92, 149–54.

17. Cowen, *Medicine and Health in New Jersey*, 6; Bell, Jr., "A Portrait of the Colonial Physician," 505.

18. Lester S. King, *The Medical World of the Eighteenth Century* (Chicago, 1958), 34–38.

19. For an excellent discussion of the physician-naturalists, see Brooke Hindle, *The Pursuit of Science in Revolutionary America, 1735–1789* (Chapel Hill, North Carolina, 1956), 36–58.

20. John Duffy, *A History of Public Health in New York City, 1625–1866* (New York, 1968), 43–45.

21. Hindle, *Pursuit of Science in Revolutionary America*, 51; Waring, *History of Medicine in South Carolina, 1670–1825*, pp. 254–60.

22. Claude E. Heaton, "Medicine in New York During the English Colonial Period, 1664–1775," *Bull. of Hist. of Med.*, XVII (1945), 36–37.

23. For a good biography of Morgan see Whitfield J. Bell, Jr., *John Morgan, Continental Doctor* (Philadelphia, 1965).

24. Benjamin Franklin, *Some Account of the Pennsylvania Hospital*, introduction by I. Bernard Cohen (Baltimore, 1954), x–xiii.

25. William Pepper, *The Medical Side of Benjamin Franklin* (Philadelphia, 1910), 11, 28.

26. *Ibid.*, 20–21, 45, 72, 81.

27. Franklin, *Some Account of the Pennsylvania Hospital*, xix–xxi.

28. Blanton, *Medicine in Virginia in the Eighteenth Century*, 181; "William Byrd to Sir Hans Sloane, Virginia, April 20, 1706," *William and Mary College Quarterly*, ser. 2, I (1921), 186; Douglass, *A Summary . . . of the British Settlements in North America*, II, 352.

29. John Oldmixon, *The British Empire in America*, 2 vols. (London, 1741), I, 429; New York Historical Society *Collections*, LXI (New York, 1928), 198, 254–55.

30. James J. Walsh, *History of the Medical Society of the State of New York* (Brooklyn, 1907), 33.

31. Thomas Ruston to Job Ruston, Edinburgh, September 30, 1764, in Thomas Rustin Papers, Library of Congress mss.

32. Bell, Jr., "A Portrait of the Colonial Physician," 507–8.

33. *Ibid.*, 516–17.

34. Thomas C. Parramore, "The Saga of 'The Bear' and the 'Evil Genius,'" *Bull. of Hist. of Med.*, XLII (1968), 321–22.

35. Blanton, *Medicine in Virginia in the Seventeenth Century*, 149–50; John E. Ransom, "The Beginnings of Hospitals in the United States," *Bull. of Hist. of Med.*, XIII (1943), 521; E. B. O'Callaghan, ed., *Register of New Netherland: 1626 to 1674* (Albany, New York, 1865), 128.

36. Samuel Wilson, Jr., "An Architectural History of the Royal Hospital and the Ursuline Convent of New Orleans," *Louisiana Historical Quarterly*, XXIX (1946), 559–60; John Duffy, ed., *The Rudolph Matas History of Medicine in Louisiana*, I (Baton Rouge, 1958), 82–103.

37. Will of Jean Louis, November 16, 1735, Document 5948 (A 35/85), Cabildo Archives, New Orleans, Louisiana; Duffy, *The Rudolph Matas History of Medicine in Louisiana*, I, 103–11.

38. Robert J. Hunter, "Benjamin Franklin and the Rise of the Free Treatment of the Poor by the Medical Profession of Philadelphia," *Bull. of Hist. of Med.*, XXXI (1957), 137.

39. Heaton, "Three Hundred Years of Medicine in New York City," *Bull. of Hist. of Med.*, XXXII (1958), 520; Joseph I. Waring, "St. Philips Hospital in Charleston in Carolina," *Annals of Medical History*, n.s., IV (1932), 284.

40. *Minutes of the Common Council of New York, 1675–1776* (New York, 1905), VI, 211, 369–70.

41. Franklin, *Some Account of the Pennsylvania Hospital*, 25.

42. *Ibid.*, 27.

43. *Ibid.*, 29; Hunter, "Benjamin Franklin and the Rise of Free Treatment of the Poor by the Medical Profession of Philadelphia," 138–40.

44. Franklin, *Some Account of the Pennsylvania Hospital*, 36.

45. Fielding H. Garrison, *Contributions to the History of Medicine from the Bulletin of the New York Academy of Medicine, 1925–1935* (New York, 1966), 806–10; Hindle, *Pursuit of Science in Revolutionary America*, 118–19; James Hardie, *The Description of the City of New York* (New York, 1827), 256–57.

CHAPTER 5

1. John E. Lane, "Daniel Turner and the First Degree of Doctor Conferred in the English Colonies of North America by Yale College in 1723," *Annals of*

Medical History, II (1919), 367.

2. Bell, Jr., *John Morgan, Continental Doctor*, 118–24.

3. Whitfield J. Bell, Jr., *Early American Science* (Williamsburg, Virginia, 1955), 25; Packard, *History of Medicine in the United States*, I, 342–66; Genevieve Miller, "Medical Schools in the Colonies," *Ciba Symposia*, VIII (1947), 522–32.

4. Walsh, *History of Medicine in New York*, I, 46, 48–49, 52.

5. Peter Middleton, *A Medical Discourse* (New York, 1769), 51; Garrison, *Contributions to the History of Medicine*, 808; Walsh, *History of Medicine in New York*, I, 48.

6. Frederick Waite, "Medicinal Degrees Conferred in the American Colonies and in the United States in the 18th Century," *Annals of Medical History*, n.s., IX (1937), 317–18.

7. Richard H. Shryock, *Medical Licensing in America, 1650–1965* (Baltimore, 1967), 3–4.

8. Edward Ingle, "Regulating Physicians in Colonial Virginia," *Annals of Medical History*, IV (1922), 248–50; Blanton, *Medicine in Virginia in the Eighteenth Century*, 399–401.

9. Shryock, *Medical Licensing in America*, 16.

10. Walsh, *History of Medicine in New York*, I, 76, 78–79; *Report of a Committee of the Medical Society of New York, on the Subject of Medical Education* (Albany, New York, 1840), 3–4; Charles B. Coventary, "History of Medical Legislation in the State of New York," *New-York Journal of Medicine and the Collateral Sciences*, IV (1845), 152.

11. Gertrude L. Annan, "The Academy of Medicine of New York, 1825–1830, and Its Contemporary, the New York Academy of Medicine," *Bulletin of the Medical Library Association*, XXXVI (1948), 117–23; Walsh, *History of Medicine in New York*, I, 57, 73; Claude E. Heaton, "Three Hundred Years of Medicine in New York City," *Bull. of Hist. of Med.*, XXXII (1958), 520.

12. Waring, *History of Medicine in South Carolina, 1670–1825*, pp. 65–66.

13. Joseph I. Waring, "Lionel Chalmers, Medical Author," *Bull. of Hist. of Med.*, XXXII (1958), 353–54.

14. Hindle, *Pursuit of Science in Revolutionary America*, 111–12, 127–28.

15. Cowen, *Medicine and Health in New Jersey*, 10–12.

16. *Ibid.*, 11–12, 19.

17. Shryock, *Medical Licensing in America*, 18–19.

CHAPTER 6

1. Philip Cash, *Medical Men at the Siege of Boston, April, 1775–April, 1776* (Philadelphia, 1973), 27, 82.

2. Louis C. Duncan, *Medical Men in the American Revolution, 1775–1783* (Carlisle Barracks, Pennsylvania, 1931), 153, 212; James Thacher, *A Military Journal*

During the American Revolutionary War, 1775–1783 . . . (Boston, 1823), 426; James Tilton, *Economical Observations on Military Hospitals; and the Prevention of Diseases Incident to an Army* (Wilmington, Delaware, 1813), 34.

3. *American Archives*, ser. 4, VI, 1036–39, 1083; Hugh Thursfield, "Smallpox in the American War of Independence," *Annals of Medical History*, ser. 3, II (1940), 312–15.

4. Blanton, *Medicine in Virginia in the Eighteenth Century*, 257–59; Thacher, *A Military Journal*, 343; *American Archives*, ser. 5, II, 1363.

5. John C. Fitzpatrick, ed., *The Writings of George Washington* (Washington, 1931), III, 433; Cash, *Medical Men in the Siege of Boston*, 34–36.

6. Waring, *A History of Medicine in South Carolina, 1670–1825*, pp. 98–99.

7. Joseph M. Toner, *Medical Men of the Revolution, with a Brief History of the Medical Department of the Continental Army* . . . (Philadelphia, 1876), 14 fn. 2.

8. Duncan, *Medical Men in the Revolution*, 60–64; Bell, Jr., *John Morgan, Continental Doctor*, 208.

9. Cash, *Medical Men at the Siege of Boston*, 118–25.

10. John Morgan, *A Vindication of His Public Character in the Situation of Director-General* (Boston, 1777), 54–59; Genevieve Miller, "Dr. John Morgan's Report to General Washington, March 3, 1776," *Bull. of Hist. of Med.*, XIX (1946), 450–54; *American Archives*, ser. 4, V, 115–16.

11. Morgan, *A Vindication*, 103; Thacher, *Military Journal*, 63, 306.

12. *American Archives*, ser. 4, V, 1024–25; Duncan, *Medical Men in the American Revolution*, 117–22.

13. David F. Hawke, *Benjamin Rush, Revolutionary Gadfly* (Indianapolis & New York, 1971), 186–87; Duncan, *Medical Men in the American Revolution*, 192–98; Bell, Jr., *John Morgan, Continental Doctor*, 222–23.

14. Hawke, *Benjamin Rush, Revolutionary Gadfly*, 206–23.

15. Duncan, *Medical Men in the American Revolution*, 333–46.

CHAPTER 7

1. Waring, *History of Medicine in South Carolina, 1670–1825*, p. 107.

2. Hawke, *Benjamin Rush, Revolutionary Gadfly*, 192–93.

3. Benjamin Rush, "An Account of the Influence of the Military and Political Events of the American Revolution Upon the Human Body," *Medical Inquiries and Observations*, I (Philadelphia, 1818), 128–32. Reprinted in *Bulletin of the New York Academy of Medicine*, XLVI (1970), 558–61.

4. No American physician has received as much attention by historians as Dr. Benjamin Rush. Genevieve Miller's *Bibliography of the History of Medicine of the United States and Canada, 1939–1960* (Baltimore, 1964) lists fifty-eight books and articles on Rush published in the twenty-one-year period. Among the most perceptive works are those by Lyman H. Butterfield, George W. Corner, and Richard H. Shryock.

5. J. H. Powell, *Bring Out Your Dead* (Philadelphia, 1949), 77–78.
6. Genevieve Miller, "Benjamin Rush's Criticism of Hippocrates," *Communication au XVIIe Congrès International d'Histoire de la Mĕdecine, Extrait du Tome i du Congrès* (Athènes, 1960), I, 128–31.
7. Powell, *Bring Out Your Dead*, 73–75, 82–84.

CHAPTER 8

1. Duffy, *The Rudolph Matas History of Medicine in Louisiana*, I, 269–80.
2. M. L. Haynie, "Observations on the Fever of Tropical Climates, and the Use of Mercury as a Remedy," *Medical Repository*, n.s., I (1813), 218–20.
3. Russell M. Jones, "American Doctors and the Parisian Medical World, 1830–1840," *Bull. of Hist. of Med.*, XLVII (1973), 40–65; Irving A. Beck, "An Early American Journal Keyed to Medical Students: A Pioneer Contribution of Elisha Bartlett," *Bull. of Hist. of Med.*, XL (1966), 124–34.
4. Joseph F. Kett, *The Formation of the American Medical Profession, The Role of Institutions, 1780–1860* (New Haven, Connecticut, 1968), 157–58.
5. For a good account of Washington's death, see Blanton, *Medicine in Virginia in the Eighteenth Century*, 305–12.
6. *Ibid.*, 305–7.
7. Jabez W. Heustis, *Physical Observations, and Medical Tracts and Researches, on the Topography and Diseases of Louisiana* (New York, 1817), 117–18.
8. Edward H. Barton, *The Application of Physiological Medicine to the Diseases of Louisiana* (Philadelphia, 1832), 38.
9. "Health in the Country," *New Orleans Medical and Surgical Journal* (hereinafter cited as *N.O.M. & S.J.*), I (1844), 247–48.
10. *N.O.M. & S.J.*, X (1853–54), 279.
11. *The Cholera Bulletin*, July 23, 1832, pp. 57–60.
12. Donald D. Vogt, "Trends in 19th Century American Cholera Therapy," *Pharmacy in History*, XVI (1974), 43–44.
13. Norman Dain, *Disordered Minds, The First Century of Eastern State Hospital in Williamsburg, Virginia, 1766–1866* (Williamsburg, Va., 1971).
14. For a good treatment of this subject, see Norman Dain, *Concepts of Insanity in the United States, 1789–1865* (New Brunswick, N.J., 1964) and Gerald N. Grob, *The State and the Mentally Ill, A History of the Worcester State Hospital in Massachusetts, 1830–1920* (Chapel Hill, North Carolina, 1966).

CHAPTER 9

1. Samuel Thomson, *New Guide to Health; or Botanic Family Physician . . . to which is prefixed, A Narrative of the Life and Medical Discoveries of the Author* (2nd ed., Boston, 1825).

2. The best source for Thomsonianism is Thomson's *New Guide to Health*, but excellent brief accounts of the movement can be found in William G. Rothstein, *American Physicians in the Nineteenth Century, From Sects to Science* (Baltimore & London, 1972); Kett, *Formation of the American Medical Profession*; and James Harvey Young, *The Toadstool Millionaires, A Social History of Patent Medicine in America before Federal Regulation* (Princeton, New Jersey, 1961).
3. Kett, *Formation of the American Medical Profession*, 105–7, 138–39.
4. *Code of Ethics of the American Medical Association, adopted May, 1847* (Philadelphia, 1848), 18–19. The best discussion of this and the following material can be found in Martin Kaufman, *The Rise and Fall of Medical Heresy* (Baltimore and London, 1971) chapters 4–6.
5. Richard H. Shryock, "Public Relations of the Medical Profession in Great Britain and the United States: 1600–1870 . . .," *Annals of Medical History*, n.s., II (1930), 317. The best discussion of Neo-Thomsonianism can be found in Alex Berman, "Neo-Thomsonianism in the United States," *Journal of the History of Medicine and Allied Sciences* (hereinafter cited as *Jnl. of Hist. of Med. & All. Sci.*), XI (1956), 133–55. See also Rothstein, *American Physicians in the Nineteenth Century*, 146.
6. Richard H. Shryock, *Medicine in America, Historical Essays* (Baltimore, 1966), 116–18.
7. Kitty Hamilton to Father, Biloxi, Mississippi, June 8, 13, 20, 1851, Hamilton (William S.) Papers, 1841–53, Louisiana State University Archives; Penelope Hamilton to Father, Biloxi, Mississippi, July 11, 19, 21, 1851, *ibid.*; Shryock, *Medicine in America*, 121–22.
8. *Ibid.*, 124.
9. *Daily Pittsburgh Gazette*, November 9, 1837; *Pittsburgh Saturday Evening Visitor*, June 22, 1839, V, 49.
10. Young, *The Toadstool Millionaires*, 17–18.
11. Henry Burnell Shafer, *The American Medical Profession, 1783 to 1850* (New York and London, 1936), 200–1; Jacques M. Quen, "Elisha Perkins, Physician Nostrum-Vendor, or Charlatan?" *Bull. of Hist. of Med.*, XXXVII (1963), 164.
12. Richard H. Shryock, "Public Relations of the Medical Profession in Great Britain and the U.S., 1600–1870," *Annals of Medical History*, n.s., II (1930), 316.
13. Young, *The Toadstool Millionaires*, covers the period up to 1906; *The Medical Messiahs* (Princeton, 1967) deals with the twentieth century.
14. Thomas Thacher, *A Brief Rule to Guide the Common People of New England how to order themselves and theirs in the Small Pocks, or Measles* (Boston, 1677); John Wesley, *Primitive Physick: or an easy and natural method of curing most diseases* (Philadelphia, 1764, 12th ed. printed by Andrew Stewart).
15. James Ewell, *The Medical Companion, or Family Physician* (Washington, 1827), xv–xix.
16. G. C. Gunn, *Gunn's Domestic Medicine, or Poor Man's Friend* (New York, 1853), 862–66.
17. J. Cam Massie, *Treatise on the Eclectic Southern Practice of Medicine* (Philadelphia, 1854), 5–8.

CHAPTER 10

1. Moses Hibbard, "Case of a Uterine Tumor—Removed by Operation," *Boston Medical and Surgical Journal*, VIII (1833), 69.
2. Valentine Mott, ed., A.-A.-L.-M. Velpeau, *New Elements of Operative Surgery*. Translated by P. S. Townsend under the supervision of, and with notes and observations by, V. Mott (New York, 1847), I, 20.
3. L. R. C. Agnew and G. F. Shelden, "Philip Syng Physick (1768–1837): 'The Father of American Surgery'," *Journal of Medical Education*, XXXV (1960), 545–46.
4. Duffy, *The Rudolph Matas History of Medicine in Louisiana*, II, 44.
5. *Ibid.*, 55; "The New Orleans Charity Hospital," *Harper's Weekly*, III (1859), 569–70.
6. Fielding H. Garrison, *An Introduction to the History of Medicine* (Philadelphia and London, 4th ed., 1929), 349; Emmet Field Horine, *Daniel Drake (1785–1852), Pioneer Physician of the Midwest* (Philadelphia, 1961), 71; Blanton, *Medicine in Virginia in the Eighteenth Century*, 17–18.
7. Samuel D. Gross, *Memorial Oration in Honor of Ephraim McDowell, "The Father of Ovariotomy"* (Louisville, Kentucky, 1879), 14ff.; *id.*, *Lives of Eminent American Physicians and Surgeons of the Nineteenth Century* (Philadelphia, 1861), 207–30.
8. T. V. Woodring, *Pioneer Medicine and Early Physicians in Nashville* (n.d., n.p.), 11–14.
9. J. Marion Sims, *Story of My Life* (New York, 1968), 115–16.
10. *Ibid.*, 138, 226–436.
11. Wyndham B. Blanton in his *Medicine in Virginia in the Eighteenth Century*, 17–18, credits Dr. Jesse Bennet of Rockingham County, Virginia, with performing the first operation of this kind in America, reputedly operating on his wife in an emergency situation during 1794. In a paper entitled "The Legend of Jesse Bennet's 1794 Caesarean Section," which was delivered at the American Association of the History of Medicine's 1975 meeting in Philadelphia, Dr. Arthur G. King of Cincinnati completely demolished the Bennet story. Dr. King also has reservations about Prévost, but I think the evidence is fairly conclusive. (St. Francisville Asylum, February 7, 1825.)
12. Rudolph Matas, "François Marie Prévost and the Early History of the Cesarean Section in Louisiana," *N.O.M. & S.J.*, LXXXIX (1937), 604–25; Robert P. Harris, "A Record of Cesarean Operations that have been Performed in the State of Louisiana during the Present Century," *ibid.*, n.s., VI (1878–79), 933–42; Robert P. Harris, "Twenty Cesarean Operations, with 15 Women Saved, in Louisiana," *ibid.*, n.s., VII (1879–80), 456, 938–41; Duffy, *The Rudolph Matas History of Medicine in Louisiana*, II, 72–74.
13. Arthur G. King, "America's First Cesarean Section," *Obstetrics and Gynecology*, XXXVII (1971), 797–802; Garrison, *Introduction to the History of Medicine*, 508.

14. Sir William Osler has an excellent account of the accident which opened the way for Beaumont's experiments in the introduction to a facsimile edition of Beaumont's book, *Experiments and Observations on the Gastric Juice and the Physiology of Digestion . . . Facsimile . . . with a Biographical Essay . . . by Sir William Osler* (New York, 1959); Victor Robinson, *The Story of Medicine* (New York, 1943), 466–68.
15. Jerome J. Bylebyl, "William Beaumont, Robley Dunglison and the Philadelphia Physiologists," *Jnl. of Hist. of Med. & All. Sci.*, XXV (1970), 3–21.
16. *Dictionary of American Biography*, 22 vols. (New York, 1946), II, 104–9.
17. Thomas E. Keys, *History of Surgical Anesthesia* (New York, 1963), 10–18.
18. Richard H. Shryock, *Development of Modern Medicine* (New York and London, 1969), 178–79; James E. Dexter, *A History of Dental and Oral Science in America* (Philadelphia, 1876), 12–13, 143–48, 180–81.
19. Keys, *History of Surgical Anesthesia*, 21–22.
20. Long's chief advocate is Frank K. Boland, *The First Anesthetic: The Story of Crawford Long* (Athens, Georgia, 1950).
21. Charles D. Meigs, *Obstetrics: The Science and the Art* (Philadelphia, 1849), 316–19.
22. John Duffy, "Anglo-American Reaction to Obstetrical Anesthesia," *Bull. of Hist. of Med.*, XXXVIII (1964), 32–37.
23. *Dictionary of American Biography*, XIX, 640–41.
24. Boland, *The First Anesthetic: The Story of Crawford Long*, 120.

CHAPTER 11

1. Edward D. Churchill, ed., *To Work in the Vineyard of Surgery, Reminiscences of J. Collins Warren (1842–1927)* (Cambridge, Massachusetts, 1958), 1–18.
2. Christine Chapman Robbins, *David Hosack, Citizen of New York* (Philadelphia, 1964), 109, 134–36.
3. Horine, *Daniel Drake, Pioneer Physician*, 96–100, 157–63, 380–81; Samuel D. Gross, *A Discourse on the Life, Character, and Services of Daniel Drake, M.D. . . . January 27, 1853* (Louisville, Kentucky, 1853), contains an excellent account of his life and work. It is especially useful if used in connection with Gross's *Lives of Eminent Physicians and Surgeons*, 614–62.
4. Howard A. Kelly and Walter L. Burrage, *American Medical Biographies* (Baltimore, 1920), 470–73.
5. John B. Blake, *Benjamin Waterhouse and the Introduction of Vaccination, A Reappraisal* (Philadelphia, 1957).
6. John L. Riddell, "On the Binocular Microscope," *N.O.M. & S.J.*, X (1853–54), 321–27; *New Orleans Medical News and Hospital Gazette*, I (1855–56), 118. See Duffy, *The Rudolph Matas History of Medicine in Louisiana*, II, 84–86, for further details.

CHAPTER 12

1. Hawke, *Benjamin Rush: Revolutionary Gadfly*, 84.
2. Robbins, *David Hosack, Citizen of New York* (Philadelphia, 1964), 102–4.
3. J. W. Francis, *An Historical Sketch of the Origin, Progress, and Present State of the College of Physicians and Surgeons, of the University of the State of New-York* (New York, 1813), 8–16; Heaton, "Three Hundred Years of Medicine in New York City," *Bull. of Hist. of Med.*, XXXII (1958), 517–30; Fred B. Rogers, "Nicholas Romayne, 1756–1817: Stormy Petrel of American Medical Profession," *Journal of Medical Education*, XXXV (March, 1960), 258–60.
4. Carleton B. Chapman, *Dartmouth Medical School: The First 175 Years* (Hanover, New Hampshire, 1973), 11–21.
5. Emmet Field Horine, "Early Medicine in Kentucky," *Jnl. of Hist. of Med. & All. Sci.*, III (1948), 265–68.
6. *The Medical Register of the City of New York, for the Year Commencing June 1, 1865* (New York, 1866), 195–97; Walsh, *History of Medicine in New York*, I, 53–54.
7. Chapman, *Dartmouth Medical School*, 19.
8. Wyndham B. Blanton, *Medicine in Virginia in the Nineteenth Century* (Richmond, Virginia, 1933), 71.
9. Horace Montgomery, "A Body Snatcher Sponsors Pennsylvania's Anatomy Act," *Jnl. of Hist. of Med. & All. Sci.*, XXI (1966), 374–93.
10. Harry C. Hull, "Professors of Surgery, an Introduction," *Bulletin*, University of Maryland at Baltimore, LVI (nos. 3 and 4, 1971).
11. Shryock, *Medical Licensing in America*, 28; W. F. Norwood, *Medical Education in the United States Before the Civil War* (Philadelphia, 1944), 430; N. S. Davis, *Medical Education and Medical Institutions in the United States of America, 1776–1876* (Washington, 1877), 41.
12. Duffy, *The Rudolph Matas History of Medicine in Louisiana*, II, 239ff.
13. John Duffy, ed., *Parson Clapp of the Strangers' Church of New Orleans* (Baton Rouge, 1957), 39–40.
14. Duffy, *The Rudolph Matas History of Medicine in Louisiana*, II, 243ff.
15. Stanford E. Chaillé, *Historical Sketch of Medical Department of University of Louisiana* (New Orleans, 1861), 5–6.
16. For a good discussion of this see Kett, *The Formation of the American Medical Profession*, 47ff.
17. Whitfield J. Bell, Jr., "The Medical Institution of Yale College, 1810–1885," *Yale Journal of Biology and Medicine*, XXXIII (1960), 172.
18. *Ibid.*; I am indebted to Dr. Martin Kaufman of the Massachusetts State College at Westfield for some of this material, having used his manuscript, *American Medical Education: The Formative Years, 1765–1910* (in preparation).
19. Proceedings of the National Medical Convention, held in New York, 1846, and Philadelphia, 1847, pp. 73–74.
20. Kaufman, *American Medical Education*, chap. 6, pp. 14–15.
21. Shryock, *Medical Licensing in America*, 35.

22. John Duffy, *A History of Public Health in New York City, 1625–1866* (New York, 1968), 65–66.
23. Walsh, *History of Medicine in New York*, I, 81–82.
24. Duffy, *The Rudolph Matas History of Medicine in Louisiana*, I, 326–40.
25. Rothstein, *American Physicians in the Nineteenth Century*, 79–80.
26. Duffy, *The Rudolph Matas History of Medicine in Louisiana*, II, 114–15; Cowen, *Medicine and Health in New Jersey*, 69–70; Shryock, *Medical Licensing in America*, 30–31.
27. Horine, *Daniel Drake, Pioneer Physician of the Midwest*, 76; Woodring, *Pioneer Medicine and Early Physicians in Nashville*, 16.
28. Shafer, *American Medical Profession*, 157–61.
29. *Ibid.*, 166–67.

CHAPTER 13

1. Rothstein, *American Physicians in the Nineteenth Century*, 34; Barnes Riznik, "The Professional Lives of Early 19th Century New England Doctors," *Jnl. of Hist. of Med. & All. Sci.*, XIX (1964), 1–16.
2. Genevieve Miller, "One Hundred Years Ago," *Bull. of Hist. of Med.*, XXI (1947), 488.
3. Philip M. Hamer, *The Centennial History of the Tennessee State Medical Association, 1830–1930* (Nashville, 1930), 22–23.
4. Genevieve Miller, "Medical Education One Hundred Years Ago—An Introductory Lecture," *Ohio Medical Journal*, LIV (1958), 1578–82; LV (1959), 40–41, 44.
5. Churchill, *To Work in the Vineyard of Surgery*, 27, fn. 16.
6. *Proceedings of the Physico-Medical Society of New Orleans in Relation to the Trial and Expulsion of Charles A. Luzenberg, with comments on the same: Published by Order of the Society* (New Orleans, 1838), 24–25.
7. See Duffy, *The Rudolph Matas History of Medicine in Louisiana*, II, 88–92.
8. New Orleans *Daily Delta*, August 28, September 10, 1859; New Orleans *Bee*, August 31, September 10, 1859.
9. Duffy, *The Rudolph Matas History of Medicine in Louisiana*, II, 95.
10. For a discussion of this, see Thomas N. Bonner, "The Social and Political Attitudes of Midwestern Physicians, 1840–1940: Chicago as a Case History," *Jnl. of Hist. of Med. & All. Sci.*, XIII (1953), 133–64; Thomas N. Bonner, *Medicine in Chicago, 1850–1950* (Madison, Wisconsin, 1957), 10–11.
11. P. S. Townsend, *An Account of the Yellow Fever, as It Prevailed in the City of New York, in the Summer and Autumn of 1822* (New York, 1823), 235; Duffy, *The Rudolph Matas History of Medicine in Louisiana*, II, 172–73, 183.
12. *New-York Medical and Physical Journal*, VII (1828), 174–75; Genevieve Miller, "Dr. John Delamater, 'True Physician'," *Journal of Medical Education*, XXXIV (1959), 24–31.

13. New Orleans *Courier*, August 8, 1839; *Planters' Banner* (Franklin Parish, Louisiana), July 15, 1847; Shryock, *Medicine in America*, 150–51.

CHAPTER 14

1. John Pintard, *Letters from John Pintard to his Daughter Eliza Noel Pintard Davidson, 1816–1833* (New York, 1940–41), 72; *Questions of the Board of Health in Relation to Malignant Cholera* (New York, 1832); Charles Rosenberg, *The Cholera Years* (Chicago, 1962), 43.
2. Barbara Guttmann Rosenkrantz, *Public Health and the State, Changing Views in Massachusetts, 1842–1936* (Cambridge, 1972), 1.
3. For a discussion of this, see Duffy, *History of Public Health in New York City, 1625–1866*, Chapter 4.
4. *Ibid.*, 82.
5. *Ibid.*, 48–50, 75–76, 195, 204–5.
6. Blake, *Public Health in the Town of Boston, 1630–1822*, p. 210.
7. For an excellent account of this epidemic, see Powell, *Bring Out Your Dead*.
8. For more information on this and the following material on New York City, see Duffy, *History of Public Health in New York City, 1625–1866*, chapter 6.
9. For the best account of Boston health conditions, see Blake, *Public Health in the Town of Boston, 1630–1822*.
10. Rosenkrantz, *Public Health and the State*, chapter 1.
11. *Ibid.*, 30.
12. Harold M. Cavins, "The National Quarantine and Sanitary Conventions of 1857 to 1860 and the Beginnings of the American Public Health Association," *Bull. of Hist. of Med.*, XIII (1943), 405–8.
13. Cavins, "The National Quarantine and Sanitary Conventions of 1857 to 1860 . . .," 409–14; Duffy, *History of Public Health in New York City, 1625–1866*, pp. 416, 530, 545.
14. Shryock, "The Early Public Health Movement," *Medicine in America*, 135–36.

CHAPTER 15

1. The two standard works on Civil War medicine are H. H. Cunningham, *Doctors in Gray: The Confederate Medical Service* (Baton Rouge, Louisiana, 1958), and George Worthington Adams, *Doctors in Blue: The Medical History of the Union Army in the Civil War* (New York, 1952). (The latter work is the more readable.)
2. The best account of the United States Sanitary Commission is the classic one by Charles J. Stillé, *History of the United States Sanitary Commission, Being the General Report of Its Work during the War of the Rebellion* (Philadelphia, 1866).

3. *Daily Pittsburgh Gazette*, June 28, 1862, July 6, 1863; New York *Times*, January 24, 1864.
4. Adams, *Doctors in Blue*, has a good account of Hammond's work. For Jonathan Letterman, see Gordon W. Jones, "The Medical History of the Fredericksburg Campaign: Course and Significance," *Jnl. of Hist. of Med. & All. Sci.*, XVIII (1963), 241–56.
5. Joseph Jones, "The Medical History of Confederate Army and Navy," *Southern Historical Society Papers*, XX (1892), 118.
6. Joseph Janvier Woodward, *Outlines of the Chief Camp Diseases of the United States Armies*, introduction by Saul Jarcho (New York and London, 1964), 267.
7. *Ibid.*, 58–59, 74–75.
8. Alvin Raymond Sunseri, "The Organization and Administration of the Medical Department of the Confederate Army of Tennessee," reprint from *Journal of the Tennessee State Medical Association*, vols. 52–53 (January–July, 1960), 167.
9. A vivid description of operating conditions in the field hospitals can be found in Adams, *Doctors in Blue*, 112–29.
10. Mary Louise Marshall, "Medicine in the Confederacy," *Bulletin of the Medical Library Association*, XXX (1942), 285; Blanton, *Medicine in Virginia in the Nineteenth Century*, 303.
11. Geroge Winston Smith, *Medicines for the Union Army, The United States Army Laboratories during the Civil War* (Madison, Wisconsin, 1962), 1.
12. For an excellent account of the Confederate side see Norman H. Franke, *Pharmaceutical Conditions and Drug Supply in the Confederacy* (Madison, Wisconsin, 1955).

CHAPTER 16

1. Shryock, *Medicine in America*, 77–78.
2. Samuel D. Gross, *History of American Medical Literature from 1776 to the Present Time* (Philadelphia, 1876), 55–56; Fielding H. Garrison, *John Shaw Billings: A Memoir* (New York and London, 1915), 15–16, 213–27.
3. Paul F. Clark, "Theobald Smith, Student of Disease," *Jnl. of Hist. of Med. & All. Sci.*, XIV (1959), 490–514.
4. Phyllis A. Richmond, "American Attitude toward the Germ Theory of Disease," *Jnl. of Hist. of Med. & All. Sci.*, IX (1954), 453–54; George T. Harrell, "Osler's Practice," *Bull. of Hist. of Med.*, XLVII (1973), 550; Duffy, *The Rudolph Matas History of Medicine in Louisiana*, II, 341.
5. For an excellent discussion of medical practice, see Charles Rosenberg, "The Practice of Medicine in New York a Century Ago," *Bull. of Hist. of Med.*, XLI (1967), 223–53.
6. Austin Flint, "Conservative Medicine," quoted in Gert H. Brieger, ed., *Medical America in the Nineteenth Century, Readings from the Literature* (Baltimore

and London, 1972), 135–36; Duffy, *The Rudolph Matas History of Medicine in Louisiana*, II, 350.

7. John S., Jr., and Robin M. Haller, *The Physician and Sexuality in Victorian America* (Urbana, Chicago, and London, 1974), 275–77; David F. Musto, *The American Disease, Origins of Narcotic Control* (New Haven and London, 1973), 1–3, 252 fn. 5.

8. Rothstein, *American Physicians in the Nineteenth Century*, 194–95.

9. Moritz Schuppert, "Blood-Letting and Kindred Questions," *N.O.M. & S.J.*, n.s., IX (1881–82), 247–56.

10. *N.O.M. & S.J.*, n.s., XII (1884–85), 36–37; XIV (1886–87), 230–31.

11. Rothstein, *American Physicians in the Nineteenth Century*, 182.

12. The Pittsburgh *Daily Post* from December 7, 1867, to February 13, 1868, reported four doctors elected to office in this two-month period; *Daily Post*, February 19, 1868.

13. A wealth of literature has appeared on this topic in the past two or three years. One of the most recent articles is H. Tristram Engelhardt, Jr., "The Disease of Masturbation: Values and Concept of Disease," *Bull. of Hist. of Med.*, XLVIII (1974), 234–48.

14. For examples of this, see John Duffy, "One Hundred Years of the *New Orleans Medical and Surgical Journal*," *Louisiana Historical Quarterly*, XL (1957), 12.

15. Eugene F. Cordell, *The Medical Annals of Maryland, 1799–1899* (Baltimore, 1900), 173.

16. The best study of the Rockefeller Institute is by George Corner, *A History of the Rockefeller Institute, 1901–1953* (New York, 1964). For general research activities, see Richard H. Shryock, *American Medical Research, Past and Present* (New York, 1947).

17. For the history of the United States Public Health Service, see Ralph C. Williams, *The United States Public Health Service, 1798–1950* (Washington, 1951) and Bess Furman, *A Profile of the United States Public Health Service, 1798–1948* (Washington, n.d.).

18. For a short history of yellow fever, see John Duffy, "Yellow Fever in the Continental United States during the Nineteenth Century," *Symposia in Clinical Tropical Medicine*, Kevin M. Cahill, ed., vol. I (New York, 1970). For the work of the Reed Commission, see John M. Gibson, *Soldier in White, the Life of General George Miller Sternberg* (Durham, North Carolina, 1958).

19. Garrison, *An Introduction to the History of Medicine*, 705; Furman, *A Profile of the United States Public Health Service*, 258–60; Raymond B. Fosdick, *The Story of the Rockefeller Foundation* (New York, 1952), 10, 24, 30ff.

20. A fascinating account of Goldberger and pellagra can be found in Elizabeth W. Etheridge, *The Butterfly Caste, A Social History of Pellagra in the South* (Westport, Connecticut, 1972). See also Milton Terris, ed., *Goldberger on Pellagra* (Baton Rouge, Louisiana, 1964).

21. A E. Casey and E. H. Hidden, "George Colmer and the Epidemiology of Poliomyelitis," *Southern Medical Journal*, XXXVII (1944), 471–77; Duffy, *A History of Public Health in New York City, 1866–1966*, pp. 273–74.

22. See John R. Paul, *A History of Poliomyelitis* (New Haven, Connecticut, 1971).
23. Saul Benison, *Tom Rivers, Recollections on a Life in Medicine and Science* (Cambridge and London, 1967), 414–15; Robert Shaplen, *Toward the Well-Being of Mankind: Fifty Years of the Rockefeller Foundation* (Garden City, New York, 1932), 39–40.

CHAPTER 17

1. Robert F. Weir, "On the Antiseptic Treatment of Wounds, and Its Results," *New York Medical Journal*, XXVI (1877), 561.
2. Duffy, *The Rudolph Matas History of Medicine in Louisiana*, II, 364–67.
3. The best account of the introduction of rubber gloves into surgery can be found in William S. Halsted, "The Employment of Silk in Preference to Catgut . . .," *Journal of the American Medical Association* (hereinafter cited as J.A.M.A.), LX (1913), 1119–26.
4. Rudolph Matas, "Post-Operative Thrombosis and Pulmonary Embolism before and after Lister, a Retrospect and Prospect," *University of Toronto Medical Bulletin*, X (1932), 10–12.
5. Keys, *The History of Surgical Anesthesia*, 65–67; Duffy, *The Rudolph Matas History of Medicine in Louisiana*, II, 374–75.
6. Walter C. Burkett, ed., *Surgical Papers by William Stewart Halsted*, 2 vols. (Baltimore, 1924), I, 167–78.
7. Duffy, *The Rudolph Matas History of Medicine in Louisiana*, II, 372–74.
8. I am indebted to one of my students, Miss Debra A. Lowe, for gathering this and other information from the *Annual Announcements of the Board of Visitors of the Baltimore College of Dental Surgery*, 1840 to 1858.
9. For a history of dentistry in Maryland see Ben Robinson, "The Foundations of Professional Dentistry," *Proceedings*, Dental Centenary Celebration, Baltimore, Maryland, March 18, 19, and 20, 1940 (Baltimore, 1940), 1000–29.
10. Chapin A. Harris, *The Dental Art, A Practical Treatise on Dental Surgery* (Baltimore, 1839).
11. William Simon, *History of the Baltimore College of Dental Surgery* (n.p., 1904), 1–15; Robinson, "The Foundations of Professional Dentistry," 1015–24; Cordell, *The Medical Annals of Maryland, 1799–1899*, p. 105.
12. Garrison, *An Introduction to the History of Medicine*, 615; Duffy, *The Rudolph Matas History of Medicine in Louisiana*, II, 383–84.
13. Ronald L. Kathren, "Early X-ray Protection in the United States," *Health Physics*, VIII (1962), 503–11; *id.*, "William H. Rollins (1852–1929): X-ray Protection Pioneer," *Jnl. of Hist. of Med. & All. Sci.*, XIX (1964), 287–94.
14. For a good brief account of late nineteenth-century American surgery, see A. Scott Earle, "The Germ Theory in America," *Surgery*, LXV (1969), 508–22.
15. Brieger, *Medical America in the Nineteenth Century*, 201, 209.
16. For brief sketches of these surgeons see Garrison, *An Introduction to the History of Medicine*.

17. Richard H. Meade, *An Introduction to the History of General Surgery* (Philadelphia, London and Toronto, 1968), 291–94; Charles A. Beard, ed., *A Century of Progress* (New York and London, 1933), 342–43.
18. *Ibid.*, 100, 111–13.
19. E. Warren, *A Doctor's Experience on Three Continents* (Baltimore, 1885), reprint in *Bulletin of the New York Academy of Medicine, XLIX* (1973), 1019–20.
20. Duffy, *The Rudolph Matas History of Medicine in Louisiana*, I, 380–81.
21. Frederick G. Kilgour, "Modern Medicine in Historical Perspective," *Bulletin of the Medical Library Association*, L (1962), 48–49.

CHAPTER 18

1. William Pepper, *Higher Medical Education, the True Interest of the Public and of the Profession* (Philadelphia, 1894), 15–16.
2. Whitfield J. Bell, Jr., "J. M. Toner (1825–1896) as a Medical Historian," *Bull. of Hist. of Med.*, XLVII (1973), 10; Peter D. Olch, "William S. Halsted's New York Period, 1874–1886," *ibid.*, XL (1966), 497–98; Martin Kaufman, "Edward H. Dixon and Medical Education in New York," *New York State History Quarterly* (1970), 405.
3. Charles McIntyre, "The Percentage of College-Bred Men in the Medical Profession," *Medical Record*, XXII (December 16, 1882), 681–84; see also Kaufman, *American Medical Education*, chap. 7, p. 1.
4. American Medical Association, *Council on Medical Education, Medical Schools in the United States, 1906* (Chicago, 1906), 46; Thomas F. Harrington, *The Harvard Medical School, A History, Narrative and Documentary, 1782–1905* (New York and Chicago, 1905), III, 1056–57.
5. Kaufman, *American Medical Education*, chap. 9, pp. 11, 21; chap. 11, pp. 2–4; Rothstein, *American Physicians in the Nineteenth Century*, 285–86.
6. The standard history is Alan M. Chesney, *The Johns Hopkins Hospital and the Johns Hopkins School of Medicine, A Chronicle*, 3 vols. (Baltimore, 1963), continued by Thomas B. Turner, *Heritage of Excellence, The Johns Hopkins Medical Institutions, 1914–1947* (Baltimore and London, 1974). An excellent analysis of Welch and his role at Hopkins can be found in Donald Fleming, *William H. Welch and the Rise of Modern Medicine* (Boston, 1954).
7. See A.M.A., Council on Medical Education, *Report of the First Annual Conference, 1905* (Chicago, 1905), and *Report of the Second Annual Conference* (Chicago, 1906).
8. Abraham Flexner, *Medical Education in the United States and Canada, A Report to the Carnegie Foundation for the Advancement of Teaching* (New York, 1910).
9. Flexner, *Medical Education*, 233, 238.
10. Shryock, *American Medical Research, Past and Present*, 119–21.
11. Abraham Flexner, "Medical Education, 1909–1924," *J.A.M.A.*, LXXXII (1924), 834–35.

12. For an elaboration of these points, see Gerald E. Markowitz and David K. Rosner, "Doctors in Crisis: A Study of the Use of Medical Education Reform to Establish Modern Professional Elitism in Medicine," *American Quarterly*, XXV (1973), 83–107.

13. A brief account of medical education in the twentieth century can be found in John Field, "Medical Education in the United States: Late Nineteenth and Twentieth Centuries," *The History of Medical Education*, C. D. O'Malley, ed. (Los Angeles, 1970), 501–30. For a more perceptive one, see Julius B. Richmond, *Currents in American Medicine, a Developmental View of Medical Care and Education* (Cambridge, Massachusetts, 1969).

14. The emergence of medical specialties is well covered in Rosemary Stevens, *American Medicine and the Public Interest* (New Haven and London, 1971).

15. T. B. Turner, "The Medical Schools Twenty Years Afterward: The Impact of the Research Programs of the National Institutes of Health," *Journal of Medical Education*, XLII (1967), 109–18.

16. There is no first-rate history of women in medicine, but John Blake's "Women and Medicine in Ante-Bellum America," *Bull. of Hist. of Med.*, XXXIX (1965), 99–123, is an excellent article. Richard H. Shryock wrote a very perceptive essay entitled "Women in Medicine," which is reprinted in his *Medicine in America*, 177–99. See also Carol Lopate, *Women in Medicine* (Baltimore, 1968), chap. 1.

17. Elizabeth Blackwell, *Pioneer Work in Opening the Medical Profession to Women, Autobiographical Sketches* (reprint, New York, 1970), 5, 46, 58ff.; *Boston Medical and Surgical Journal*, XXXVII (1847), 405.

18. Thomas A. Ashby, "Abstract of an Address on the Medical Education of Women . . .," *Maryland Medical Journal*, IX (1882), 272.

19. Lopate, *Women in Medicine*, 7.

20. *Boston Medical and Surgical Journal*, XLI (1850), 520–22; XLVIII (1853), 66; LIII (1855), 292–94; LIV (1856), 168–74.

21. Martin Kaufman, "John Stainback Wilson and Female Medical Education," *Jnl. of Hist. of Med. & All. Sci.*, XXVIII (1973), 397.

22. Charles D. Meigs, *Females and Their Diseases* (Philadelphia, 1848), 47; Morris Fishbein, *A History of the American Medical Association, 1847 to 1947* (Philadelphia and London, 1969), 82–83; *Medical and Surgical Reporter*, II (1859), 275–76.

23. *Medical and Surgical Reporter*, II (1859), 295–96; XVI (1867), 335; *N.O.M. & S.J.*, XVII (1860), 908–11.

24. *Boston Medical and Surgical Journal*, LXXXIV (1871), 350–54; Fishbein, *History of the American Medical Association*, 91; Lopate, *Women in Medicine*, 17.

25. Ashby, "Abstract of An Address on the Medical Education of Women . . .," 273–74.

26. Ashby, "Abstract of An Address on the Medical Education of Women . . .," 271–72; *Boston Medical and Surgical Journal*, C (1879), 727–30, 789–91.

27. Simon Flexner and James Thomas Flexner, *William Henry Welch and the Heroic Age of American Medicine* (New York, 1941), 215–21.

28. Lopate, *Women in Medicine*, 193; *Journal of Medical Education*, LIX (1974), 303.

29. Duffy, *The Rudolph Matas History of Medicine in Louisiana*, I, 89–91.

30. The two best histories of nursing are Richard H. Shryock, *The History of Nursing, An Interpretation of the Social and Medical Factors Involved* (Philadelphia, 1959), and Lavinia L. Dock and Isabel M. Stewart, *A Short History of Nursing* (New York and London, 1920). Minnie Goodnow, *Nursing History in Brief* (Philadelphia and London, 1939), has some additional information.

31. Fishbein, *History of the American Medical Association,* 77–78.

32. Duffy, *History of Public Health in New York City, 1866–1966,* pp. 187–88.

33. Shryock, *The History of Nursing,* 300.

34. Helen E. Marshall, *Mary Adelaide Nutting, Pioneer of Modern Nursing* (Baltimore and London, 1972), 33–39, 51.

35. *Ibid.,* 135–36; Goodnow, *Nursing History in Brief,* 229.

36. Goodnow, *Nursing History in Brief,* 133–34.

37. Shryock, *The History of Nursing,* 309–15.

38. Kelly Miller, "The Historic Background of the Negro Physician," *Journal of Negro History,* I (1916), 99–109; Harold E. Farmer, "An Account of the Earliest Colored Gentlemen in Medical Science in the United States," *Bull. of Hist. of Med.,* VIII (1940), 599–618; M. O. Bousfield, "An Account of Physicians of Color in the United States," *ibid.,* XVII (1945) 61–84.

39. Herbert M. Morais, *The History of the Negro in Medicine* (New York, Washington, and London, 1967), 8–10.

40. Duffy, *The Rudolph Matas History of Medicine in Louisiana,* I, 324–25.

41. New Orleans *Daily Picayune,* March 12, 1890.

42. Morais, *History of the Negro in Medicine,* 36–37.

43. Henry A. Bullock, *A History of Negro Education in the South from 1619 to the Present* (Cambridge, Massachusetts, 1967), 33–34; Flexner, *Medical Education in the United States and Canada,* 202, 230, 232, 280–81, 303–5, 307.

44. Bousfield, "An Account of Physicians of Color in the United States," 70.

45. L. A. Falk and N. A. Quaynor-Malm, "Early Afro-American Medical Education in the United States: The Origins of Meharry Medical College in the Nineteenth Century," *Proceedings* of the XXIII International Congress of the History of Medicine, London, September 2–9, 1972, I (London, 1974), 346–56; Morais, *History of the Negro in Medicine,* 68–69.

46. Bousfield, "An Account of Physicians of Color in the United States," 72–73; Morais, *History of the Negro in Medicine,* 85–86, 127.

47. Morais, *History of the Negro in Medicine,* 110, 128.

48. Benjamin R. Epstein and Arnold Foster, *Some of My Best Friends* (New York, 1962), 178–79.

49. New York *Times,* June 23–24, 1922; "Harvard's Sifting Committee on Racial Proportion," *School and Society,* XVI (July, 1922), 12–13; *Nation,* CXIV (June, 1922), 108.

50. R. P. Boas, "Who Shall Go to College," *Atlantic,* CXXX (October, 1922) 441–48.

51. *Literary Digest,* CV (May, 1930), 32; CVI (September, 1930), 20; *School and Society,* XL (December, 1934), 836.

52. See "Anti-Semitism at Dartmouth," *New Republic,* CXIII (August, 1945), 208–9.

53. Nathan C. Belth, ed., *Barriers, Patterns of Discrimination Against Jews* (New York, 1958), 74–76.

CHAPTER 19

1. The best historical study of American medical licensure is Shryock, *Medical Licensing in America*.
2. Long, *Medicine in North Carolina*, I, 215–22.
3. Waring, *History of Medicine in South Carolina, 1825–1900*, pp. 144–45.
4. Duffy, *The Rudolph Matas History of Medicine in Louisiana*, II, 403–12.
5. An excellent account of New York's licensure problems can be found in Kaufman, *American Medical Education*.
6. Duffy, *The Rudolph Matas History of Medicine in Louisiana*, II, 409–10.
7. Shryock, *Medical Licensing in America*, 58–59.
8. Duffy, *The Rudolph Matas History of Medicine in Louisiana*, II, 355.
9. For the development of specialties in the nineteenth century, see Rothstein, *American Physicians in the Nineteenth Century, from Sects to Science*, 207–16; and for the twentieth century, see Stevens, *American Medicine and the Public Interest*.
10. Young, *Medical Messiahs*, 184–88; James G. Burrow, *AMA: Voice of American Medicine* (Baltimore, 1963), 67ff.
11. Young, *Medical Messiahs*, 415–18.
12. Shryock, *Medical Licensing in America*, 80–83.
13. Robert C. Derbyshire, *Medical Licensure and Discipline in the United States* (Baltimore and London, 1969), 163–68.
14. Rosenberg, "The Practice of Medicine in New York A Century Ago," 229.
15. *Proceedings of the Orleans Parish Medical Society, 1898* (New Orleans, 1898), "Meeting of February 12, 1898," pp. 51–54; George Rosen, *Fees and Fee Bills, Some Economic Aspects of Medical Practice in Nineteenth Century America* (Baltimore, 1946), 88–89.
16. New Orleans *Bee*, June 22, 1875; New Orleans *Daily Picayune*, June 29, 1875.
17. Shryock, *Medical Licensing in America*, 30.
18. Blanton, *Medicine in Virginia in the Nineteenth Century*, 91.
19. Stanford E. Chaillé, *Address on State Medicine and Medical Organization* (New Orleans, 1879); Cowen, *Medicine and Health in New Jersey*, 59–60.
20. *J.A.M.A.*, XXXVI (1901), 1601.
21. Fishbein, *A History of the American Medical Association, 1847 to 1947*, 108–13, 201–13.
22. For the emergence of the AMA as an effective medical lobby, see Jonathan D. Wirtschafter, "The Genesis and Impact of the Medical Lobby, 1898–1906," *Jnl. of Hist. of Med. & All. Sci.*, XIII (1958), 15–49.
23. Burrow, *AMA: Voice of American Medicine*, 146–51.
24. Fishbein, *A History of the American Medical Association, 1847 to 1947*, p. 331. See also his section "The War Against Socialized Medicine—1925–1929," pp. 358–80

25. Burrow, *AMA: Voice of American Medicine*, 198–99.
26. *Ibid.*, 214–15.

CHAPTER 20

1. Duffy, *History of Public Health in New York City, 1866–1966*, p. 231.
2. Bonner, *Medicine in Chicago, 1850–1950*, pp. 20–21; *Annual Report of the Louisiana State Board of Health, 1881* (New Orleans, 1882), 242–44.
3. Stanford E. Chaillé, *Life and Death-Rates. New Orleans and Other Cities Compared*. Reprinted from *N.O.M. & S.J.*, August, 1888, p. 13.
4. Duffy, *History of Public Health in New York City, 1866–1966*, pp. 208–11.
5. Erwin H. Ackerknecht, *Malaria in the Upper Mississippi Valley, 1760–1900* (Baltimore, 1945); Shapiro and Miller, *Physician to the West*, 379; Stuart Galishoff, *Safeguarding the Public Health: Newark, 1895–1918* (Westport, Conn., 1975), 70.
6. Duffy, "Yellow Fever in the Continental United States During the Nineteenth Century," 687–701.
7. For some insight into conditions, see J. Thomas May, "The Medical Care of Blacks in Louisiana during Occupation and Reconstruction, 1862–1868; Its Social and Political Background," Ph.D. dissertation, Tulane University, 1970.
8. Alan Raphael, "Health and Social Welfare of Kentucky Black People, 1865–1870," *Societas, A Review of Social History*, II (1972), 143–57.
9. See John H. Ellis, "Businessmen and Public Health in the Urban South During the Nineteenth Century, New Orleans, Memphis, and Atlanta," Bull. of Hist., & Med.; XLIV (1970), 197–212.
10. Gillson, *Louisiana State Board of Health, The Formative Years*, chaps. 3 and 4; Rosenkrantz, *Public Health and the State, Changing Views in Massachusetts, 1842–1936*, p. 52.
11. Michael L. Berger, "The Influence of the Automobile on Rural Health Care, 1900–1929," *Jnl. of Hist. of Med. & All. Sci.*, XXVIII (1973), 319–35.
12. A good short account can be found in Kramer, "Agitation for Public Health Reform in the 1870s," *Jnl. of Hist. of Med. & All. Sci.*, IV (1949), 75–89. For a detailed study, see Peter Bruton, "The National Board of Health, 1879–1893," Ph.D. dissertation, University of Maryland, 1974.
13. A brief survey of Federal health measures prior to 1930 can be found in William G. Carleton, "Government and Health before the New Deal," *Current History*, XLV (August, 1963), 71–76.
14. Roy Lubove, "The New Deal and National Health," *ibid.*, 77–86.
15. Cecil G. Sheps and Daniel L. Drosness, "Medical Progress, Prepayment for Medical Care," *New England Journal of Medicine*, CCLXIV (1961), 390–96, 444–48, 494–99.

CHAPTER 21

1. For an excellent discussion of this and other ethical questions, see H. Tristram Engelhardt, Jr., "The Philosophy of Medicine: A New Endeavor," *Texas Reports on Biology and Medicine*, XXXI (Fall, 1973), 443–52. I am obligated to Dr. James P. Morris of the Texas A & M School of Medicine for his assistance with this chapter.
2. Lewis Thomas, "Guessing and Knowing, Reflections on the Science and Technology of Medicine," *Saturday Review*, LV (December 23, 1972), 52–57.
3. For a provocative article on this subject see Daniel S. Greenberg, "The 'War on Cancer': Official Fictions and Harsh Facts," *Science and Government Report*, December 1, 1974.
4. Mike Gorman, in "The Challenge of Change," *MH*, LIX (Fall, 1975), 10–12, discusses some possible solutions.
5. *Health Resources Statistics, 1974*, U.S. Department of Health, Education and Welfare (Washington, D.C., 1974), 3.
6. *Forbes*, III cxi (March 15, 1973), 28–29.

BIBLIOGRAPHY

There is no definitive history of American medicine, but Francis R. Packard's *History of Medicine in the United States*, 2 vols. (New York, 1931), does contain a good deal of useful information. The only other work to which one can turn for details is that encyclopedic medical history by Fielding H. Garrison, *An Introduction to the History of Medicine* (fourth edition, Philadelphia and London, 1929). A useful small work which contains a series of essays of varying quality is Felix Martí-Ibañez, ed., *History of American Medicine, a Symposium* (New York, 1958). A definitive history of American medicine cannot be written until far more work is done at the state and local level. Medical and public health histories for many states and cities are simply not available, and, where such histories do exist, a good share of them are out of date.

Among the best of the older state histories are Wyndham B.

Blanton's three volumes, *Medicine in Virginia in the Seventeenth Century* (Richmond, Va., 1930), *Medicine in Virginia in the Eighteenth Century* (Richmond, Va., 1931), *and Medicine in Virginia in the Nineteenth Century* (Richmond, Va., 1933); Eugene F. Cordell, *The Medical Annals of Maryland* (Baltimore, 1903); Samuel A. Green, *History of Medicine in Massachusetts* (Boston, 1881); Philip M. Hamer, *The Centennial History of the Tennessee State Medical Association* (Nashville, Tenn., 1930); Henry R. Viets, *A Brief History of Medicine in Massachusetts* (Boston, 1930); James J. Walsh, *History of Medicine in New York, Three Centuries of Medical Progress*, 3 vols. (New York, 1919); and Stephen Wickes, *History of Medicine in New Jersey* (Newark, 1879).

Among the more recent state and municipal histories are: Thomas N. Bonner, *Medicine in Chicago, 1850–1950, A Chapter in the Social and Scientific Development of a City* (Madison, Wisc., 1957), and *The Kansas Doctor: A Century of Pioneering* (Lawrence, Kansas, 1959); David L. Cowen, *Medicine and Health in New Jersey: A History* (Princeton, New York, Toronto, and London, 1964); John Duffy, ed., *The Rudolph Matas History of Medicine in Louisiana*, 2 vols. (Baton Rouge, La., 1958–62); Dorothy Long, ed., *Medicine in North Carolina, Essays in the History of Medical Science and Medical Service, 1524–1960*, 2 vols. (Raleigh, N.C., 1972); Reginald C. McGrane, *The Cincinnati Doctors' Forum* (Cincinnati, 1957); Pat Ireland Nixon, *A History of the Texas Medical Association, 1853–1953* (Austin, Texas, 1953); and Joseph I. Waring's two volumes, *A History of Medicine in South Carolina, 1670–1825* (Columbia, S.C., 1964), and *A History of Medicine in South Carolina, 1825–1900* (Columbia, S.C., 1967).

As with the history of medicine, there is no satisfactory history of public health in the United States, but there are a number of good local and regional studies: John B. Blake, *Public Health in the Town of Boston, 1630–1822* (Cambridge, Mass., 1959); John Duffy's two volumes, *A History of Public Health in New York City, 1625–1866* (New York, 1968), and *A History of Public Health in New York City, 1866–1966* (New York, 1974); Stuart Galishoff, *Safeguarding the Public Health, Newark, 1895–1918* (Westport, Conn., and London, 1975); Gordon E. Gillson, *Louisiana State Board of Health, The Formative Years* (Baton Rouge, La., 1968); Philip D. Jordan, *The People's Health, A History of Public Health in Minnesota to 1948* (St. Paul, Minn., 1953); and Barbara G. Rosenkrantz, *Public Health and the State, Changing Views in Massachusetts, 1842–1936* (Cambridge, Mass., 1972). Four other useful works in the history of public health are: Louis I. Dublin and Alfred J. Lotka, *Twenty-Five Years of Health Progress . . . the Metropolitan Life Insurance Company 1911 to 1935* (New York, 1937); Bess Furman, *A Profile of the United States Health Service, 1798–1948* (Washington, n.d.); Mazyck P. Ravenel, ed., *A Half Century of Public Health* (New York, 1921); and Ralph C. Williams, *The United States Public Health Service, 1798–1950* (Washington, 1951).

For the colonial period, the following works are especially useful: Whitfield J. Bell, Jr., *Early American Science* (Williamsburg, Va., 1955), and *John Morgan, Continental Doctor* (Philadelphia, 1965); Otho T. Beall, Jr., and Richard H. Shryock, *Cotton Mather, First Significant Figure in American Medicine* (Baltimore, 1954); Ernest Caulfield, *The Throat Distemper of 1735–1740 . . .* (New Haven, Conn., 1939); John Duffy, *Epidemics in Colonial America* (Baton Rouge, 1953); Benjamin Franklin, *Some Account of the Pennsylvania Hospital*, introduction by I. B. Cohen (Baltimore, 1954); Brooke Hindle, *The Pursuit of Science in Revolutionary America, 1735–1789* (Chapel Hill, N.C., 1956); Cotton Mather, *The Angel of Bethesda*, introduction by Gordon W. Jones (Barre, Mass., 1972); Lester S. King, *The Medical World of the Eighteenth Century* (Chicago, 1958); Richard H. Shryock, *Medical Licensing in America, 1650–1965* (Baltimore, 1967); ———, *Medicine and Society in America, 1660–1860* (New York, 1960); ———, *Medicine in America, Historical Essays* (Baltimore, 1966); Joseph M. Toner, *Contributions to the Annals of Medical Progress and Medical Education . . .* (Washington, 1874); E. Wagner and Allen E. Stearn, *The Effect of Smallpox on the Destiny of the Amerindian* (Boston, 1945).

For the American Revolution, see Philip Cash, *Medical Men at the Siege of Boston, April, 1775–April, 1776* (Philadelphia, 1973); Louis C. Duncan, *Medical Men in the American Revolution, 1775–1783* (Carlisle Barracks, Pa., 1931); David F. Hawke, *Benjamin Rush, Revolutionary Gadfly* (Indianapolis and New York, 1971); and Joseph M. Toner, *Medical Men of the Revolution, with a Brief History of the Medical Department of the Continental Army . . .* (Philadelphia, 1876). The lack of a first-rate history of medicine in the Revolutionary War makes three sources indispensable: John Morgan, *A Vindication of His Public Character in the Situation of*

Director-General (Boston, 1777); James Thacher, *A Military Journal During the American Revolutionary War, 1775–1783 . . .* (Boston, 1823); and James Tilton, *Economical Observations on Military Hospitals; and the Prevention of Diseases Incident to an Army* (Wilmington, Del., 1813).

For the period from the Revolution to the present, the better printed sources include: Louisa May Alcott, *Hospital Sketches* (New York, 1957); William Beaumont, *Experiments and Observations on the Gastric Juice and Physiology of Digestion . . . Facsimile . . . with a Biographical Essay . . . by Sir William Osler* (New York, 1959); *Elizabeth Blackwell, Pioneer Work in Opening the Medical Profession to Women, Autobiographical Sketches* (reprint, New York, 1970); Kate Cumming, *Kate, The Journal of a Confederate Nurse,* R. B. Harwell, ed. (Baton Rouge, La., 1959); N. S. Davis, *Medical Education and Medical Institutions in the U.S.A., 1776–1876* (Washington, 1877); James Ewell, *The Medical Companion, or Family Physician* (Washington, 1827); Abraham Flexner, *Medical Education in the United States and Canada, A Report to the Carnegie Foundation for the Advancement of Teaching* (New York, 1910); Timothy Flint, *The History and Geography of the Mississippi Valley* (Cincinnati, 1833); Samuel D. Gross, *History of American Medical Literature from 1776 to the Present Time* (Philadelphia, 1876); ———, *Lives of Eminent American Physicians and Surgeons of the Nineteenth Century* (Philadelphia, 1861); G. C. Gunn, *Gunn's Domestic Medicine, or Poor Man's Friend* (New York, 1853); Chapin A. Harris, *The Dental Art, a Practical Treatise on Dental Surgery* (Baltimore, 1839); Jabez W. Heustic, *Physical Observations, and Medical Tracts and Researches, on the Topography and Diseases of Louisiana* (New York, 1817); Gert Brieger, ed., *Medical America in the Nineteenth Century, Readings from the Literature* (Baltimore and London, 1972); Oliver Wendell Holmes, *Currents and Counter-Currents in Medical Science, An Address Delivered before the Massachusetts Medical Society . . . May 30, 1860 . . .* (Boston, 1860); J. Cam Massie, *Treatise on the Eclectic Southern Practice of Medicine* (Philadelphia, 1854); Charles D. Meigs, *Obstetrics: The Science and the Art* (Philadelphia, 1849); William Pepper, *Higher Medical Education, the True Interest of the Public and of the Profession* (Philadelphia, 1894); J. Marion Sims, *The Story of My Life* (New York, 1968); Charles J. Stillé, *History of the United States Sanitary Commission, Being the General Report of Its Works during the War of Rebellion*

(Philadelphia, 1866); Samuel Thomson, *New Guide to Health; or Botanic Family Physician . . . to which is prefixed, A Narrative of the Life and Medical Discoveries of the Author* (2nd ed., Boston, 1825); and Joseph J. Woodward, *Outlines of the Chief Camp Diseases of the United States Armies,* introduction by Saul Jarcho (New York and London, 1964).

The following is a list of the better secondary works: Erwin H. Ackerknecht, *Malaria in the Upper Mississippi Valley, 1760–1900* (Baltimore, 1945); George Worthington Adams, *Doctors in Blue, The Medical History of the Union Army in the Civil War* (New York, 1952); Charles A. Beard, ed., *A Century of Progress* (New York and London, 1933); Saul Benison, *Tom Rivers, Recollections on a Life in Medicine and Science* (Cambridge, Mass., and London, 1967); John B. Blake, *Benjamin Waterhouse and the Introduction of Vaccination, A Reappraisal* (Philadelphia, 1957); Frank K. Boland, *The First Anesthetic: The Story of Crawford Long* (Athens, Ga., 1950); Henry A Bullock, *A History of Negro Education in the South from 1619 to the Present* (Cambridge, Mass., 1967); James G. Burrow, *AMA: Voice of American Medicine* (Baltimore, 1963); Edward D. Churchill, ed., *To Work in the Vineyard of Surgery, Reminiscences of J. Collins Warren (1842–1927)* (Cambridge, Mass., 1958); George Corner, *A History of the Rockefeller Institute, 1901–1953* (New York, 1964); H. H. Cunningham, *Doctors in Gray, The Confederate Medical Service* (Baton Rouge, La., 1958); Robert C. Derbyshire, *Medical Licensure and Discipline in the United States* (Baltimore and London, 1969); James E. Dexter, *A History of Dental and Oral Science in America* (Philadelphia, 1876); Lavinia L. Dock and Isabel M. Stewart, *A Short History of Nursing* (New York and London, 1920); John Duffy, *The Sword of Pestilence, The New Orleans Yellow Fever Epidemic of 1853* (Baton Rouge, La., 1966); Elizabeth W. Etheridge, *The Butterfly Caste, A Social History of Pellagra in the South* (Westport, Conn., 1972); Morris Fishbein, *A History of the American Medical Association, 1847 to 1947* (Philadelphia and London, 1969); Donald Fleming, *William H. Welch and the Rise of Modern Medicine* (Boston, 1954); Simon Flexner and James Thomas Flexner, *William Henry Welch and the Heroic Age of American Medicine* (New York, 1941); Raymond B. Fosdick, *The Story of the Rockefeller Foundation* (New York, 1952); Norman H. Franke, *Pharmaceutical Conditions and Drug Supply in the Confederacy* (Madison, Wisc., 1955); Fielding

H. Garrison, *Contributions to the History of Medicine from the Bulletin of the New York Academy of Medicine, 1925–1935* (New York, 1966); John M. Gibson, *Soldier in White, the Life of General George Miller Sternberg* (Durham, N.C., 1958); Minnie Goodnow, *Nursing History in Brief* (Philadelphia and London, 1939); John S., Jr., and Robin M. Haller, *The Physician and Sexuality in Victorian America* (Urbana, Chicago and London, 1974); Emmet Field Horine, *Daniel Drake (1785–1852), Pioneer Physician of the Midwest* (Philadelphia, 1961); Martin Kaufman, *American Medical Education, The Formative Years, 1765–1910* (in publication); Martin Kaufman, *Homeopathy in America, The Rise and Fall of a Medical Heresy* (Baltimore and London, 1971; Joseph E. Kett, *The Formation of the American Medical Profession, The Role of Institutions, 1780–1860* (New Haven, Conn., 1968); Thomas E. Keys, *History of Surgical Anesthesia* (New York, 1963); Carol Lopate, *Women in Medicine* (Baltimore, 1968); Helen E. Marshall, *Mary Adelaide Nutting, Pioneer of Modern Nursing* (Baltimore and London, 1972); Richard H. Meade, *An Introduction to the History of General Surgery* (Philadelphia, London and Toronto, 1968); Herbert M. Morais, *The History of the Negro in Medicine* (New York, Washington and London, 1967); W. F. Norwood, *Medical Education in the United States Before the Civil War* (Philadelphia, 1944); John R. Paul, *A History of Poliomyelitis* (New Haven, Conn., 1971); William Pepper, *The Medical Side of Benjamin Franklin* (Philadelphia, 1910); J. H. Powell, *Bring Out Your Dead* (Philadelphia, 1949); Julius B. Richmond, *Currents in American Medicine, A Developmental View of Medical Care and Education* (Cambridge, Mass., 1969); Christine Chapman Robbins, *David Hosack, Citizen of New York* (Philadelphia, 1964); Victor Robinson, *The Story of Medicine* (New York, 1943); George Rosen, *Fees and Fee Bills, Some Economic Aspects of Medical Practice in Nineteenth Century America* (Baltimore, 1946); Charles Rosenberg, *The Cholera Years* (Chicago, 1962); William G. Rothstein, *American Physicians in the 19th Century, from Sects to Science* (Baltimore and London, 1972); Henry Burnell Shafer, *The American Medical Profession, 1783 to 1850* (New York and London, 1936); Robert Shaplen, *Toward the Well-Being of Mankind: Fifty Years of the Rockefeller Foundation* (Garden City, New York, 1932); Henry D. Shapiro and Zane L. Miller, eds., *Physician to the West, Selected Writings of Daniel Drake on Science and Society* (Lexington, Ky., 1970); Richard H. Shryock, *Development of*

Modern Medicine (New York and London, 1969); Richard H. Shryock, *The History of Nursing, An Interpretation of the Social and Medical Facts Involved* (Philadelphia, 1959); Richard H. Shryock, *American Medical Research, Past and Present* (New York, 1947); George Winston Smith, *Medicines for the Union Army, The United States Army Laboratories during the Civil War* (Madison, Wisc., 1962); William Simon, *History of the Baltimore College of Dental Surgery* (n.p., 1904); Rosemary Stevens, *American Medicine and the Public Interest* (New Haven and London, 1971); James J. Walsh, *History of Medicine in New York, Three Centuries of Medical Progress*, 3 vols. (New York, 1919); James Harvey Young, *The Medical Messiahs* (Princeton, 1971); James Harvey Young, *The Toadstool Millionaires: A Social History of Patent Medicines in America Before Federal Regulation* (Princeton, 1961).

I have not listed newspapers, medical and lay journals, historical society collections, pamphlets, and the miscellaneous secondary and source materials cited in the footnotes. They will be of help for those wishing to pursue any particular facet of American medical history.

INDEX

ABOUT THE AUTHOR

John Duffy is Priscilla Alden Burke Professor of History at the University of Maryland, and was formerly Professor of the History of Medicine at Tulane University. He is one of the country's foremost writers on the history of medicine in the United States, is President of the American Association for the History of Medicine, was Acting Editor of *The American Historical Review*, and is active in groups and societies concerned with the evolving state of medicine.